Problems in

small animal

neurology

Cheryl L. Chrisman, D.V.M.

College of Veterinary Medicine
University of Florida
Gainesville, Florida

Problems in small animal neurology

Second edition

Lea & Febiger

1991

Philadelphia · London

Lea & Febiger
2000 Chester Field Parkway
Malvern, Pennsylvania   19355
U.S.A.
(215) 251-2230
1-800-444-1785

Reprints of chapters may be purchased from Lea & Febiger in quantities of 100 or more.

Library of Congress Cataloging in Publication Data

Chrisman, Cheryl L.
    Problems in small animal neurology / Cheryl L. Chrisman.—2nd ed.

        p.   cm.
    ISBN 0-8121-1349-7
        1. Dogs—Diseases. 2. Cats—Diseases. 3. Veterinary neurology.
I. Title. II. Title: Small animal neurology.
    SF992.N3C48 1991   90-5881
    636.089′68—dc20   CIP

PRINTED IN THE UNITED STATES OF AMERICA

Print Number   3   2   1

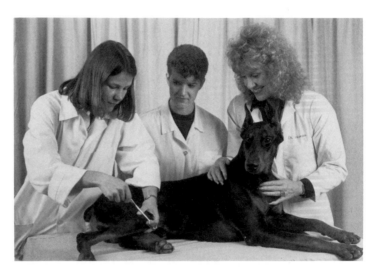

Preface

This text is a brief, concise handbook of small animal clinical neurology. It was designed to serve as a guide to general practitioners who have had little neurology training in school and beginning neurology students. The aim of the book is to provide a simple, rational diagnostic approach and therapeutic regimen for common neurologic complaints dealt with in veterinary practice.

The problem-oriented format of this book evolved over the past 20 years from practicing and teaching clinical neurology to veterinary students at the Ohio State University and University of Florida and from teaching neurology continuing education courses to veterinarians. The contents of the book are the small animal portion of the clinical neurology course presently part of the core veterinary curriculum at the University of Florida.

Part I of the book contains a brief overview of neuroanatomy, information pertinent to the evaluation of an animal with a neurologic problem, and some general principles of therapy.

Part II of the book is divided into 14 chapters. Each chapter deals with a common primary complaint that might be posed to a veterinarian in clinical practice. At the beginning of each chapter is a list of possible locations of lesions and mechanisms of disease and differential diagnosis for that particular problem. A discussion of pertinent regional anatomy, patient evaluation, and a basic diagnostic approach for the problem follows. The clinical diagnosis, management, and prognosis of each disease listed in the differential diagnosis at the beginning of the chapter are then discussed.

Some approaches to diagnosis, management regimens, and prognoses for certain problems may be controversial. The opinions presented in this book evolved from the experience of the author and may not be equally shared by all practicing neurologists.

The reader is referred to other texts for in-depth discussions of neuroanatomy, neurophysiology, pathophysiology, neurosurgical techniques, and pathology. The number of footnotes and references are purposely limited to a pertinent few.

It is my wish that the format and concise nature of the text will help veterinarians deal more effectively with neurologic problems in their daily practices. The text may also inform general practitioners of special diagnostic tools available in neurology specialty practices when referral of a case is desired. Lastly, it is my wish that the text will provide a simple approach to teaching clinical neurology to veterinary students that will give them a basic foundation for the diagnosis and management of neurologic problems.

The second edition has been undated to include current information on new diagnostic techniques, previously described diseases, and recently reported new diseases. More specific therapeutic regimens have been added to make this textbook more useful to veterinary practitioners.

Cheryl L. Chrisman, D.V.M.
Gainesville, Florida

Acknowledgments

I especially acknowledge Dr. Laurie Pearce, who has been a joy and inspiration to me. Her continual encouragement, great ideas, and delightful sense of humor have been a positive force in my life, and gave me the strength to finish the second edition of this book. I am grateful our paths have crossed.

C.L.C.

Contents

Part I

Evaluation and management of the neurologic patient

Chapter 1

Introduction to the nervous system

Prior to neurologic evaluation of animals and solving of problems, a review of the structure and function of the nervous system and its components is necessary. Detailed descriptions of functional neuroanatomy of dogs and cats are presented elsewhere.[2, 5-7] Regional anatomy will be discussed further with each problem, but an overview of some basic concepts is given in this chapter.

The cells of the nervous system

Two basic types of cells make up the nervous system: neurons and glial cells.

Neurons

Neurons are the cells capable of transmitting an electrical impulse and are responsible for the master control the nervous system provides for activities of the body. All other elements of the nervous system provide support, protection, and nutrition for the neurons. Neurons may be unipolar, bipolar, or multipolar in shape, but they all have one or more afferent processes called dendrites, which transmit information to the cell body, and at least one efferent process called an axon, which transmits information away from the cell body. Groups of cell bodies outside the central nervous system (CNS) in the peripheral nervous system (PNS) are called ganglia. Groups of cell bodies within the central nervous system are referred to as nuclei. Gray matter of the central nervous system contains cell bodies, or groups of nuclei. White matter is composed of groups of axons separated into bundles called tracts. Many of the axons are covered with a sheath of myelin, thus the name white matter. Neurons, when arranged in networks and provided with adequate informational input, can store information and respond in many ways to a stimulus.

Unipolar neurons have a common dendrite and axon stalk leading to and from the cell body (Fig. 1–1). The single dendrite is very long and is located in peripheral cranial and spinal sensory nerves. Most of the cell bodies are located in ganglia exterior to the spinal cord or brain stem. Unipolar neuron cell bodies are also located in the mesencephalic nucleus of the trigeminal nerve in the brain stem.

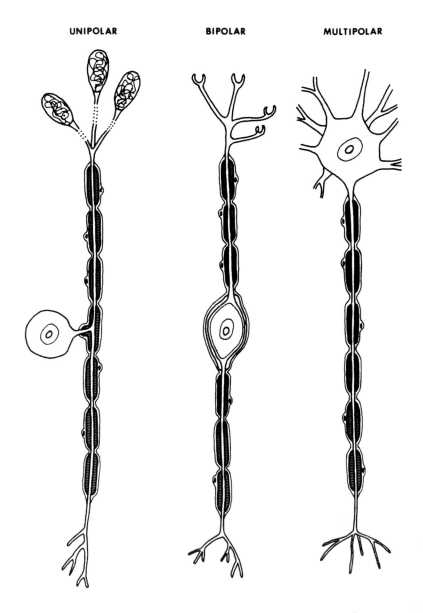

UNIPOLAR   BIPOLAR   MULTIPOLAR

Figure 1–1. Types of neurons.

From the cell bodies in the peripheral nerve ganglion, the axons enter the spinal cord or brain stem and synapse on other neurons. The unipolar neurons carry sensory or afferent information such as proprioception, touch, and pain from the exterior body into the central nervous system.

Bipolar neurons have one dendrite and one axon from separate areas of the cell body, and transmit information from the body into the nervous system (Fig. 1–1). These types of neurons carry sensory information for olfaction, vision, audition, and equilibrium.

Most neurons are multipolar with multiple dendrites and one major axon that may branch (Fig. 1–1). Multipolar neurons can be sensory, or afferent neurons, and transmit information from the spinal cord and brain stem to the higher centers of the cerebellum and cerebrum. Multipolar neurons can also be motor, or efferent neurons, and carry information from higher brain centers to lower brain stem and spinal cord centers and from the spinal cord through peripheral nerves to glands and muscles. These types of neurons may have a variety of dendrite shapes, and may vary in size. Multipolar neurons with short axons form internuncial neurons of the CNS, which transmit information short distances. Multipolar neurons with long axons form the tracts of the CNS and the peripheral nerves. The multipolar type neurons are given different names in various anatomic regions, such as pyramidal cells in the cerebral cortex and Purkinje cells in the cerebellum.

The dendrites of the multipolar neurons receive most of the synapses, or connections, with other axons. Information then is transmitted from the dendrite to the cell body. If a sufficient amount of dendritic stimulation is received and reaches a threshold level, an action potential will develop at the initial portion of the axon and be transmitted down the main axon to the nerve terminal.

An action potential is transmitted by an alteration in the polarity of the membrane of the axon (Fig. 1–2). In the normal resting state, the interior of the cell is negative compared with the exterior because of large anionic proteins. The membrane is semipermeable, and sodium ion (Na^+) is actively extruded and potassium ion (K^+) is taken into the cell. The potassium ion (K^+) concentration is high and the sodium ion (Na^+) concentration is low on the inside as compared with the outside of the cell. When the membrane is stimulated to a threshold level by an electrical, chemical, or mechanical stimulus, a spontaneous series of events results. The cell membrane becomes permeable to Na^+, which rushes into the cell, making the inside positive and the outside negative, and depolarization results (Fig. 1–2). Shortly thereafter, the membrane again becomes impermeable to Na^+, and K^+ ion leaves the cell. The interior of the cell returns to a relatively negative charge as compared with the exterior, and repolarization is achieved (Fig. 1–2). In the repolarized state, Na^+ is actively extruded once again and K^+ is taken back into the cell, so the original ion concentration is reestablished. Depolarization continues along the axon to the terminal portion that contains vesicles of neurotransmitter substance. When the depolarization reaches the nerve terminal, neurotransmitter substance is released. The neurotransmitter substance chemically stimulates or inhibits a receptor on another neuron, gland, or muscle. Messages are transmitted throughout the nervous system networks in this manner.

The diameter of the axon and the thickness of the myelin sheath determine the speed of conduction. Myelin covers the axon in segments, and the areas between the segments are referred to as nodes of Ranvier (Fig. 1–2). The multiple myelin segments act as insulators, and deplorization occurs only at the node of Ranvier instead of along the entire axon. Depolarization from node to node is called salta-

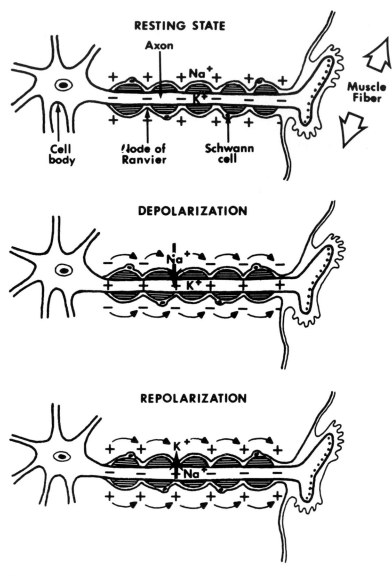

Figure 1–2. Anatomy and physiology of a multipolar motor neuron.

tory conduction and greatly speeds up the transmission of the electrical impulse (Fig. 1–2). Large diameter, heavily myelinated axons transmit the fastest impulses.

Neurons may be facilitory and produce depolarization of the cells they contact, or be inhibitory and prevent depolarization of the cell. The effects of a neurotransmitter compound are dependent on the type of postsynaptic receptor they contact and not simply due to the chemical effects of the neurotransmitter itself. Acetylcholine is the most common neurotransmitter. Other neurotransmitters are norepinephrine, epinephrine, dopamine, serotonin, glutamine, glycine, taurine, and gamma aminobutyric acid (GABA).

A lower motor neuron (LMN) is a multipolar neuron with its dendrites and cell body in a brain stem nucleus or in the gray matter of the spinal cord. The axon of the

LMN travels out of the central nervous system through the peripheral nerves to synapse on a gland or muscle. Spinal cord and brain stem reflexes are composed of two or more neurons (Fig. 1–3). A unipolar neuron carries information from the body through the peripheral nerve into the nervous system, and stimulates a lower motor neuron directly or indirectly through an internuncial neuron. If all portions of the reflex are intact, the reflex will be present. If any portion of the reflex is diseased, the reflex will be depressed or abolished.

The upper motor neurons (UMN) have their dendrites and cell bodies in the cerebral cortex gray matter or nuclei of the brain stem. Their axons travel through the brain stem and spinal cord in bundles of fibers called tracts, which form part of the white matter of the brain stem and spinal cord (Fig. 1–4). The functions of the major tracts are reviewed later in this section. Some UMN initiate voluntary movement and influence the LMN, usually through an internuncial neuron that either stimulates or inhibits them. The UMN

has an overall inhibitory, or calming, effect on the LMN reflexes. If the UMN cell bodies or tracts are diseased, there is a release of the inhibitory influence on the LMN. If the LMN is not also diseased, the cranial or spinal nerve reflex with which it is associated becomes exaggerated or hyperactive.

The longer a cranial and spinal nerve reflex is without the influence of the UMN, the more hyperactive the reflex becomes. It is suspected that sprouting of axons from afferent and internuncial neurons fills in the synaptic sites left empty from degenerated UMN. Consequently, when the reflex is elicited, impulses from the sprouted axons stimulate the lower motor neuron at different time intervals. The reflex is brisk and often repeats itself in a series referred to as clonus.

Reflex extension and flexion of the limbs can occur in dogs and cats with UMN paralysis when excessive axon sprouting has occurred. Such a paralyzed animal may appear to take some steps although there is no voluntary movement or conscious perception of limb position. This

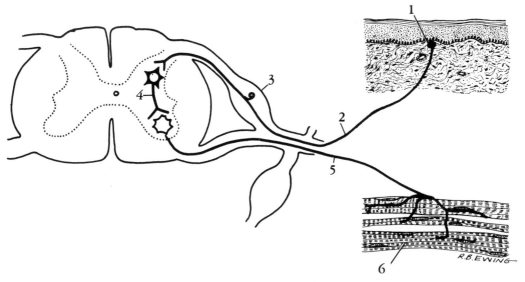

Figure 1–3. An example of a three-neuron spinal reflex. The components are (1) the skin receptor, (2) the sensory neuron, (3) the dorsal root ganglion, (4) the internuncial neuron, (5) the lower motor neuron, and (6) the muscle. (From Jenkins, T.: Functional Mammalian Neuroanatomy. Philadelphia, Lea & Febiger, 1978.)

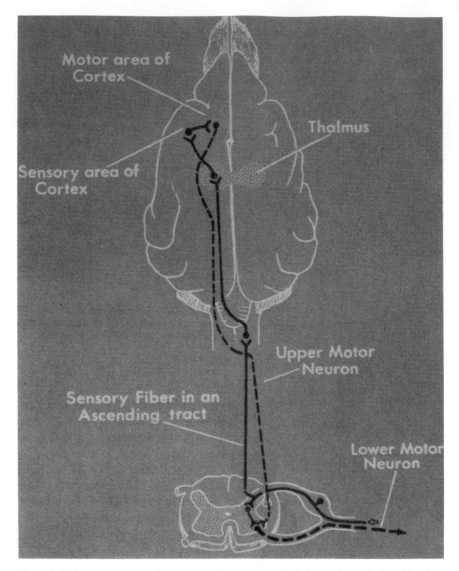

Figure 1–4. The arrangement of an upper motor neuron (UMN) descending spinal cord tract and the lower motor neuron (LMN) in the peripheral nerve, and one sensory ascending spinal cord tract for the conscious perception of pain.

spinal walking is due to hyperactive spinal reflex activity, and may be seen even when the spinal cord is severed, so long as the reflex pathways of the pelvic limbs are intact. Testing the spinal cord and brain stem reflexes, and knowing which peripheral nerves and spinal cord or brain stem segments are involved in the reflex, can be used to locate lesions (Chapter 3). An ex-aggerated spinal reflex often means a disease process is located above the level of the reflex. An absent cranial or spinal nerve reflex means the lesion is located within the reflex arc.

Neurons neither reproduce nor have mitotic activity. The precursor of the neuron, the neuroblast, can form a tumor, the neuroblastoma, in young animals.

Neuroglia

There are billions of neurons in the CNS and PNS, but there are five to six times more supporting cells, called neuroglia. Oligodendroglia are found in gray and white matter of the CNS, and form and maintain myelin on various segments of several axons in white matter. The loss of one oligodendroglia may result in the segmental demyelination of several axons. Oligodendroglia are found in close proximity to neurons even where there is no myelin, and are suspected of providing some type of functional support. In the PNS, the myelin is produced by Schwann cells. One Schwann cell produces one segment of myelin and the neurolemmal sheath on one axon.

Oligodendrogliomas are neoplasms produced by oligodendroglia. Schwannomas, neurolemmomas, and neurinomas are neoplasms produced by Schwann cells. Neurofibromas and neurofibrosarcomas are neoplasms of fibroblasts that support peripheral nerves. CNS and PNS myelin are antigenically different, so that a disease process resulting in destruction of CNS myelin may not affect PNS myelin and vice versa.

Astrocytes are of two types, protoplasmic and fibrous, which are located primarily in gray and white matter, respectively. Astrocytes maintain substance and support to the nervous system. Astrocytes form a complete membrane on the external surface of the brain, referred to as the external glial limiting membrane. They also fuse with ependymal cell processes, and form an internal glial limiting membrane. Astrocyte processes tend to separate neuronal processes and form the internal skeleton of the nervous system. Astrocyte feet surround all blood vessels and regulate the ion and water environment of the neurons. During disease processes, astrocytes may proliferate and produce a scar where neurons died. In severe destruction, astrocyte scars may not be able to fill in the defect and an astrocyte-lined cavity results. Astrocytomas are the neoplasms produced by astrocytes.

Microglia are small cells located throughout the nervous system that become active during disease and are capable of phagocytosis. Microglia are also called gitter cells when they are phagocytic.

Ependymal cells line the ventricular system of the brain and spinal cord and provide a barrier between the brain and CSF in the ventricular system. In the lateral, third, and fourth ventricles, specialized ependymal cells and capillaries form the choroid plexus and produce cerebrospinal fluid. Ependymomas and choroid plexus papillomas are neoplasms produced by these cells.

Mixed glial cell neoplasms are referred to as gliomas. Immature forms are referred to as glioblastomas or spongioblastomas.

Blood–brain barrier

The endothelial cells of the blood vessels of the nervous system contain no porous openings, but have tight junctions between them. The basement membrane of the vascular endothelial cells merges with an amorphous coating and the astrocyte end feet to form the anatomic basis of the blood–brain barrier. The blood–brain barrier acts to protect and control the environment of the neurons for proper function.[1]

For some compounds the blood–brain barrier acts similarly to semipermeable cell membranes in general. Permeability is directly proportional to lipid solubility, and inversely proportional to degree of ionization of a substance. The blood–brain barrier is impermeable to large macromolecules such as proteins. There is active transport into and extrusion of materials out of the brain across the barrier.

Glucose, but none of its isomers, and

amino acids have a carrier-mediated transport system that is specific and bidirectional. Potassium ion concentration is controlled within narrow limits by bidirectional active processes. Hydrogen ion concentration remains rather constant within the brain and CSF during systemic acidosis and alkalosis by active exchange processes. Carbon dioxide (CO_2) and oxygen (O_2) pass the blood–brain barrier freely, but bicarbonate ion (HCO_3^-) does not. A rapid correction of metabolic acidosis may drive CO_2 across the blood–brain barrier and not HCO_3^- and result in a severe selective acidosis in the CNS.[1] The pH of the cerebrospinal fluid can aid in the diagnosis of CNS acidosis.

Some organic acids, such as penicillin, are actively extruded from CSF into the blood. A review of the anatomy and function of the blood–brain barrier is found in Figure 1–5.

The blood vessels of the brain and spinal cord are also sensitive to blood CO_2 concentration. The blood vessels dilate with increased CO_2 levels, and cerebral edema can result. In cases of low CO_2 tension, blood vessels may constrict and produce ischemia of an area.

Neural energetics

The major source of energy production in neurons is aerobic glycolysis through the tricarboxylic acid or Kreb's cycle, producing 38 moles of adenosine triphosphate (ATP).[1] Therefore oxygen and glucose are necessary for proper energy production. Within neurons, there is also a diversion

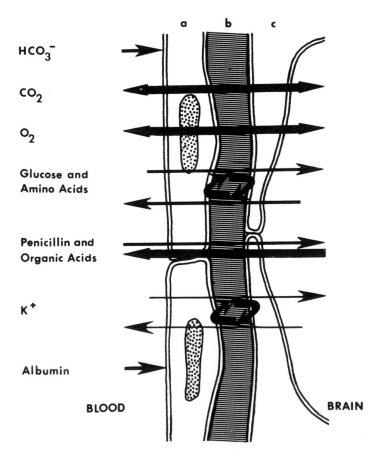

Figure 1–5. Overview of the anatomy and physiology of the blood–brain barrier (BBB): (a) blood vessel endothelial cells with tight junctions, (b) basement membrane, (c) astrocyte end feet. Arrows indicate direction substances flow across BBB: heavy arrows indicate large amounts; thin arrows indicate controlled amounts.

HCO$_3^-$

CO$_2$

O$_2$

Glucose and Amino Acids

Penicillin and Organic Acids

K$^+$

Albumin

BLOOD

BRAIN

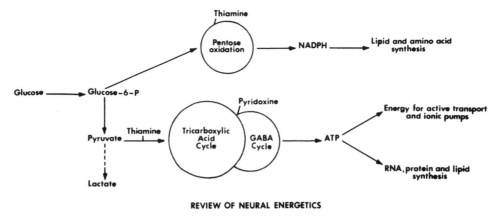

Figure 1–6. An overview of biochemical pathways most commonly used for energy in the CNS.

of the tricarboxylic acid cycle to form gamma amino butyric acid (GABA), often used as an inhibitory neurotransmitter. The GABA shunt also provides conversion of carbohydrates to glutamic acid, which forms glutamine and other amino acids.

Another source of energy is the direct oxidation of glucose-6-phosphate to form a pentose phosphate, whose metabolism results in the formation of nicotinamide adenine dinucleotide phosphate (NADP). The glucose-6-phosphate oxidative pathway requires no oxygen and can provide pentose for nucleic acid synthesis and energy for amino acids and lipid synthesis.

Thiamine (B_1) is needed to enter pyruvate in the tricarboxylic acid cycle. Thiamine is also needed in pentose oxidation. Hypoxia, hypoglycemia, and thiamine deficiency all produce central nervous system deficit by altering neural energetics.

Pyridoxine is a cofactor necessary for the GABA cycle. In pyridoxine deficiency there is a decrease in GABA production, and seizures can result. Neural energetics is reviewed in Figure 1–6.

Divisions of the central nervous system

The central nervous system is divided into four gross structures, the cerebrum, the brain stem, the cerebellum, and the spinal cord. The cerebrum and brain stem can also be divided into regions based on embryonic development. The cerebrum is the telencephalon and the brain stem is divided into the diencephalon, mesencephalon, metencephalon, and myelencephalon (Fig. 1–7). The cerebellum is an outgrowth of the metencephalon.

Telencephalon

The telencephalon consists of the cerebral cortex and basal nuclei. The cerebral cortex is divided into four main sections, the frontal, parietal, occipital, and temporal lobes (Fig. 1–8). Each lobe has characteristic functions (Table 1–1).

Intellectual activities and learning are processed in the frontal lobe. The animal is mentally alert and responsive to its environment with normal frontal lobe function. Fine motor abilities, such as those tested by hopping and placing reactions during the neurologic examination, depend on the frontal lobe. Gross motor activities do not depend on the frontal lobe in animals as they do in humans.

The parietal lobe processes sensory information such as pain, touch, and proprioception. The thalamus may process more of the sensory information in animals than in man, as animals do not seem

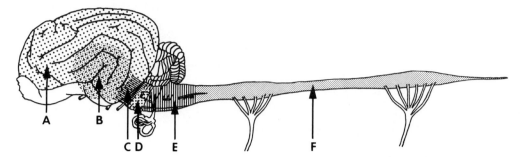

Figure 1–7. The major divisions of the central nervous system. (A) cerebral cortex, (B) diencephalon covered by the cerebral cortex, (C) mesencephalon, (D) metencephalon, (E) myelencephalon, and (F) spinal cord.

to depend on the parietal lobe for processing many sensations.

The occipital lobe is necessary for proper vision and processing visual information.

The temporal lobe processes auditory information and aids in the localization of sound. Animals do not appear to depend on the temporal lobe for the complete ability to hear. Auditory information is also processed in brain stem structures (Chapter 13).

The temporal lobe is also responsible for some complex behavior. Parts of the temporal and frontal lobe cortex are included in the limbic system. The limbic system is responsible for many emotions and for innate survival behavior such as protective, maternal, and sexual reactions. The pyriform area of the temporal lobe is one area responsible for aggressiveness. The amygdala is a large nucleus beneath the temporal lobe that is also part of the limbic system and is responsible for many fear responses. Parts of the hypothalamus are also included in the limbic system. The sensory (ascending) and motor (descending) tracts passing to and from the cerebral

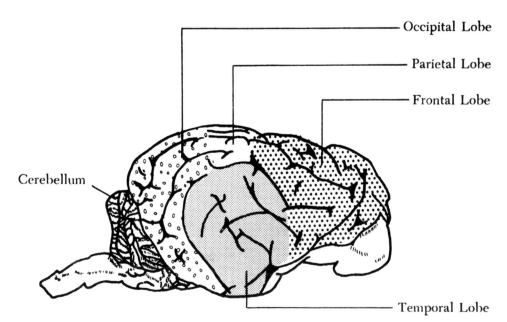

Occipital Lobe

Parietal Lobe

Frontal Lobe

Cerebellum

Temporal Lobe

Figure 1–8. The divisions of the cerebral cortex. (From McGrath, J.T.: Neurologic Examination of the Dog. Philadelphia, Lea & Febiger, 1960.)

Table 1–1
Divisions of the central nervous system

Major structures	Functions
Telencephalon	
Cerebral Cortex	
Frontal lobe	Intellect, behavior, fine motor activity
Parietal lobe	Touch, nociception (pain), conscious proprioception
Occipital lobe	Vision
Temporal lobe	Behavior, hearing
Basal Nuclei	
Caudate, putamen, globus pallidus	Muscle tone, initiation and control of motor activity
Internal Capsule	Ascending and descending sensory and motor activities
Diencephalon	
Hypothalamus	
Many nuclei	Autonomic control, appetite, thirst, temperature, electrolyte and water balance, sleep, and behavior
Pituitary gland	Endocrine functions
Thalamus	
Many nuclei	Touch, nociception (pain), proprioception
Reticular activating system	Consciousness
Subthalamus	
Reticular activating system	Consciousness
Olfactory System	
Cranial nerve I	Olfaction
Optic nerves, chiasm, and tracts (cranial nerve II)	Vision, pupillary light reflex
Mesencephalon	
Midbrain	
Reticular activating system—reticular formation	Consciousness and sleep
Oculomotor nerves (cranial nerve III)	Extraocular muscles, pupil constriction
Trochlear nerves (cranial nerve IV)	Extraocular muscle
Red nucleus	Motor activity, origin of rubrospinal tract
Ascending and descending tracts	Sensory and motor activities
Metencephalon	
Pons	
Trigeminal nerves (cranial nerve V)	Sensation from head, motor to muscles of mastication
Reticular formation	Vital centers—respiration and sleep
Ascending and descending tracts	Sensory and motor activities

(continued)

Table 1–1
Divisions of the central nervous system (Continued)

Major structures	Functions
Cerebellum	
Vermis and hemispheres	Coordination of movement and muscle tone; unconscious proprioception
Flocculonodular lobe	Equilibrium
Myelencephalon	
Medulla Oblongata	
Acending and descending tracts	Sensory and motor activities
Abducent nerves (cranial nerve VI)	Extraocular muscles
Facial nerves (cranial nerve VII)	Motor for facial expression, glands, and taste
Vestibular and cochlear nerves (cranial nerve VIII)	Equilibrium, hearing, vestibulospinal tract
Glossopharyngeal nerves (cranial nerve IX)	Sensation caudal tongue, laryngeal muscles, glands, and taste
Vagus nerves (cranial nerve X)	Motor and sensory for thoracic and abdominal viscera, laryngeal muscles
Accessory nerves (cranial nerve XI)	Motor to neck muscles
Hypoglossal nerves (cranial nerve XII)	Motor to tongue
Spinal Cord	
Gray Matter	
Dorsal horn	Sensory neurons and reflexes
Ventral horn	Lower motor neurons and reflexes
Intermediolateral	Autonomic neurons
White Matter	
Spinocerebellar tracts	Unconscious and conscious proprioception
Dorsal columns	Conscious proprioception, sharp nociception (pain)
Spinothalamic tracts	Nociception (pain) and temperature
Propriospinal tract	Communication between spinal cord segments
Rubrospinal tract	Voluntary motor (fine movements)
Corticospinal tract	Voluntary motor (fine movements)
Vestibulospinal tracts	Postural motor
Reticulospinal tracts	Postural motor and voluntary motor

cortex in the subcortical white matter form the internal capsule.

The basal nuclei are several groups of cell bodies beneath the cerebral cortex. The caudate, putamen, and globus pallidus are part of the telencephalon and are the main basal nuclei. Many authors also include the diencephalic structures, the amygdala, claustrum, and subthalamus, and the mesencephalic structures, the substantia nigra and red nuclei, as part of the basal nuclei. All these nuclei contribute to muscle tone and initiation and control of voluntary motor activity. Although disease in these nuclei produces important clinical syndromes in man such as Parkinson's disease and Huntington's chorea, the signs in animals attributed to disease in these nuclei are not well established.

Diencephalon

The diencephalon is the most rostral part of the brain stem and includes the hypothalamus, thalamus, subthalamus, and metathalamus. The hypothalamus modulates autonomic nervous system control throughout the body. Many of the sympathetic and parasympathetic UMN originate here. Appetite, thirst, temperature regulation, electrolyte balance, sleep, and behavior responses are some of the hypothalamic functions. The pituitary gland is attached by a stalk to the ventral surface of the hypothalamus. The pituitary gland controls many of the endocrine functions of the body.

The thalamus is a complex of many nuclei with intricate functions. The ventral caudal lateral and medial nuclei constitute the nociceptive (pain) and proprioception sensory relay system to the cerebral cortex. As was discussed earlier, much of the processing of sensory information in animals probably occurs in the thalamus rather than in the parietal lobe cerebral cortex. Part of the reticular activating system (RAS) projects from the midbrain through the thalamus diffusely to the cerebral cor-

tex, and is responsible for alerting the cerebral cortex and keeping the animal awake. Another part of the RAS projects through the subthalamus region to the cerebral cortex. Although there are many structures located there, the diencephalon can have large lesions with relatively few clinical signs (Table 3–2).

The olfactory nerves (cranial nerve I) are responsible for smell, and are located rostral to the hypothalamus (Fig. 1–9). Olfactory fibers project into the hypothalamus and other parts of the limbic system to produce a proper behavioral response to smell.

The optic nerves and optic chiasm (cranial nerve II), necessary for vision and pupillary light reflexes, are located on the ventral surface of the hypothalamus near the pituitary gland (Fig. 1–9). The lateral geniculate nucleus is part of the metathalamus and is the sensory relay nucleus to the cerebral cortex for vision.

Mesencephalon

The mesencephalon, or midbrain, has many important structures (Table 1–1), which result in severe neurologic deficits when diseased (Table 3–2). The reticular activating system (RAS) passes through the tegmentum (lower half) of the midbrain through the thalamus and subthalamus to the cortex. When the RAS is stimulated by visual, auditory, painful, and tactile inputs, the animal maintains an alert state. When the RAS does not receive or process these inputs, the animal goes to sleep. Lesions of the cerebral cortex, diencephalon, and midbrain can produce coma (Chapter 10).

The oculomotor nerves (cranial nerve III) are located in the midbrain, and constrict the pupil during the pupillary light reflex (Fig. 1–9). The oculomotor nerves innervate the medial rectus, dorsal rectus, ventral rectus, and inferior oblique muscles of the eyeball, and are responsible for proper eyeball movement. They also in-

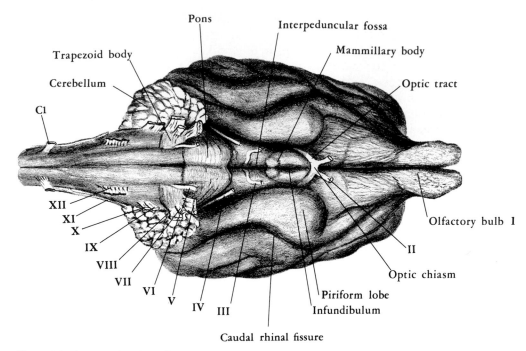

Figure 1–9. The ventral surface of the dog brain, demonstrating the location of the cranial nerves. (I) olfaction, (II) optic, (III) oculomotor, (IV) trochlear, (V) trigeminal, (VI) abducens, (VII) facial, (VIII) vestibular, (IX) glossopharyngeal, (X) vagus, (XI) accessory, (XII) hypoglossal. (From Jenkins, T.W.: Functional Mammalian Neuroanatomy. Philadelphia, Lea & Febiger, 1978.)

nervate a small muscle in the upper eyelids that aids in keeping the eyelids open. The trochlear nerves (cranial nerve IV) are located in the midbrain and innervate the superior oblique extraocular muscles (Fig. 1–9).

The red nucleus is located in the midbrain and is the origin of the rubrospinal tract, which assists in fine motor movements. Disease processes from the midbrain caudally are capable of producing paralysis. Other sensory and motor tracts pass through the midbrain, and will be reviewed below.

Metencephalon

The metencephalon contains the pons and cerebellum. The trigeminal nerves (cranial nerve V) and part of the nucleus are located in the pons (Fig. 1–9). The trigeminal nerves transmit sensations such as pain and proprioception from the entire head, and supply motor activity to the muscles of mastication (Table 1–1). Some vital centers associated with respiration are also located in the pons. Sensory and motor tracts passing through the pons are reviewed below.

The cerebellum is situated on three pairs of structures, called peduncles, over the fourth ventricle at the junction of the pons and the medulla oblongata. The cerebellum coordinates all motor activity of the head, neck, trunk, and limbs. The cerebellum also controls muscle tone in animals. The flocculonodular lobe of the cerebellum is part of the vestibular system and maintains equilibrium in an animal. Cerebellar function and dysfunction are further discussed in Chapter 15.

Myelencephalon

The myelencephalon, or medulla oblongata, is also composed of many ascending and descending pathways and nuclei. The abducent, facial, and vestibulocochlear nerves (cranial nerves VI, VII, and VIII, respectively) are located in the rostral portion at the junction with the pons (Fig. 1–9). The glossopharyngeal, vagus, spinal accessory, and hypoglossal nerves (cranial nerves IX, X, XI, and XII) are located in the caudal portion (Fig. 1–9).

Abducent nerves (cranial nerve VI) innervate the lateral rectus and retractor oculi muscles, and produce lateral and retractor movements of the eyeball, respectively. The facial nerves (cranial nerve VII) produce movement of the lips and ears and close the eyelids. The facial nerves also innervate tear glands and the mandibular and sublingual salivary glands, and provide taste from the anterior two thirds of the tongue. The vestibular nerves (cranial nerve VIII) maintain the equilibrium of the animal. The cochlear nerves (cranial nerve VIII) are needed for hearing.

The glossopharyngeal nerves (cranial nerve IX) innervate muscles of the larynx and pharynx as well as the zygomatic and parotid salivary glands. The glossopharyngeal nerve also provides sensation from the caudal tongue and pharynx as well as taste from the caudal tongue. The vagus nerves (cranial nerve X) innervate the thoracic and abdominal glands, cardiac and smooth muscle to the colon. They also innervate the skeletal muscles of the larynx, pharynx, and soft palate. In addition, vagus nerves transmit sensory information from the pharynx, larynx, thoracic and abdominal viscera. The spinal accessory nerves (cranial nerve XI) innervate the sternocleidomastoid and trapezius muscles. The hypoglossal nerves (cranial nerve XII) innervate the skeletal muscles of the tongue. Further discussions of function and dysfunction of cranial nerves are found in Chapters 3 and 11.

Vital centers that control respiration, blood pressure, and heart rate are located throughout the central core of the medulla oblongata. Functions of the medulla oblongata are listed in Table 1–1. Signs of dysfunction are found in Table 3–2.

Spinal cord

The spinal cord is composed of a central core of gray matter containing cell bodies of sensory, internuncial, and lower motor neurons. The gray matter has a dorsal horn that contains synapses from many peripheral sensory neurons and cell bodies of internuncial and ascending sensory neurons. The ventral horn gray matter contains many of the cell bodies of the LMN to skeletal muscle. An intermediary gray matter area contains cell bodies of sympathetic LMN. The external portion of the spinal cord is composed of white matter divided into ascending and descending groups of axons called tracts. The relative location of these tracts is shown in Figure 1–10, and their function is described in the next section. Signs of spinal cord dysfunction with lesions at various sites are outlined in Table 3–2.

Ascending and descending pathways through the spinal cord and brain stem

The pathways in the brain stem and spinal cord can be divided into those that ascend to the brain and are sensory in function, and those that descend from the brain and are motor to flexor and extensor muscles (Fig. 1–10). The tracts are generally named from where they begin to where they end. Only the main pathways considered to have the greatest clinical significance are reviewed.

Sensory tracts

In domestic animals, the sensory modalities of proprioception, touch, temperature, and nociception (pain) may ascend in more than one of the sensory tracts in the spinal cord. The four ascending systems are the spinocerebellar, spinothalamic, and spinoreticular tracts and the dorsal columns.

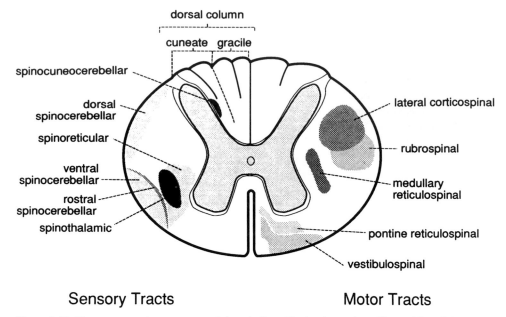

dorsal column
cuneate gracile

spinocuneocerebellar

dorsal spinocerebellar

spinoreticular

ventral spinocerebellar

rostral spinocerebellar

spinothalamic

lateral corticospinal

rubrospinal

medullary reticulospinal

pontine reticulospinal

vestibulospinal

Sensory Tracts   Motor Tracts

Figure 1–10. The sensory and motor tracts of the spinal cord in the dog and cat. The position of these tracts is approximate. In the motor tracts, axons to the pelvic limbs are lateral to those to the thoracic limbs (Adapted from King, A.S.: Physiological and Clinical Anatomy of the Domestic Mammals. Vol. 1, Central Nervous System. New York, Oxford University, 1987.) The rostral spinocerebellar tract is the cranial spinocerebellar tract.

The spinocerebellar tracts carry proprioceptive information to the cerebellum to provide the input needed to coordinate muscle movement. The dorsal and ventral spinocerebellar tracts carry proprioceptive information from the pelvic limbs, and are located in the most superficial region of the lateral funiculus of the spinal cord (Fig. 1–10). The rostral or cranial spinocerebellar and cuneocerebellar tracts carry proprioceptive information from the thoracic limbs. The rostral or cranial spinocerebellar tract is located medially to the dorsal and ventral spinocerebellar tracts (Fig. 1–10). The cuneocerebellar tracts ascend in the fasciculus cuneatus. Most fibers from the dorsal and rostral or cranial spinocerebellar and cuneocerebellar tracts enter the cerebellum via the ipsilateral caudal cerebellar peduncle. Fibers from the ventral and remaining rostral or cranial spinocerebellar tracts enter through the rostral cerebellar peduncle. The ventral spinocerebellar tract crosses in the spinal cord and crosses again before entering the

rostral cerebellar peduncle to the cerebellum on the ipsilateral side. These tracts are affected in mild superficial spinal cord compressions, and produce ataxia, an incoordinated gait (Table 3–2).

Some proprioceptive fibers travel in the spinocerebellar tracts and, instead of going to the cerebellum, exit to synapse in a nucleus in the caudal medulla oblongata. Fibers from the caudal medulla oblongata nucleus join the ipsilateral medial lemniscus, go to the thalamus, and contribute to conscious proprioception discussed below.

A second sensory system is the dorsal column system located in the dorsal funiculus of the spinal cord. This pathway contains fibers that carry proprioception, touch, and localized nociception (pain). The dorsal columns are divided into two main tracts. The fasciculus gracilis carries information from the tail and pelvic limbs (Cd to T6), and the fasciculus cuneatus carries information from the thoracic segments, the thoracic limbs, and neck (T6 to C1). Axons enter the spinal cord, ascend in their respective fasciculus, and synapse either in the nucleus of the gracilis or cuneatus at the junction of the spinal cord and medulla oblongata. The second group of neurons crosses to the opposite side and ascends in a contralateral pathway called the medial lemniscus and synapses in the ventral caudal lateral nucleus of the thalamus. A third group of neurons leaves the thalamus, passes through the internal capsule, and synapses in the somatosensory cortex of the parietal lobe of the cerebral cortex.

Conscious proprioception is tested by standing the dog or cat knuckled onto the dorsum of the paw and observing its ability to correct this malposition. Lesions of the spinal cord, medulla oblongata, and pons produce ipsilateral conscious proprioceptive deficits as determined by this test. Cerebral cortex lesions produce contralateral proprioceptive deficits. This type of proprioceptive information must ascend in the ipsilateral medial lemniscus and then cross the midline at some level above the pons before projecting to the cerebral cortex.

The spinothalamic and spinoreticular systems carry nociception (pain). These tracts are located deep in the white matter of the lateral and ventral funiculus of the spinal cord (Fig. 1–10). Fibers in these tracts project to both sides of the spinal cord, forming a multisynaptic, bilateral nerve network. The modality of deep pain, a dull, aching, nonlocalized pain, travels in these systems. To destroy the modality of deep pain, there must be a severe bilateral deep spinal cord lesion. Testing for deep pain is a useful prognostic guide in a paralyzed animal. The absence of deep pain 72 hours or more following spinal cord injury is generally considered an indication of a severe lesion in many animals.

The propriospinal tract carries information up and down the spinal cord between pelvic and thoracic limbs and is located around the gray matter of the lateral and ventral funiculus.

Motor tracts

Four main motor tract systems are considered here. The motor tracts may be divided into two groups: those for voluntary movement (flexor tracts) and those for posture and supporting weight against gravity (extensor tracts).[7,8] The cerebellum modulates the activity in the flexor and extensor systems and produces smooth, coordinated flexion and extension. The motor tracts are also named by where they begin and where they end.

The corticospinal tract (pyramidal tract) originates from the motor area of the frontal lobe of the cerebral cortex, descends through the internal capsule and the brain stem, then crosses to the opposite side in the caudal medulla oblongata (decussation of the pyramids) and descends in the spinal cord near the rubrospinal tract (Fig. 1–10). The corticospinal tract is very important in man, and when a lesion of the motor cortex or internal capsule occurs, contralateral hemiparesis or hemiplegia results. When a lesion of the motor cortex or internal capsule occurs in dogs and cats, little or transient weakness is present, but a contralateral placing and hopping deficit are observed (Table 3–2).

The rubrospinal tract begins in the red nucleus of the midbrain, crosses to the opposite side immediately, and descends through the brain stem to the spinal cord. The tract is located in the lateral funiculus of the spinal cord medial to the spinocerebellar tracts and next to the corticospinal tract (Fig. 1–10). Like the corticospinal tract, the rubrospinal tract is suspected as being important for the initiation of fine motor movements as tested during hopping and placing (Chapter 3).

The vestibulospinal tracts are important for maintaining posture and supporting weight against gravity in the dog and cat. They originate in the vestibular nuclei of the pontine medullary junction of the brain stem and descend uncrossed through the medulla oblongata and spinal cord. The vestibulospinal tracts are located in the ventral funiculus of the spinal cord. Early in the course of spinal cord compression, the animal may lose the ability to support weight on the limbs due to the involvement of these spinal cord tracts.

The reticulospinal tracts begin in the reticular formation of the midbrain, pons, and medulla and descend in the brain stem and spinal cord. The reticulospinal tract system is believed to be the most important motor system for voluntary movement, as specific lesions of the red nucleus and cerebral cortex produce only transient weakness. The medullary reticulospinal tract, like the rubrospinal and corticospinal tracts, is mainly associated with voluntary motor activity, and is primarily located in the lateral funiculus of the spinal cord. The pontine reticulospinal tract, like the vestibulospinal tract, is located in the ventral funiculus and influences postural motor activity. As the rubrospinal, corticospinal, vestibulospinal, and reticulospinal tracts all become involved due to spinal cord compression, the limbs are paralyzed and unable to produce voluntary movements or support weight.

The peripheral nervous system

The peripheral nervous system includes the 12 pairs of cranial nerves arising from the various parts of the brain stem, and the 36 pairs of spinal nerves arising from the spinal cord.

The sensory and motor functions of the cranial nerves are described earlier in this chapter and also in Chapter 3. The dorsal rootlets of the spinal cord are composed primarily of sensory neuron processes. The ganglia of the dorsal roots are the cell bodies of unipolar sensory neurons. The ventral rootlets of the spinal cord are composed of lower motor neuron axons. The dorsal and ventral roots fuse to form a peripheral spinal nerve that contains a combination of motor and sensory processes (Fig. 1–11).

In two sections of the spinal cord, C6 to T2 and L4 to S2, the peripheral spinal nerves form a plexus of nerves to and from the limbs, called the brachial and lumbosacral plexuses, respectively.

The spinal cord ends within the spinal canal at vertebrae L6 in the dog and S1 in the cat. The spinal nerves continue within the canal and exit after the vertebrae of the same number. These spinal nerves are also called the cauda equina and commonly consist of L7 and the sacral and caudal (Cd) nerves.

The autonomic nervous system

The autonomic nervous system is divided into two systems, the parasympathetic and the sympathetic (Fig. 1–12). The cranial portion of the hypothalamus contains cell bodies of the parasympathetic neurons that descend and synapse in brain stem nuclei associated with the oculomotor, facial, glossopharyngeal, and vagus cranial nerves and in spinal cord gray matter at sacral segments S1 to 3. The caudal portion of the hypothalamus contains cell bodies of the sympathetic neurons, which descend and synapse in the intermediolateral gray column of the spinal cord at thoracolumbar segments T1 to L3. These descending autonomic neurons have been referred to as first order neurons (UMN), and serve to moderate the activity of the peripheral autonomic neurons (LMN). Local reflex stimuli also modulate the activity of the peripheral autonomic neurons.

The peripheral autonomic nervous system (LMN) is composed of a two-neuron chain. The preganglionic neuron (second order neuron) cell bodies are located in the brain stem or spinal cord gray matter, and their axons exit the spinal cord through motor cranial nerves or ventral roots of the spinal nerves to synapse on

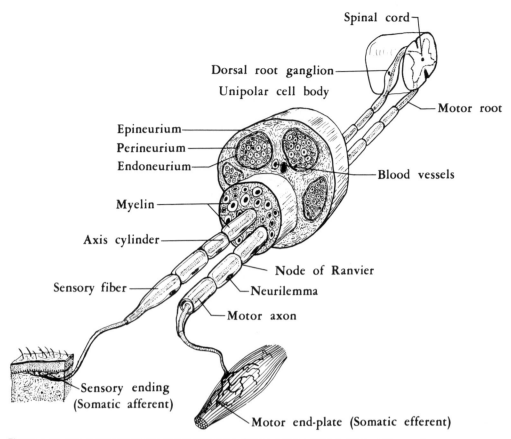

Figure 1–11. The components of a peripheral nerve. (From Jenkins, T.W.: Functional Mammalian Neuroanatomy. Philadelphia, Lea & Febiger, 1978.)

postganglionic neuron (third order neuron) cell bodies in outlying ganglia. The postganglionic neurons then innervate their target tissue, either smooth or cardiac muscle or glands of the body.

The parasympathetic peripheral nervous system has a cranial nerve outflow that exits the nervous system through oculomotor, facial, glossopharyngeal, and vagus nerves, and innervates smooth muscles and glands of the head and thoracic and abdominal viscera (Fig. 1–12). The parasympathetic system also has a sacral outflow (S1-S3), which innervates the urinary and reproductive tracts, colon, and rectum. The axons of the preganglionic neurons are very long, and synapse in ganglia near or in plexuses within the walls of the target organ. The postganglionic neuronal

axons are short. Acetylcholine is the neurotransmitter of the preganglionic and postganglionic parasympathetic neurons, and the parasympathetic system is referred to as a cholinergic system. The basic functions of the parasympathetic nervous system are related to long-term survival such as cardiovascular function, digestion, and excretion of waste products.

The peripheral sympathetic nervous system has a thoracolumbar outflow, which originates from cell bodies in the intermediolateral gray column of the spinal cord from T1 to L3 and exits the spinal cord through the ventral roots. The preganglionic axons are relatively short, and many synapse in the paravertebral ganglion of the sympathetic chain or trunk. The cervical part of the sympathetic chain

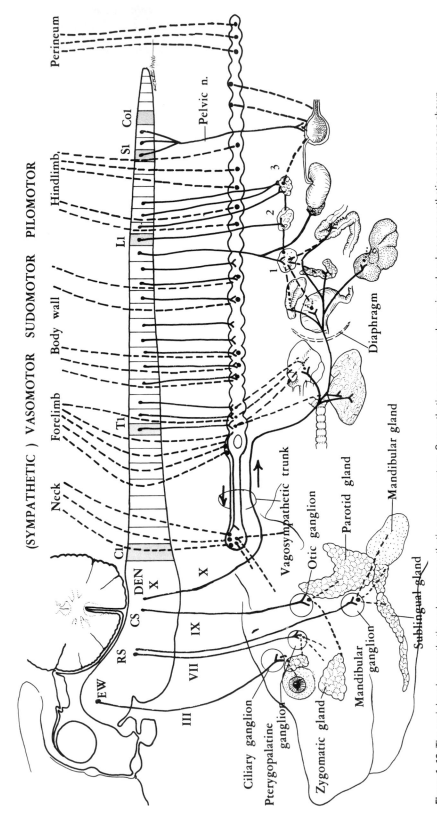

(SYMPATHETIC) VASOMOTOR SUDOMOTOR PILOMOTOR

Figure 1–12. The peripheral sympathetic and parasympathetic nervous system. Sympathetic neurons are shown in red and parasympathetic neurons are shown in blue. Solid lines are preganglionic neurons and broken lines are postganglionic neurons. (EW) Edinger-Westphal nucleus, (RS) rostral salivatory nucleus, (CS) caudal salivatory nucleus, (DEN X) dorsal efferent nucleus of the vagus; (C1) cervical-1 level, (T1) thoracic-1 level, (L1) lumbar-1 level, (S1) sacral-1 level, (Cdl) caudal level; (III) oculomotor nerve, (VII) facial nerve, (IX) glossopharyngeal nerve, (X) vagus nerve; (1) celiac ganglion, (2) cranial mesenteric ganglion, (3) caudal mesenteric ganglion.

22

contains several ganglia composed of cell bodies of postganglionic neurons for blood vessels, sweat glands, and other smooth muscles and glands of the head and thoracic viscera. Other preganglionic axons synapse in prevertebral ganglia of the abdomen, and postganglionic axons innervate abdominal viscera. The sympathetic preganglionic neurons release acetylcholine, while postganglionic neurons release norepinephrine and the system is classified as adrenergic. Preganglionic sympathetic neurons also innervate the medulla of the adrenal gland. Stimulation of these neurons results in the release of epinephrine from the adrenal medulla and the classic "fight or flight," or short-term survival activity, associated with the sympathetic nervous system.

Autonomic function and problems are discussed further in Chapter 19 with urinary incontinence, and wherever autonomic dysfunction complicates other nervous system problems.

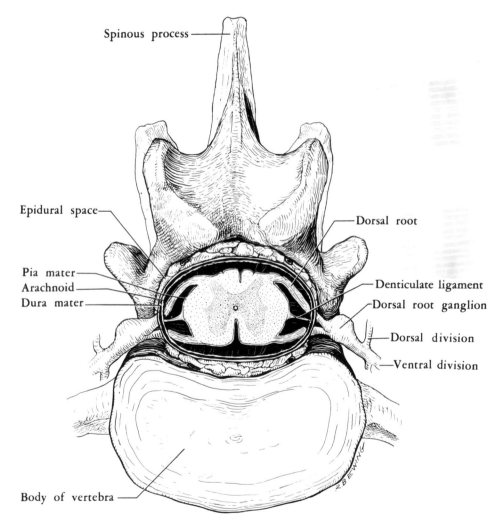

Figure 1–13. Transverse section of spinal cord within the vertebral canal to show the formation of a spinal nerve in relation to the vertebra and meninges. Note the adipose tissue and blood vessels in the epidural space. (From Jenkins T. W.: Functional Mammalian Neuroanatomy. Philadelphia, Lea & Febiger, 1978.)

The meninges

Three membranes cover the brain and spinal cord, and serve to protect the nervous tissue in the bony cavities of the cranium and vertebral column.

The outermost layer is a tough membrane called the dura mater. It closely adheres to the periosteum of the cranial vault, but is surrounded by an epidural fat layer within the vertebral column.

The next layer is the arachnoid membrane, so called for the web-like projections connecting this layer to the innermost membrane, the pia mater. The dura mater and arachnoid membrane are in close contact. Cerebrospinal fluid flows in the space between the arachnoid membrane and the pia mater. The pia mater is a delicate membrane that makes intimate contact with the brain and spinal cord and follows the contours of the gyri, sulci, and fissures. The relationship of the spinal cord, meninges, nerve roots, and vertebral column is shown in Figure 1–13. The epidural space is filled with fat.

Cerebrospinal fluid

Cerebrospinal fluid (CSF) is formed by the choroid plexuses of the lateral and the third and fourth ventricles as well as from the external and internal lining of the CNS. The CSF fills the ventricular system of the brain, the central canal of the spinal cord, and the subarachnoid spaces, suspending the nervous system in a fluid medium. The CSF serves as a shock absorber and protects the nervous tissue. CSF also aids in the maintenance of a constant environment for the nervous tissue. CSF is continually produced and circulates throughout the ventricular system and central canal and exits into the subarachnoid space through the lateral foramen (foramen of Luschka) in the fourth ventricle. CSF is then reabsorbed, mostly by arachnoid villi associated with the dorsal sagittal venous sinus. A large collection of CSF in the subarachnoid space is located between the caudal cerebellum and medulla oblongata, and is called the cerebellomedullary cistern. CSF can be collected in animals from this cistern. Abnormalities in CSF production, flow, or reabsorption can result in excess accumulation and hydrocephalus (Chapter 7).

References

1. Allen, N.: The chemical basis of neurologic disorders. Clin Neurosurg, *4*:386, 1967.
2. Breazile, J.E.: Textbook of Veterinary Physiology. Philadelphia, Lea & Febiger, 1971.
3. Clark, R.G.: Manter and Gatz's Essentials of Clinical Neuroanatomy and Neurophysiology. 5th Ed. Philadelphia, F.A. Davis Company, 1975.
4. Curtis, B.A., Jacobsen, S., and Marcus, E.: An Introduction to the Neurosciences. Philadelphia, W.B. Saunders, 1972.
5. DeLahunta, A.: Veterinary Neuroanatomy and Clinical Neurology. Philadelphia, W.B. Saunders, 1983.
6. Jenkins, T.W.: Functional Mammalian Neuroanatomy. Philadelphia, Lea & Febiger, 1978.
7. King, A.S.: Physiological and Clinical Anatomy of the Domestic Mammals. Vol. 1, Central Nervous System. New York, Oxford University Press, 1987.
8. Latshaw, W.K.: Neural control of locomotion. Am Anim Hospital Assoc J, *10*:598, 1974.
9. Miller, M.E., Christensen, G.C., and Evans, H.E.: Anatomy of the Dog. Philadelphia, W.B. Saunders, 1968.

Chapter 2

The neurologic history

The basic information collected on all animals regardless of the presenting complaint consists of history, physical and neurologic examinations, and initial clinicopathologic tests, and is referred to as the data base. One of the most invaluable parts of the data base is the history.[1] The types of problems an animal has and the possible mechanisms of disease processes that could produce the problems can be obtained from an analysis of the history. The basic mechanisms of disease include congenital or familial, inflammatory (infection, immune-mediated, or other), metabolic, toxic, nutritional, traumatic, vascular, degenerative, neoplastic, or idiopathic disorders. Information collected in the history can also be used by the clinician to decide whether the problem originates within the nervous system or in some other body system secondarily affecting the nervous system. If it is suspected that the lesion is located within the nervous system, the clinician can form an initial impression of the anatomic location and severity of the lesion. A rational diagnostic plan can then be outlined, so that diagnostic tests can be used to evaluate specific parts of the nervous system as well as other body systems. The clinician can also use historical information to plan an appropriate therapeutic regimen and provide an accurate prognosis. An outline of informa-

Table 2–1
Neurologic history

Signalment   Species _____ Breed _____ Age _____
              Sex _____ Color _____
Primary complaint _____
              Duration _____ Status _____
Mechanism of disease
  Familial problems _____
  Past illness (onset, course, duration) _____
  _____

  Present illness _____
    General attitude _____ Sneezing _____
    Body condition _____ Exercise tolerance _____
    Water consumption _____ Body discharges _____
    Urinations _____ Bleeding _____
    Vomiting _____ Abortions _____
    Diarrhea _____ Deaths _____
    Constipation _____ Vaccinations _____
    Coughing _____
  Toxicity _____
  Diet _____
  Past trauma _____ Recovery _____
  Recent trauma _____
  Past or present neoplasia _____
Owner's neurologic evaluation
  Behavior and personality changes _____
  _____

  Description of the seizures: Aura or localizing sign _____
    Ictus _____ Ictus length _____
    Recovery _____ Recovery length _____
    Date of onset _____ Frequency of occurrence _____
    Patterns _____ Duration of condition _____
              Total number of seizures _____

tion to be obtained in the history is represented by the neurologic history form in Table 2–1.

Signalment

The signalment, which includes species, age, breed, sex, and color, should be initially considered, and basic principles re-

garding the common mechanisms of disease associated with a given signalment should be reviewed.

Age

Specific age ranges often have certain disease mechanisms associated with them. Congenital malformations usually produce clinical signs in dogs and cats under 1 year

Table 2–1
Neurologic history (Continued)

Head coordination and posture _____
Cranial nerves
    Smell _____   Dropped jaw _____
    Vision _____   Paralysis of face _____
    Pupils _____   Deafness _____
    Strabismus _____   Head tilt _____
    Nystagmus _____   Swallowing _____
    Loss of facial sensation _____   Regurgitation _____
    Head muscle atrophy _____   Dyspnea _____
                                       Tongue _____
Past limb involvement (onset, course, duration) _____

Present limb involvement
    Onset _____   Side or limb involved first _____
    Course _____
    Duration _____
    Present involvement (side, limb or limbs) _____
    Bowels _____   Bladder _____
Past or present pain and location _____

Therapeutic attempts
    Medications (dose, duration, response) _____

    Surgery _____
Conclusions
    Possible disease mechanisms (differential diagnosis) _____

    Location of lesion _____
    Severity of involvement _____

of age. Toxicities, infections, or trauma have no specific age predilection, but are most common in young animals, which have a tendency to chew on foreign objects and become intoxicated, have improper immunizations, or have little experience with moving vehicles.

The first seizures from inherited epilepsy usually begin in animals 9 months to 3 years of age. Seizures occurring in animals younger than 9 months of age are most often due to some other cause.

Seizures associated with hypoglycemia in toy breed dogs and dogs with portacaval shunts and hepatic encephalopathy most commonly begin when the animal is less than 1 year of age.

Seizures due to hypoglycemia from an insulinoma usually occur in dogs over 5 years of age. Other neoplastic processes are frequently seen in adult dogs and cats over 5 years of age.

Degenerative diseases such as degenerative myelopathy in German Shepherd

Table 2-2
Breeds, age ranges, and specific disorders

Breed	Age of onset or presentation	Disorder
Afghan	6–9 mos	Afghan myelopathy
Akita	Under 6 mos	Idiopathic vestibular disorder
Australian heeler	Birth	Deafness
Australian shepherd	Birth	Deafness
Australian Silky terrier	Under 1 yr	Glucocerebrosidosis
Bassett hound	Adult	Intervertebral disc disease
	6–9 mos	Globoid leukodystrophy
Beagle	3–6 mos	Deafness and idiopathic vestibular disorder
	3–6 mos	GM_1 gangliosidosis
	3–6 mos	Cerebellar neuronal abiotrophy
	3–6 mos	Glycoproteinosis
	6–9 mos	Globoid leukodystrophy
	1–3 yrs	True epilepsy
	Adult	Intervertebral disc disease
Bernese mountain dog	3–6 mos	Cerebellar abiotrophy
Border collie	Birth	Deafness
	3 mos	Cerebellar degeneration
Boston terrier	From birth	Hydrocephalus
	From birth	Deafness
	Young	Hemivertebrae, myelodysplasia
	Over 5 yrs	Primary brain tumors
Bouvier des Flandres	Under 1 yr	Laryngeal paralysis
Boxer	6–12 wks	Dysmyelinogenesis
	Less than 6 mos	Boxer neuropathy
	Over 5 yrs	Primary brain tumors
Brittany Spaniel	Adult	Cerebellar degeneration
	Under 1 yr	Spinal muscular atrophy
Bull mastiff	3–6 mos	Cerebellar neuronal abiotrophy
Bull terrier	Birth	Deafness
Bulldog	Birth	Sacrocaudal agenesis
	Birth	Spina bifida, hemivertebrae, and myelodysplasia
Cairn terrier	6–9 mos	Globoid leukodystrophy
Chihuahua	6–12 mos	Hydrocephalus
	Adult	Ceroid lipofuscinosis
Chow Chow	Birth	Myotonia
	Birth	Cerebellar hypoplasia
	Birth	Myotonia
	6–12 wks	Dysmyelinogenesis
Cocker spaniel	Birth	Deafness
	Adult	Idiopathic facial paralysis
	Adult	Intervertebral disc disease
	Adult	Ceroid lipofuscinosis

Table 2–2
Breeds, age ranges, and specific disorders (Continued)

Breed	Age of onset or presentation	Disorder
Collie	Birth	Deafness
	3–6 mos	Cerebellar neuronal abiotrophy
	3–6 mos	Dermatomyositis
Dalmatian	Birth	Deafness
	3–6 mos	Dalmatian leukodystrophy
	3–6 mos	Hypomyelination
	3–6 mos	Spinal dysraphism
Dachshund	Birth	Sensory neuropathy
	Adult	Intervertebral disc disease
	Adult	Narcolepsy
	Adult	Ceroid lipofuscinosis
Doberman pinscher	3–6 mos	Idiopathic vestibular disorder
	6–9 mos	Narcolepsy
	Young and over 5 yrs	Cervical vertebral malformation
	Over 5 yrs	Cervical disc disease
	Adult	Sensory neuronopathy
	Adult	Myositis of head muscles, polymyopathy, Dancing Doberman disease
Domestic shorthair cats	6 mos–1 yr	Neuroaxonal dystrophy
English bullterrier	From birth	Sacrocaudal malformations
English pointer	3–6 mos	Sensory neuronopathy
English setter	From birth	Deafness
	3–6 mos	Ceroid lipofuscinosis
Fox terrier	3–6 mos	Spinocerebellar degeneration
	3–6 mos	Myasthenia gravis
	3 mos	Deafness and vestibular disorder
	6 mos	Lissencephaly
German shepherd	3–6 mos	Idiopathic vestibular disorders
	3–6 mos	Megaesophagus
	1–3 yrs	True epilepsy
	Adult	Myositis of head muscles, polymyopathy,
	Adult	Myasthenia gravis
	Adult	Fibrocartilaginous infarct
	Adult	Giant axonal neuropathy
	Adult	Lumbar intervertebral disc disease
	Adult	Lumbosacral malformation
	Over 5 yrs	Degenerative myelopathy

(continued)

Table 2–2
Breeds, age ranges and specific disorders (Continued)

Breed	Age of onset or presentation	Disorder
German shorthaired pointer	3–6 mos	Gangliosidosis
Golden retriever	3–6 mos	Myotonic myopathy
	Adult	Sensory neuronopathy
Gordon setter	6–9 mos	Cerebellar neuronal abiotrophy
Great Dane	6 mos—2 yrs	Cervical vertebral malformation
	3–6 mos	Megaesophagus
	Adult	Fibrocartilaginous infarct
	Adult	Intervertebral disc disease
Hounds	Adult	Acute polyradiculoneuritis
Irish setter	Birth	Quadriplegia and amblyopia
	3–6 mos	Cerebellar neuronal abiotrophy
	3–9 mos	Lissencephaly
	1–3 yrs	True epilepsy
Irish terrier	3–6 mos	Myotonic myopathy
Jack Russell terrier	6–12 mos	Myasthenia gravis
	3–6 mos	Spinocerebellar degeneration
Keeshound	Adult	Idiopathic epilepsy
Kerry blue terrier	3–6 mos	Cerebellar neuronal abiotrophy
Labrador retriever	Birth	Familial reflex myoclonus
	3–6 mos	Familial myopathy
	3–6 mos	Spongiform degeneration
	3–6 mos	Narcolepsy
	3–9 mos	Fibrinoid leukodystrophy
Lhasa Apso	3–6 mos	Lissencephaly
	3–6 mos	Hydrocephalus
	Adult	Epilepsy
Maltese terrier	Birth–3 mos	Hydrocephalus
Manx cat	Birth	Sacrocaudal malformations
Old English sheepdog	Birth	Sacrocaudal malformations
	Birth	Deafness
Pekingese	Adult	Intervertebral disc disease
Poodle	Less than 1 yr	Hypoglycemia
	3–6 mos	Cerebellar hypoplasia
	3–9 mos	Hydrocephalus
		Globoid leukodystrophy
		Glycoproteinosis
		Sphingomyelin lipidosis
		Demyelinating myelopathy
	Less than 1 yr	Atlantoaxial subluxation
	Less than 1 yr	Narcolepsy
	6–9 mos	Globoid leukodystrophy
	1–3 yrs	True epilepsy
	Adult	Intervertebral disc disease

Table 2-2
Breeds, age ranges, and specific disorders (Continued)

Breed	Age of onset or presentation	Disorder
Pug	Adult	Encephalitis
Rottweiler	3–9 mos	Polyneuropathy
	Adult	Neuroaxonal dystrophy
	Adult	Leukomyelopathy
Saint Bernard	3–9 mos	Narcolepsy
	1–3 yrs	True epilepsy
	Adult	Fibrocartilaginous infarct
Saluki	Adult	Ceroid lipofuscinosis
Samoyed	3–6 mos	Cerebellar neuronal abiotrophy
Schnauzer	6 mos–2 yrs	Hyperlipidemia and seizures
	6 mos–2 yrs	"Flybiting" and "stargazing" seizures
	Adult	Fibrocartilaginous infarct
Scottish terrier	6 mos–3 yrs	Scottie cramp
	Adult	Sensory neuronopathy
Shetland sheepdog	3–6 mos	Dermatomyositis
Siamese cat	Birth	Congenital strabismus and nystagmus
	3–6 mos	Deafness or vestibular disorder
	3–6 mos	Gangliosidosis
	3–6 mos	Sphingomyelinosis
	Adult	Ceroid lipofuscinosis and mucopolysaccharidosis
Siberian husky	6–9 mos	Laryngeal paralysis
	Adult	Degenerative myelopathy
	Adult	Sensory neuronopathy
Silky terrier	3 mos	Spongiform degeneration
	3–6 mos	Glucocerebrosidosis
Springer spaniel	3 mos	Hypomyelinogenesis
	3–6 mos	Myasthenia gravis
	Adult	Fucosidosis
	Adult	Rage syndrome
Swedish Lapland	3 mos	Spinal muscular atrophy
Tervuren shepherd	Adult	Epilepsy
Tibetan mastiff	3–6 mos	Hypertrophic neuropathy
Weimaraner	Birth	Spinal dysraphia
West Highland white terrier	3–6 mos	Globoid leukodystrophy
Whippet	Adult	Sensory neuronopathy
Yorkshire terrier	3–6 mos	Hydrocephalus
	Less than 1 yr	Atlantoaxial subluxation

dogs occur most frequently after 5 years of age.

Breed

Many neurologic disorders have an age and breed predilection that should be considered when forming a differential diagnosis for a particular problem (Table 2–2).

Sex

Few neurologic disorders have a specific sex predilection. Hypocalcemia associated with whelping and mammary adenocarcinoma with metastasis to the nervous system are two disorders seen in females. Prostatic adenocarcinomas can also metastasize to the nervous system in male dogs.

Coat Color

In a few instances, genetic neurologic disorders may be related to coat color. Blue-eyed white cats are commonly deaf. Congenital deafness in English Setters and other breeds of dogs can also be related to a predominance of white in the coat color.

Primary complaint

The clinician should assume control of the conversation with a client and ask specific questions in a consistent order, so that a logical sequence of events can be developed and no information overlooked (Table 2–1). Histories can be misleading if the owner rambles on and the veterinarian only listens and then tries to fit the pieces of information into a logical sequence.

A clear, concise description of the primary complaint should first be derived. Most of the primary complaints of neurologic patients can fit into one or more of the problems listed in Table 2–3. From the primary complaint, the clinician can de-velop an initial opinion on which part of the nervous system is involved and if the signs are symmetric or asymmetric (Table 2–3). The duration of the signs and the present status of the disease process should be established to determine whether the disease is acute or chronic, and whether it is progressive, static, or regressive.

Mechanism of disease

Examples of neurologic disorders associated with the various mechanisms of disease are listed in Table 2–4. The mechanisms of disease often have a typical signalment, onset, and progression of signs and symmetry or asymmetry of neurologic deficit. The mechanisms of disease and their typical histories are listed in Tables 2–5 and 2–6. A logical approach in questioning may be used to explore the possibility of each one.

Congenital and familial disorders

A history of similar problems in litter mates and animals of the same blood line may support the possibility of a problem due to a congenital malformation or to true epilepsy. Many animals with congenital and familial disorders manifest clinical signs before 1 year of age, except those with epilepsy, which is seen usually between 9 months and 3 years of age. Clinical signs manifested at birth may be static or progressive.

Infections and other inflammations and metabolic disorders

A history of past or present illnesses might support a diagnosis of a multiple-system inflammatory or metabolic disorder. Information about the general attitude, body growth or condition, appetite, water consumption, urinations, vomiting, diarrhea,

Table 2–3
Problems and location of lesions causing them

Problems	Location
Behavior and personality disorders	Telencephalon, diencephalon
Seizures	Telencephalon, diencephalon
Visual dysfunction	Optic nerve, visual pathways, and telencephalon
Coma and altered states of consciousness	Telencephalon, diencephalon, mesencephalon
Signs related to other autonomic and somatic cranial nerve dysfunction	Other autonomic or somatic cranial nerves
Anisocoria	Sympathetic, parasympathetic
Strabismus	Oculomotor, trochlear, abducent
Dropped jaw and head muscle atrophy	Trigeminal, muscle
Increased or decreased facial sensation	Trigeminal
Paralysis of eyelid, lip, and/or ear	Facial
Dysphagia	Glossopharyngeal, vagus
Megaesophagus	Vagus
Laryngeal paralysis	Vagus
Paralysis of tongue	Hypoglossal
Head tilt, circling, and nystagmus	Vestibular system
Deafness	Auditory system
Opisthotonus, tetanus, tetany, tremors, myoclonus, and other muscle spasms	Multiple sites in CNS, PNS, and muscle
Incoordination of the head and limbs	Cerebellum
Hemiplegia, hemiparesis, quadriplegia, quadriparesis, ataxia of all four limbs, and episodic weakness	Brain stem, spinal cord, peripheral nerve, neuromuscular junction, and muscle
Paraplegia, paraparesis, and ataxia	Spinal cord
Paralysis or paresis of one limb	Peripheral nerve
Dilated anus, atonic tail, and distended bladder	Cauda equina
Self-mutilation	Multiple sites in CNS and PNS

Table 2–4
Mechanisms of disease and examples of specific diseases

Congenital and familial disorders

Hydrocephalus
Lissencephaly
Lysosomal storage diseases
Congenital nystagmus
True epilepsy
Congenital deafness
Dysmyelinogenesis

Virally induced cerebellar hypoplasia
Vertebral malformations (hemivertebra, spina bifida, cervical vertebral malformation)
Spinal cord malformations (spinal dysraphia, meningomyelocele)
Afghan myelopathy

Infections and other inflammations

Viral—Distemper, adenovirus 1, panleukopenia, feline infectious peritonitis, rabies, herpes
Bacterial—meningitis, discospondylitis
Fungal—cryptococcosis, blastomycosis, histoplasmosis, aspergillosis
Protozoal—toxoplasmosis
Rickettsia—Rocky Mountain spotted fever and Erlichiosis
Parasites—dirofilaria immitis
Granulomatous meningoencephalitis (reticulosis)

Steroid-responsive meningoencephalomyelitis
Pug encephalitis
Allergic encephalomyelitis
Acute polyradiculoneuritis
Myasthenia gravis
Polymyositis
Temporal and Masseter myositis

Metabolic disorders

Hypoglycemia
Hyperglycemia
Hypocalcemia
Hypercalcemia
Hyperkalemia
Hypokalemia
Hypernatremia
Hyponatremia
Hypoxia
Hypoadrenocorticism
Hyperadrenocorticism

Hypothyroidism
Hyperthyroidism
Uremic encephalopathy
Hepatic encephalopathy
Osmolality disturbances
Acid–base disturbances

Table 2-4
Mechanisms of disease and examples of specific diseases (Continued)

Toxicity

Lead   Aminoglycoside antibiotics
Organophosphates   Ethylene glycol
Chlorinated hydrocarbons   Ivermectin

Nutritional disorders

Thiamine deficiency

Trauma

Head injury   Intervertebral disc herniation
Spinal cord injury   Peripheral nerve injury

Vascular disorders

Infarction from thrombus or embolus
Septicemia
Vasculitis
Hemorrhage from bleeding disorders

Degeneration

German Shepherd myelopathy
Senile deafness
Cerebellar degeneration
Intervertebral disc degeneration

Neoplasia

Gliomas, glioblastoma   Choroid plexus papilloma
Astrocytoma   Neurofibrosarcoma,
Oligodendroglioma   neurofibroma
Meningioma   Neurinoma
Ependymoma   Metastatic neoplasia

Idiopathic disorders

Vestibular syndromes
Self-mutilation syndromes
Idiopathic epilepsy

Table 2-5
Mechanisms of disease and typical history

Mechanism of disease	Signalment	Onset and progression	Neurologic deficits
Congenital and familial	Young, often purebred	Present since birth Chronic progressive	Symmetric or asymmetric
Infections and other inflammations	Any age, breed, or sex	Acute progressive Chronic progressive	Symmetric or asymmetric
Metabolic disorders	Any age, breed, or sex	Acute progressive Chronic progressive Episodic (seizures)	Usually symmetric
Toxicity	Any age, breed, or sex	Acute progressive, usually	Usually symmetric
Nutritional disorders	Cats—thiamine deficiency	Acute progressive	Usually symmetric
Trauma	Any age, breed, or sex	Acute nonprogressive	Symmetric or asymmetric
Vascular disorders	Any age, breed, or sex	Acute nonprogressive	Symmetric or asymmetric
Degeneration	Any age, breed, or sex	Chronic progressive (Type I IV disc—see trauma)	Symmetric or asymmetric
Neoplasia	Often over 5 years of age	Chronic progressive	Symmetric or asymmetric
Idiopathic	Vary with each syndrome	Vary with each syndrome	Vary with each syndrome

constipation, coughing, sneezing, exercise tolerance, abnormal body discharges, bleeding tendencies, abortions, illness, and death of animals in the environment should be obtained. The types, numbers, and frequency of vaccinations should be recorded, and the likelihood of inadequate protection or vaccination reactions may be considered as a cause of the neurologic disorder. This information is not only important to aid in the diagnosis of problems in the nervous system, but also to detect concurrent problems in other systems that might be potentially life-threatening and should be considered prior to neurologic diagnostic tests. Infections may be acute or chronic, but usually progress without treatment. Infections can produce symmetric or asymmetric neurologic deficits. Metabolic disorders are usually acute, progress without treatment, and produce symmetric neurologic deficits.

Toxicity

The type of environment should be described further to detect potential sources of intoxicating substances or malicious neighbors who might intoxicate the animal. The animal's tendency to chew and pick up foreign objects should be established. Exposure to household chemicals,

Table 2–6
Mechanisms of disease that usually have a similar history in adult dogs and cats

Acute progressive with asymmetric neurologic deficits
   1. Infections or other inflammations
   2. Neoplasia
Acute progressive with symmetric neurologic deficits
   1. Infections or other inflammations
   2. Metabolic disorders
   3. Toxicity
   4. Nutritional disorders
Acute nonprogressive
   1. Trauma (Type I IV disc)
   2. Vascular disorders
Chronic progressive with asymmetric neurologic deficit
   1. Infections or other inflammations
   2. Degeneration (Type II IV disc)
   3. Neoplasia

paint, other sources of lead, lawn and tree sprays, external parasite sprays and dips, and deworming medication should be evaluated in relation to the onset of the clinical signs. Any chronic drug therapy the animal has received should be considered for possible neurotoxicity. Toxicities often produce acute neurologic signs that either worsen or improve with or without treatment over time. Toxicities usually produce symmetric neurologic deficits.

Nutritional disorders

The type of diet and the amount and frequency of feedings should be evaluated to determine whether adequate nutritional requirements are being met for the animal. All dietary supplements should be described. Clinical signs associated with nutritional disorders are often acute and symmetric.

Trauma

The possibility of past or recent trauma should be questioned. If a specific event is known, the onset and progression or regression of signs should be ascertained. If no specific event is known, the type of environment should be described to determine if the animal could receive a traumatic insult to the nervous system without the owner's knowledge. Traumatic and vascular disorders usually have an acute onset that either remains static or improves over time. Traumatic and vascular lesions may produce symmetric or asymmetric signs.

Neoplasia

Any surgical removal and histologic diagnosis of neoplasms should be determined, and their potential for metastasis to the nervous system considered. Neurologic deficit associated with neoplasia is usually chronic and progressive and often asymmetric.

Idiopathic

Idiopathic disorders of the nervous system often have an acute onset of clinical signs that may regress. Idiopathic disorders may produce asymmetric or symmetric neurologic deficits. The history of most idiopathic disorders varies with the specific disorder.

Owner's neurologic evaluation

Questions concerning the owner's evaluation of the neurologic status of the animal are asked in the same sequence as the neurologic examination will later be performed, beginning at the head and ending at the limbs, tail, and anus (Chapter 3). The onset, course, duration, and symmetry of each past and present neurologic sign is considered for its relationship to the primary complaint and mechanism of disease.

Changes in personality, habits, house training, eating, sleeping, and water consumption may indicate a disease process in the cerebrum or rostral brain stem.

Seizure description

Seizures are also a sign of cerebral or rostral brain stem disease. An accurate description and classification of the type of seizure should be obtained. Seizures can be simply classified into three basic types: generalized seizures, partial seizures, and partial seizures that secondarily generalize. The type of seizure the animal is having can be indicative of the mechanisms of the disease process producing the seizure (Chapter 8). There are four basic parts to a seizure. The preictal phase, or prodromal period, may occur several days or hours prior to the actual seizure, and may be manifested by restlessness and pacing, insecurity, and seeking out the owner for consolation, or some other abnormal be-

havior. An aura or localizing sign may be the actual beginning of the seizure. An aura is a feeling, and the animal may display abnormal behavior similar to the prodromal period. A localizing sign is often manifested by some involuntary contractions of certain muscle groups on one side of the face or body. The ictus, fit, or seizure can vary greatly in description, depending on the focal or diffuse nature of the seizure discharge (Table 8–1). The level of consciousness, body position, jaw and limb movements, and autonomic signs of salivation, urination, and defecation should be elicited from the owner. The length of the seizure should be noted. During the recovery, or postictal phase, the animal may be hyperactive and continually pace, or be very tired and sleep. Some animals are very hungry and thirsty, and may want to urinate or defecate if they did not do so during the seizure. The length of recovery should be noted. The onset of the first seizure, the frequency of seizures, any seizure patterns or changes in appearance, and total number of seizures should also be determined.

Head coordination and posture

Head coordination and posture should be discussed to detect cerebellar or vestibular dysfunction, respectively.

Cranial nerve disorders

Signs relating to cranial nerve abnormalities should be discussed. Difficulties in finding food can indicate a problem with olfaction. Bumping into objects might reflect a visual deficit. Dilated pupils or downward and outward eyeball deviations may indicate oculomotor nerve damage. Other abnormal eyeball deviations can indicate involvement of the trochlear, abducent, or vestibular nerves. Nystagmus or spontaneous jerking of the eyeballs can be the result of vestibular dysfunction. Loss of facial sensation, difficulty in closing the mouth or chewing, and masseter and temporalis muscle atrophy all indicate a trigeminal nerve problem. Asymmetry of the face with inability to close the eyelid or move the lip or ear can result from facial nerve paralysis. Deafness can be caused by cochlear nerve disease. Difficulties in swallowing can relate to glossopharyngeal and vagus nerve dysfunction. Regurgitation from megaesophagus can be caused by brain stem or vagus nerve disease. Inspiratory dyspnea and increased upper airway sounds may be caused by laryngeal paresis or paralysis. Difficulty in lapping water and atrophy of the tongue muscles indicate hypoglossal nerve problems.

Limb disorders

Signs of past or present limb incoordination, paresis, or paralysis should be discussed. The time of onset, the side first involved, the most affected limb, the duration, the course, and recovery, if applicable, should be ascertained for all past and present limb problems. Past or present back and neck pain may be manifested by reluctance to go up and down stairs, sit up to beg, jump off furniture, move the neck, or bend down to the food bowl.

The function of the bowels and bladder should be discussed to determine the severity of the lesion and whether the animal needs assistance with the urination and defecation processes.

Therapeutic attempts

The drugs, dosages, duration of, and response to, previous medical therapy should be discussed. Any previous surgical therapy should also be discussed. From this information, the clinician may formulate an initial therapeutic plan.

Conclusions

From the determination of the primary complaint and from answers to questions concerning signs of neurologic dysfunction, the clinician can formulate an initial impression of the location and the severity of the lesion or lesions, and of whether the disease process is focal, multifocal, or diffuse. The initial impression can later be reevaluated after the neurologic examination findings are considered (Chapter 3).

A description of the onset, course, duration, and symmetry of the primary complaint and other neurologic signs gives important insight into the possible disease mechanism. Congenital and familial disorders may produce clinical signs at birth or shortly after, and may remain the same or become progressively worse. Some congenital problems such as dysmyelinogenesis and vestibular disorders spontaneously improve or are compensated for. Inflammations, nutritional deficiencies, and metabolic disorders have an acute or chronic onset, but usually progress unless therapy is instituted. Nutritional and metabolic disorders produce symmetric signs. Traumatic and vascular disorders have an acute onset, and signs remain static or improve over time, but rarely progress. Toxicities often have an acute onset, and can progress if the intoxicating agent is not removed from the animal and the environment. Toxicities produce symmetric signs. Degenerations and neoplastic diseases often have a slower onset and progressive course, regardless of therapy. Neoplastic disorders often produce asymmetric signs. Many idiopathic disorders begin acutely, and then improve after a short time. From the information collected from the questions pertaining to the mechanisms of disease and the onset, course duration, and symmetry of the neurologic signs, the clinician can formulate an initial differential diagnosis (Tables 2–5, 2–6).

The initial differential diagnosis may be altered after the physical and neurologic examination, and initial clinicopathologic test results are considered.

Reference

1. DeLahunta, A.: Small Animal and Equine Neurologic Examinations. *In* Veterinary Neuroanatomy and Clinical Neurology. Philadelphia, W.B. Saunders, 1983.

Chapter 3

The physical and neurologic examinations

Physical and neurologic examinations are a series of observations used to evaluate the general health of the body systems and, specifically, the nervous system. Both examinations support information collected in the history, and aid in determining the mechanism, location, and severity of the disease process.[1-3]

Physical examination

A complete physical examination is an important part of the basic information collected on all animals. Most clinicians have their own approaches to the physical examination, which will not be reviewed here. The findings on the physical examination that might be pertinent to animals with neurologic disorders are discussed by body systems.

Visual system

The eyes should be examined closely during the physical examination. Vision and pupil reflex evaluations are an important part of the neurologic examination.

Conjunctivitis may occur with distemper virus infections in dogs, and less frequently with rabies infections. Corneal edema may be associated with canine adenovirus infections, which may also occasionally produce encephalopathy. Corneal ulcers may result from improper tear production or inability to properly close the eyelid because of facial nerve disease.

Anterior uveitis is often a nonspecific sign associated with feline infectious peritonitis (FIP) and feline leukemia (FeLV) viruses and toxoplasmosis infections. Anterior uveitis may occur in fungal infections and granulomatous meningoencephalitis in dogs, which also may affect the nervous system of cats.

The ocular fundus of dogs may have a chorioretinitis associated with fungal, distemper virus, and toxoplasmosis infections and granulomatous meningoencephalitis (inflammatory reticulosis). Chorioretinitis of the ocular fundus may occur in cats with FIP and FeLV viruses and toxoplasmosis infection.

Papilledema or optic nerve swelling may be noted with increased intracranial pressure or optic neuritis, respectively.

Respiratory system

A nasal discharge can be an important observation. Infections with canine distemper virus produce a serous to mucopurulent nasal discharge. Cats and dogs with cryptococcosis infections often have a chronic nasal discharge. The fungal infection can erode through the nasal cribriform plate and produce a meningoencephalitis. Nasal tumors such as mucoepidermoid carcinomas may or may not begin with a nasal discharge. The tumor may also erode through the nasal cribriform plate and affect the olfactory bulbs and prefrontal cerebral cortex.

Gross examination of the larynx and pharynx may yield important information when laryngeal hemiplegia, cricopharyngeal achalasia, other swallowing problems, and middle and inner ear infections are believed present.

Canine distemper virus, feline infec-

tious peritonitis virus, toxoplasmosis, and many of the systemic fungus infections involve the respiratory system as well as the nervous system, and may produce pneumonia or pleural effusion.

Some neoplastic processes may metastasize to the lungs before the spinal cord or brain, but thoracic radiographs are often needed to demonstrate this (Chap. 4). Some dogs and cats may develop neurogenic pulmonary edema following prolonged seizures.

Animals with pulmonary disease or severe respiratory distress and cyanosis might appear generally weak because of the secondary effects of hypoxia on the nervous system. It is important to evaluate pulmonary function in all animals before the administration of anesthesia for further diagnostic tests of nervous system function.

Cardiovascular system

Evaluation of the cardiovascular system is useful to differentiate syncopal attacks from seizures with little motor activity (Chap. 8).

Severe heart failure and cyanosis can result in weakness and collapse due to hypoxia. The diagnosis of heart failure is supported by abnormal heart and lung sounds on auscultation of the chest, blue-tinged mucous membranes, and a pendulous, fluid-filled abdomen. Arrhythmias also can produce collapse or syncope, but electrocardiographic monitoring may be necessary to definitely diagnose these. Septicemia can result in bacterial endocarditis and emboli and microabscesses diffusely in the brain. Embolization and thrombosis of the caudal aorta may produce an ischemic neuromyopathy and pelvic limb paralysis in cats with cardiomyopathy (Chap. 17).

The cardiovascular system is often further evaluated using thoracic radiographs and ultrasonography in the neurologic patient over 5 years of age (Chap. 4).

Gastrointestinal system

Canine distemper virus, feline infectious peritonitis virus, and systemic fungi infections and lymphosarcoma may affect the gastrointestinal system as well as the nervous system, producing vomiting, diarrhea, and weight loss. Esophageal dilatation and regurgitation may be seen in any disorder affecting the brain stem or vagus nerve, but are common findings in neuromuscular diseases such as polymyositis and myasthenia gravis (Chap. 16). Rarely, certain chronic gastrointestinal disturbances may be due to a lesion in the limbic portions of the brain and actually may be a type of seizure that responds to anticonvulsant therapy (Chap. 8).

Liver disorders can result in hepatic encephalopathy (Chap. 7). Palpation of liver size can help to assess the presence of disease, but clinicopathologic tests, abdominal radiographs, and biopsy often are necessary for complete evaluation of the liver. Pancreatic beta-cell neoplasia and hypoglycemia produce seizures in dogs over 5 years of age, but must be diagnosed with clinicopathologic tests, as there are usually no palpable masses in the abdomen. Diabetes mellitus can produce a hyperosmolar syndrome or severe acidosis and coma. Diabetic dogs may have cataracts, be debilitated, paretic, or paralyzed (Chap. 16). The abdomen should be thoroughly palpated for evidence of any masses that might secondarily metastasize to the nervous system.

Hemolymphatic system

Anemic animals often display generalized weakness caused by an improper oxygen supply to the nervous system as well as to other systems. Enlarged lymph nodes might suggest lymphosarcoma or systemic infection, which may also be affecting the nervous system. Petechiae and ecchymoses on the skin and mucous membranes may indicate a bleeding disorder. Spontaneous bleeding into the nervous system can produce an acute onset of paraplegia, quadriplegia, coma, or other neurologic signs.

Urinary system

Palpation of the urinary system may reveal some abnormalities, but clinicopathologic tests are often routinely performed to evaluate the urinary system (Chap. 4).

Chronic uremia may produce severe acidosis and electrolyte imbalances and encephalopathy characterized by dementia, seizures, or coma (Chaps. 7, 8, and 10). Chronic uremia can also produce polyneuropathy (Chap. 16). In quadriplegic and paraplegic dogs and cats, the ability to reflexively or voluntarily urinate must be assessed by observation or palpation and manual bladder expression.

Reproductive system

Mammary adenocarcinomas and prostatic adenocarcinomas can both metastasize to the spinal cord and brain and produce neurologic signs. Pyometra can lead to septicemia and embolization to the brain with the formation of microabscesses.

Integumentary system

Examination of the external ear canals and tympanic membranes is important, particularly, when a middle and/or inner ear infection is believed to be present. Further examination of the tympanic membranes should be performed under anesthesia if there is any question about their integrity or appearance.

Endocrinopathies associated with thyroid and adrenal malfunction may produce characteristic skin and hair coat changes, and be a symptom of hypothalamic or pituitary disease. Neuromuscular disease occasionally is associated with endocrinopathies (Chap. 16). Chronic draining abscesses or other masses, which could be associated with fungal or bacterial infections or neoplasia, might be secondarily affecting the cranium, vertebrae, and nervous tissue. Dermatitis is often associated with polymyositis in man, but is rarely seen except on the faces and tails of Collies and Shetland Sheepdogs (Chap. 16). Lacerations and bruising of the skin or scars may indicate recent or past trauma, respectively.

Quadriparetic dogs with depressed or absent spinal reflexes should be examined for evidence of an engorged tick (tick paralysis) or raccoon bite (acute polyradiculoneuritis [Chap. 16]).

Skeletal system

The skeletal system, including the cranium and vertebrae, should be palpated thoroughly for fractures, masses, or any other processes that might secondarily affect nervous system structures. The joints should be carefully palpated for swelling and pain as early polyarthritis cases may be confused with neuromuscular or spinal cord disease. The muscular system is considered with the nervous system in this text, and is evaluated as part of the neurologic examination.

Neurologic examination

The neurologic examination is used to support or confirm information collected from the history. The clinician may be able to determine if the nervous system dysfunction is primary, such as an infectious process, or secondary to disease in some other system, such as a metabolic disorder. If nervous system disease is present, the site or sites of involvement can be located using the neurologic exam. The location(s) of the lesion(s) may be used to determine if the disease process is focal, multifocal,

or diffuse. The symmetry or asymmetry of the neurologic deficit should be noted, as toxic, metabolic, and nutritional mechanisms of disease usually produce symmetric signs (see Table 2–5). Inflammatory, neoplastic, traumatic, and vascular mechanisms often are asymmetric, but on occasion can produce symmetric signs (see Table 2–5). The severity of the neurologic deficit also can be ascertained. Once the lesion is localized, or determined to be multifocal or diffuse, and the severity of involvement is known, a rational diagnostic approach can be developed. Serial neurologic examinations often are the most accurate guide to therapeutic success and prognosis.

The neurologic examination may be organized into a sequence of observations made on the animal, beginning at the head and ending at the tail.[1–4] The same series of observations are performed in the same order on each patient regardless of the neurologic complaint, unless detrimental to the condition of the animal. With a standard approach on all animals, certain tests are not forgotten and less obvious deficits are not overlooked. With an anatomic location in mind for each observation, at the completion of the examination the abnormal findings can be put together to correctly localize the lesion. Initially, an attempt should be made to relate all deficits found to a focal anatomic lesion. If this is impossible, then a multifocal or diffuse disease process must be present. The outline of the neurologic examination is shown in Table 3–1 and is divided into four sections: evaluation of the head, evaluation of the gait and strength, evaluation of the thoracic limbs and neck, and evaluation of the pelvic limbs, tail, and anus.

Evaluation of the head

Evaluation of the head is performed using observations and tests that specifically evaluate anatomic structures above the level of

Table 3–1
Outline of the neurologic examination

Evaluation of the head

Personality and mentation _____

History of seizures?   Yes _____   No _____

Endocrinopathies _____

Head posture _____

Head coordination _____

Cranial nerves:

Olfaction (I) _____	Temporal and masseter (V) _____
Menace (II, VII) _____	Special vestibular (VIII) _____
Pupil reflex (II,III) _____	Hearing (VIII) _____
Pupil size (II,PS, Symp)* _____	Swallowing (IX,X) _____
Pupil symmetry (PS, Symp)* _____	Regurgitation (X) _____
Strabismus (III,IV,VI,VIII) _____	Larynx (X) _____
Vestibular nystagmus (III,IV,VI,VIII) ____	Trapezius (XI) _____
Spontaneous nystagmus (VIII) _____	Tongue (XII) _____
Ear, eye, lip reflex (V,VII) _____	Vital signs _____

Evaluation of gait and strength (Walk, trot, turn, hemiwalk)†

Evaluation of thoracic limbs and neck

Wheelbarrow† _____
Hopping: L _____ R _____
Placing: L _____ R _____
Proprioception: L _____ R _____
Extensor strength: L _____ R _____
Biceps reflex‡: L _____ R _____
Triceps reflex‡: L _____ R _____
Extensor carpi radialis‡: L _____ R _____
Flexor reflex‡: L _____ R _____
Crossed extension: L _____ R _____
Deep pain: L _____ R _____
Babinski sign: L _____ R _____
Superficial sensation _____
Neck pain _____
Muscle atrophy _____

Evaluation of pelvic limbs, tail, and anus

Wheelbarrow† _____
Hopping: L _____ R _____
Placing: L _____ R _____
Proprioception: L _____ R _____
Extensor strength: L _____ R _____
Patellar reflex‡: L _____ R _____
Cranial tibial reflex‡: L _____ R _____
Gastrocnemius reflex‡: L _____ R _____
Flexor reflex: L _____ R _____
Crossed extension: L _____ R _____
Deep pain: L _____ R _____
Babinski sign: L _____ R _____
Anal reflex‡ _____
Tail response _____
Panniculus _____
Sensory level _____
Muscle atrophy _____

Location of lesion(s): _____
Severity of lesion(s): _____

* PS = parasympathetic; Symp = sympathetic.

†0 = paralysis	‡0 = absent
1 = some movement	1+ = depressed
2 = support weight	2+ = normal
3 = support and few steps	3+ = hyperactive
4 = stumbles occasionally	4+ = hyperactive, with
5 = normal	clonus

the foramen magnum, such as the cerebral cortex, thalamus, hypothalamus, midbrain, pons, medulla, oblongata and their respective cranial nerves, and the cerebellum. Any abnormalities found on this section of the neurologic examination are referred to as "head signs."

Personality and behavior problems. Abnormalities in personality, mentality, or intellectual abilities either observed or related in the history must also be considered "head signs," and indicate lesions of the cerebral cortex, limbic system, hypothalamus, or midbrain (Chap. 2).

Lesions of the frontal lobe cerebral cortex and internal capsule projections related to the frontal lobe produce an animal that is demented, no longer recognizes the owner, and is unable to learn. Affected animals often pace compulsively, get lost in corners and press their heads against objects. If the lesion is unilateral, the animal often compulsively paces in wide or tight circles toward the side of the lesion. This can be differentiated from circling due to a vestibular lesion because the head is not tilted, and the animal is demented and often circles until it collapses from exhaustion. In unilateral vestibular lesions, the animal's head is tilted, it is mentally normal, and the circling is not compulsive.

Lesions in the temporal lobe cortex, limbic system, and hypothalamus also can produce bizarre behavior disorders such as aggression, hyperexcitability, extreme passiveness, and hypersexuality (Chap. 7).

Lesions in the midbrain usually produce animals that are sleepy, semicomatose, or comatose (Chap. 10).

Seizures. A history of seizures is a "head sign," and indicates a disease process affecting the cerebral cortex or subcortical projection systems through the thalamus or reticular formation of the rostral brain stem to the cerebral cortex. A lesion is most commonly located rostral to the midbrain. Seizures may be due to metabolic and toxic disorders. If the disorder is mild, there may be only dysfunction of the cortex and subcortical projection systems with no structural lesion. Information collected from the history must be considered when localizing the lesion during the neurologic examination (Chap. 2). The type of seizure can further aid in localizing the lesion and determining the mechanism of disease (Chap. 8).

Endocrinopathies. A history of endocrine disturbances and signs of polyuria, polydipsia, and polyphagia might be "head signs" and indicate a lesion in the hypothalamus or pituitary gland. This information should be considered when localizing the lesion.

Head posture and coordination. With lesions of the frontal cerebral cortex, internal capsule, and basal nuclei, the dog or cat may turn the head and eyes toward the lesion when lying down or standing. They usually circle toward that side as well. Turning toward the side of the lesion is called an adversion syndrome. Observation of the head posture and coordination can also be useful in evaluating vestibular and cerebellar function. A head tilt is usually a sign of unilateral dysfunction of the vestibular nerve, vestibular nucleus of the brain stem, or flocculonodular lobe of the cerebellum. Wide excursions of the head may be seen in bilateral vestibular disease. Head bobbing and head tremors are often due to a cerebellar lesion. The animal may be suspended in the air by the pelvis (Fig. 3-1). The normal head posture is to extend the neck and lift the head. A mild head tilt may be accentuated with this test and may be further accentuated if the animal is also blindfolded. In bilateral vestibular dysfunction, when suspended by the pelvis the animal's neck will flex. If the animal is lowered to the ground, instead of extending the forelimbs to support weight it will land at the dorsum of the head and neck.

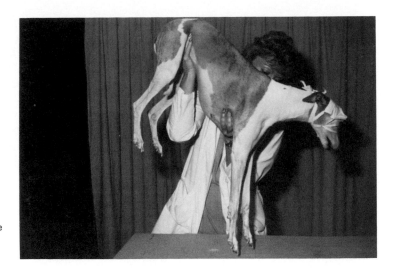

Figure 3–1. Blindfolded and suspended by the pelvic region, the animal must rely on the vestibular system for correct head, neck, and body posture.

Cranial nerves. Cranial nerve tests evaluate the function of cranial peripheral nerves and specific anatomic regions of the brain stem, from the prefrontal cortex and hypothalamus caudally to the medulla. Brain stem lesions often produce cranial nerve deficits that greatly aid in localizing the lesion to a particular segment. Cranial nerves should all be tested bilaterally, and the sides examined for asymmetry.

Cranial nerve I is *the olfactory nerve.* Lesions from the cribriform plate to the hypothalamus may affect this nerve and pro-duce problems with olfaction. There is often a history of the animal's having difficulty finding its food, and not eating until food is placed in its mouth. The presence of olfaction is suggested when the animal explores the examination room sniffing where other animals have been. Olfaction may be crudely tested by blindfolding the animal, placing food in front of it, and observing whether it can find the food by smell (Fig. 3–2). The sense of smell should not be tested with irritating substances such as ammonia or ether, as these irritate

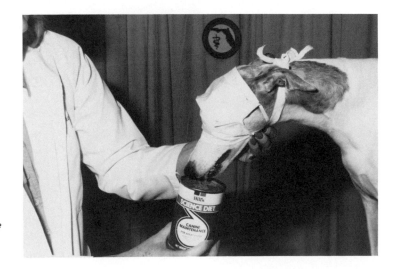

Figure 3–2. Testing *olfactory nerve* (cranial nerve 1) function by offering the blindfolded animal food.

the nasal mucosa and actually test sensation supplied by *cranial nerve V, the trigeminal nerve.*

Cranial nerve II is *the optic nerve* and is used for vision. It is located ventral to the hypothalamus (Chap. 1). Lesions involving any part of the visual pathway, the retina, the optic nerves, the optic tract, the lateral geniculate nucleus, optic radiations, and occipital lobe cortex can produce blindness (Chap. 9). A blind animal will bump into objects in an unfamiliar examination room. The examiner can toss cotton balls into the air and observe whether the animal watches them fall silently to the ground. The menace response is another test commonly used to evaluate vision. A hand is slowly advanced toward the eye, and the animal should blink in response to the threatening gesture (Fig. 3-3). Care is taken not to touch the eyelashes or to create air currents that might stimulate sensations of the face and test *cranial nerve V, the trigeminal nerve.* The menace response is not specific for vision, but an animal with a lesion in the visual system will lose the response. The menace response is also absent in young or severely demented animals, and in animals with cerebellar or facial nerve disease. If an an-

imal blinks the eyes in response to a strong light, there is at least some vision present. If it is established that the animal has a visual deficit, the pupillary light reflex is used to localize the part of the visual system affected. Light shown into the pupil normally causes the pupil to constrict, or become smaller (direct response) (Fig. 3–4). At the same time, the pupil on the opposite side that received no direct light also will constrict (consensual response). A lesion of the retina, optic nerve, optic chiasm, or optic tract produces an eye that is blind and a pupil that does not constrict properly to light. If an animal is blind, with pupils that respond normally to light, the lesion is most likely in the optic radiations or occipital lobe cortex. The specific pupillary changes and the location of the lesions are discussed in detail in Chapter 9.

Cranial nerve III is *the oculomotor nerve,* which constricts the pupil, moves the eyeball medially, dorsally, and ventrally, and elevates the eyelid. The pupils should also be observed for size and symmetry (Fig. 3–5). Widely dilated (mydriatic) pupils can result from excessive sympathetic influences such as in a terrified or hyperexcitable animal, or from the lack of parasympathetic innervation from *cranial nerve III,*

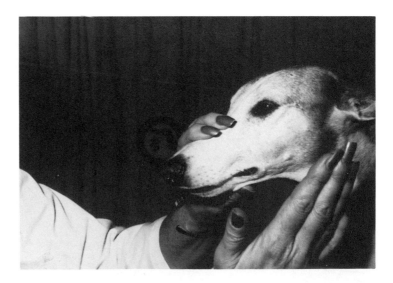

Figure 3–3. Testing *optic nerve* (cranial nerve 2) function with the menace response.

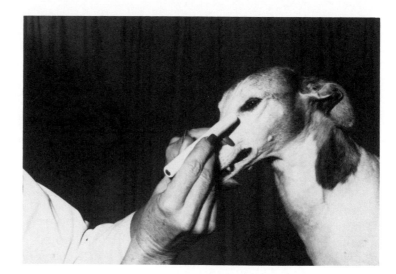

Figure 3–4. Using a penlight, a blink to a bright light *(optic nerve)* and the pupillary light reflexes *(optic* and *oculomotor nerves)* are tested.

the oculomotor nerve. The oculomotor nerve nucleus (Edinger–Westphal nucleus) is located in the midbrain. If there is a unilateral lesion of the midbrain or peripheral nerve, the pupil on the same side will be dilated and unresponsive to light during pupillary light reflex testing. This can be differentiated from optic nerve disease because the eye will have normal vision.

Constricted (miotic) pupils can result from excessive parasympathetic influences, as seen with organophosphate toxicity, or from lack of sympathetic innerva-tion. A unilateral constricted pupil can be due to a lesion in the sympathetic inner-vation to that pupil. The classic Horner's syndrome is due to the loss of sympathetic innervation to the pupil, orbit, and eyelid, resulting in a ptosis (drooped eyelid) and enophthalmus (sinking in of the globe) along with the constricted pupil (miosis). The sympathetic innervation to the pupil courses from the hypothalamus to the cau-dal cervical spinal cord (first-order neu-ron), from T2 spinal segments and nerve roots up the sympathetic chain to the su-

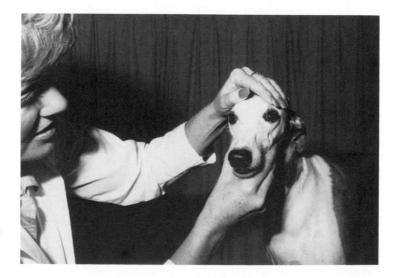

Figure 3–5. The pupils are examined for size and symmetry in normal light and the eyeballs are examined for strabismus or nystagmus.

perior cervical ganglion (second-order neuron) and then from the superior cervical ganglion through the middle ear to the pupil (third-order neuron). A lesion at any one of these sites could produce a miotic pupil; therefore, other neurologic signs must be considered with the pupil changes to localize the lesion. When asymmetric pupils are present, it must be decided whether the more constricted or dilated side is abnormal. Asymmetric pupils are referred to as anisocoria and are discussed in more detail in Chapter 11. If both the parasympathetic and sympathetic innervation is affected, as in deep midbrain lesions, the pupils are fixed in a midpoint range and do not respond to light.

The eyeballs are examined for abnormal deviations, referred to as strabismus (see Fig. 3–5). *Cranial nerve III, the oculomotor nerve,* innervates the medial rectus, inferior oblique, dorsal rectus, and ventral rectus muscles of the eyeball. Lesions of the oculomotor nerve can produce a lateral and downward deviation of the eyeball. The pupil will be dilated only if the parasympathetic fibers in the oculomotor nerve also are affected. The oculomotor nerve also innervates smooth muscle in the upper eyelid, and a lesion of this nerve may result in a ptosis, or droopy eyelid.

Cranial nerve IV is *the trochlear nerve* and innervates the superior oblique muscle of the eyeball. Trochlear nerve lesions produce a mild lateral rotation of the eyeball. Because of the round pupil in dogs, this rotation is not easily observed, but the dorsal portion of the normal vertical pupil in cats will be deviated laterally. The oculomotor and trochlear nerve nuclei are located in the midbrain (Chap. 1).

Cranial nerve VI, is *the abducent nerve* and innervates the lateral rectus and retractor oculi muscles of the eyeball. A lesion of the abducent nerve results in medial deviation of the eyeball (Chap. 11). Retraction of the globe when the cornea is touched is a reflex between *cranial nerve V, the trigeminal nerve,* and the abducent nerve. The abducent nucleus and nerve are located at the pontine medullary junction of the brain stem (Chap. 1).

Deviation of the eyeballs when the head is moved into various positions has been called the doll's eye phenomenon or oculocephalogyric reflex, and should be symmetric in both eyes. Animals can alter this response by changing their focus on objects, so the test must be carefully evaluated. Positional strabismus may be observed by holding the head straight and lifting the nose in the air. The eyeballs should deviate ventrally equally as the nose is elevated. Disturbances of *cranial nerve VIII, the vestibular nerve,* produce an excessive downward deviation of the eyeball on the affected side, referred to as an "eye drop." Other asymmetric eye positions can suggest disease of the oculomotor, trochlear, or abducent nerves. Strabismus is discussed further in Chapter 11.

During movement of the head, a few involuntary, jerky eyeball movements are seen, which stop when the motion is discontinued. This eyeball movement is a normal response, referred to as vestibular nystagmus. As the head moves to the side, a horizontal nystagmus develops, with the fast phase of the nystagmus toward the side the head is turned. As the head is moved upward, a few beats of vertical nystagmus are seen, with the fast phase upward, and when the head is moved downward, the fast phase is downward. For vestibular nystagmus to be present, the vestibular system, the medial longitudinal fasciculus from the pontine–medullary junction to the midbrain, and the oculomotor, trochlear, and abducent nerves must be functioning properly (Chap. 12).

The animal should be observed for spontaneous nystagmus. If no spontaneous nystagmus is present, the animal is placed on its side and back to see if nystagmus can be induced (positional nystagmus).

Either type of nystagmus is usually an abnormal finding associated with an imbalance within the vestibular system. The types of nystagmus and their clinical significance in locating lesions are further discussed in Chapter 12.

Cranial nerve V, the trigeminal nerve, has a sensory component that transmits sensation from the entire head, including the face, eyelids, corneas, nasal mucosa, the tongue, and inside of the mouth. *Cranial nerve VII, the facial nerve,* innervates the muscles of facial expression. Cranial nerves V and VII are tested together with a series of reflexes. The inside of the ear is tickled (Fig. 3–6), the medial canthus of the eye is touched (Fig. 3–7), and the lip is pinched (Fig. 3–8). If the ear, eye, and lip move, the sensory portion of the trigeminal nerve and the motor portion of the facial nerve are functioning. If there is no response, the examiner must decide whether the sensory or motor part is deficient. If the facial nerve is damaged, the ear and lip may droop, the nose may be deviated, and the eye will not close to the menace response (Chap. 11). If the face is pricked with a pin or pinched with a hemostat, the animal will pull its head away or cry out if sensation is present. If the animal is very stoic, the nasal mucosa may be pricked with a pin; even the most stoic dogs will pull their heads away or sneeze

if the trigeminal nerve is functioning properly (Chap. 11). Corneal sensitivity and globe retraction may be tested by holding the eyelids apart and touching the cornea and observing the retraction of the globe. This tests the sensory portion of the trigeminal nerve and the motor portion of the abducent nerve. The sensory portion of the trigeminal nucleus and nerve are located in the pons. The facial nucleus and nerve are located at the pontine medullary junction of the brain stem (Chap. 1).

Cranial nerve V, the trigeminal nerve, has a motor division that innervates the temporalis and masseter muscles of mastication. A lesion in the motor nucleus or motor portion of the nerve results in temporalis and masseter muscle atrophy and a decrease in jaw tone (Fig. 3–9). An animal with bilateral trigeminal nerve lesions may demonstrate an inability to close the mouth. The motor nucleus of the trigeminal nerve is located in the pons (Chap. 1).

Cranial nerve VIII is *the vestibulocochlear nerve.* Unilateral vestibular nerve disease can produce head tilt, circling, positional strabismus, and spontaneous nystagmus (see Fig. 3–5). Special vestibular tests are discussed in Chapter 12. The cochlear portion of the nerve is necessary for hearing.

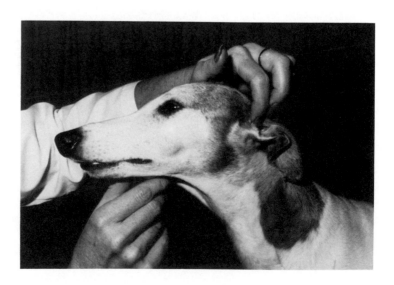

Figure 3–6. If the ear twitches when tickled, *trigeminal nerve* (cranial nerve 5), sensory, and *facial nerve* (cranial nerve 7) motor functions are intact.

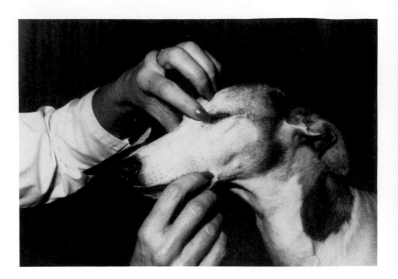

Figure 3–7. If the eyelid closes when the medial canthus is touched, *trigeminal nerve* (cranial nerve 5), sensory, and *facial nerve* (cranial nerve 7) motor functions are intact.

Deafness is usually associated with bilateral lesions of the cochlear nerves and nucleus and the ascending pathways through the brain stem to the midbrain. Deafness often is noticed by the owner and the complaint ascertained from the history. Hearing may be tested grossly by blindfolding the animal and dropping objects like keys nearby, or clapping the hands and whistling, to observe whether the animal turns its head in the direction of the sound. When the animal is asleep, loud noises without vibrations can be made in an attempt to awaken it. In temporal lobe cerebral cortex lesions, the animal might be able to hear, but can have difficultly in localizing sounds. Specific hearing testing and lesions are discussed in Chapter 13.

Cranial nerve IX, the glossopharyngeal nerve, and *cranial nerve X, the vagus nerve,* can be tested by the swallow or gag reflex (Fig. 3–10). Swallowing can be elicited by gentle external pressure on the throat in the region of the hyoid bones. The gag reflex can be elicited by insertion of the finger into the caudal pharynx. Loss of the

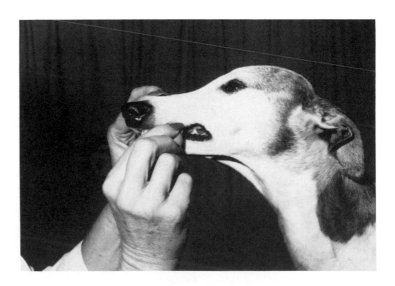

Figure 3–8. If the animal curls the lip as it is pinched, *trigeminal nerve* (cranial nerve 5), sensory, and *facial nerve* (cranial nerve 7) motor functions are intact.

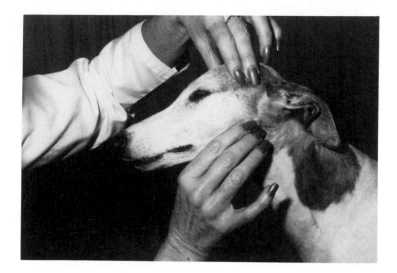

Figure 3–9. Palpation of the temporalis and masseter muscles is done to evaluate *trigeminal nerve* (cranial nerve 5) motor function.

ability to swallow can be due to damage of either nerve. The nuclei of both the glossopharyngeal and vagus nerves are located in the caudal medulla oblongata. Lesions producing swallowing difficulties, regurgitation, and laryngeal paralysis are discussed further in Chapter 11.

Cranial nerve XI, the accessory nerve, arises from the rostral cervical spinal cord segments and caudal medulla oblongata, and innervates the sternocleidomastoid and trapezius muscles of the neck (Fig. 3–11). In the rare instances of accessory nerve disease, atrophy of these muscles can be observed and palpated.

Cranial nerve XII, the hypoglossal nerve, innervates the muscles of the tongue. The tongue can be observed and palpated for asymmetry and atrophy (Fig. 3–12) (Chap. 11). The hypoglossal nucleus is also located in the caudal medulla oblongata.

Vital signs. Abnormalities in cardiac and respiratory rate and rhythm, detected on the physical examination, can be due to lesions in the brain stem control centers

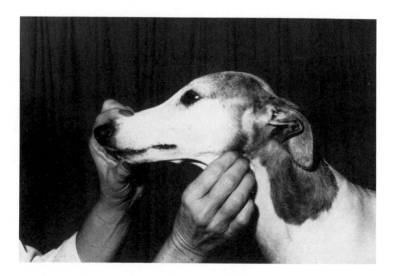

Figure 3–10. Gentle pressure on the hyoid bones will usually ellicit a swallowing reflex if *glossopharyngeal* (cranial nerve 9) and *vagus* (cranial nerve 10) nerves are intact.

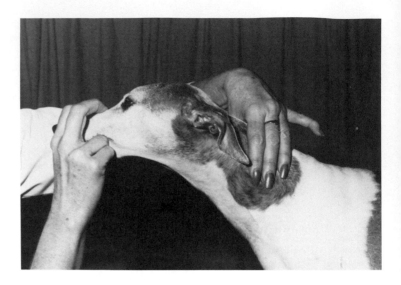

Figure 3–11. The sternocleidomastoid and trapezius muscles are palpated for atrophy associated with *accessory nerve* (cranial nerve 11) dysfunction.

in the reticular formation from the hypothalamus to the medulla. Lesions of the medulla and pons in animals are most noted for their effects on cardiac and respiratory rate and rhythm. Abnormalities in these systems must be considered during the final localization of the lesion.

Localization of lesions. An outline of the location of lesions and "head signs" is found in Table 3–2. The presence of "head signs" indicates a lesion at the ap-

propriate anatomic site within the cerebral cortex, cerebellum, or brain stem. This site should be considered as a possible cause of subsequent abnormalities found in the other three parts of the neurologic examination, i.e., the gait, the thoracic limbs, and the pelvic limbs. If it is impossible to relate other abnormalities to this initial lesion, a multifocal disease process probably is present.

If there are multiple "head signs" that cannot be explained by a focal anatomic

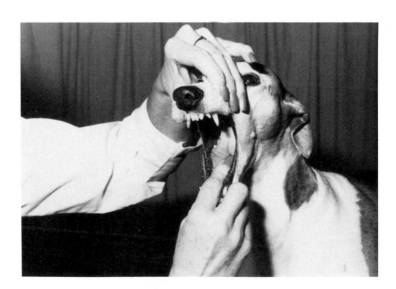

Figure 3–12. *Hypoglossal nerve* (cranial nerve 12) function is evaluated by observing and palpating the tongue.

lesion, such as a combination of behavior changes (cerebral cortex, limbic system, hypothalamus, or midbrain), head incoordination and tremor (cerebellum), and inability to swallow (medulla oblongata and cranial nerves IX and X), then it can be assumed that a multifocal cerebral cortex, cerebellar, and brain stem disease is present. This information is invaluable in determining possible mechanisms of disease and formulating a correct differential diagnosis.

When no "head signs" are discovered from the history or neurologic examination, a lesion, if it exists, must be below the foramen magnum in the spinal cord, peripheral nerves, or muscles.

Evaluation of gait and strength

The gait is examined for strength and coordination. Normal limb strength and movement is dependent on the proper functioning of upper motor neuron tracts that originate in the cerebral cortex and brain stem and descend through the brain stem and spinal cord, internuncial and lower motor neurons of the spinal cord, the neuromuscular junction, and skeletal muscles (Chap. 1). Coordination of gait is primarily dependent on the sensory peripheral nerves, the spinal cord tracts ascending to the cerebellum, and the cerebellum (Chap. 1).

The animal is observed during walking, trotting, and turning to the left and right. The posture of the limbs and trunk are observed while the animal moves and stands. A wide base posture or standing with the limbs at abnormal angles to the body may indicate a proprioceptive deficit. If the animal stands with a limb knuckled onto the dorsum of the paw, this also indicates a proprioceptive deficit. By lifting and supporting the limbs on one side, standing and walking on each side may be evaluated and compared. This is referred to as *hemistanding* and *hemiwalking*, and aids

in detecting asymmetries between the left and right limbs. Gait strength is graded from 0 to 5: 0 is complete paralysis; 1, paresis with some movement; 2, paresis with the ability to support weight, but not take steps; 3, paresis with the ability to support weight and take some steps; 4, slight paresis with only occasional stumbling; and 5, normal strength.

Localization of lesions. If "head signs" are present, an attempt is made to relate any gait deficits to the lesions suspected in the cerebral cortex, cerebellum, or brain stem. Very little gait deficit is associated with lesions rostral to the midbrain. Hemiparesis, hemiplegia, quadriparesis, and quadriplegia can be produced by lesions of the midbrain, pons, and medulla oblongata, but there also should be deficits in the cranial nerves of the affected region. Brain stem lesions below the midbrain generally produce ipsilateral signs with the deficit on the same side as the lesion.

Incoordination of the gait, or dysmetria, is manifested by excessive, exaggerated, jerky movements of the limbs and may be produced by lesions of the cerebellum, caudal cerebellar peduncles, and medulla oblongata. Head incoordination or cranial nerve deficits also may be observed. Unilateral lesions produce ipsilateral signs.

Polyneuropathies and polymyopathies can produce gait deficits and multiple cranial nerve signs, owing to the generalized involvement of many peripheral cranial and spinal nerves and muscles. These disorders can be differentiated from focal brain stem disease by testing limb spinal reflexes and palpating the limb muscles for atrophy. These points are discussed further in this chapter.

Gait deficits of all four limbs in the absence of "head signs" are most likely due to focal cervical spinal cord, diffuse or multifocal spinal cord, diffuse peripheral

Table 3–2
Location of lesions and clinical signs

Location of lesion	Clinical signs
Cerebral cortex	
Frontal lobe	Dementia; compulsive pacing; unilateral lesions: circling toward lesion, contralateral hopping and placing deficit; little gait deficit; seizures, with motor activity; acute lesions, transient contralateral hemiparesis; decreased consciousness, miotic pupils
Parietal lobe	Few signs; contralateral proprioceptive deficit; seizures, with sensory signs; possible contralateral facial hypalgesia
Occipital lobe	Contralateral visual deficit, with normal pupillary light reflexes; seizures, with visual hallucinations
Temporal lobe	Seizures, psychomotor; behavior abnormalities; hearing problems
Internal capsule	Possible frontal and parietal lobe signs
Basal nuclei	Few clinical signs in animals; possibly compulsive pacing or circling toward the lesion
Thalamus	Few clinical signs; possible irritability when handled; contralateral proprioceptive deficit; decreased consciousness; circling
Hypothalamus	Can be clinically silent or produce endocrinopathies; behavior abnormalities; temperature regulation problems; appetite and thirst disorders
Midbrain	Decreased states of consciousness; loss of pupil response to light; dilated pupils; ventrolateral strabismus; extensor rigidity in all four limbs; hemiparesis or hemiplegia, hopping, placing, and conscious proprioception deficits with unilateral lesions (contralateral with rostral lesions and ipsilateral with caudal lesions)
Pons	Quadriparesis; ipsilateral hemiparesis; hopping, placing, and conscious proprioception deficits; muscle atrophy of head; loss of facial sensation; vital sign changes; depressed, miotic pupils
Cerebellum	Ataxia of all four limbs and head; intention tremors; opisthotonus
Peripheral vestibular	Unilateral lesions: ipsilateral head tilt, circling, leaning, rolling, horizontal or rotary nystagmus (facial paralysis and Horner's syndrome in middle ear and petrous temporal bone disease), disoriented, but gait basically normal; bilateral lesions: lateral excursions of head, and ataxia, with falling to either side
Central vestibular and cranial medulla oblongata	Unilateral: head tilt, circling, leaning, rolling, horizontal, rotary, or vertical nystagmus, ipsilateral hemiparesis, with hopping, placing, and conscious proprioceptive deficits; facial paralysis; medial strabismus
Caudal medulla oblongata	Ataxia and hypermetria unilateral or bilateral; quadriparesis; ipsilateral hemiparesis, with hopping, placing, and conscious proprioception deficits; difficulty swallowing; regurgitation; laryngeal paralysis; atrophy of tongue; vital sign changes
Spinal cord	
C1 to 5	Ataxia (pelvic limbs often worse); quadriparesis, quadriplegia; ipsilateral hemiplegia, with hopping, placing, and conscious proprioceptive deficits; hyperactive spinal reflexes; neck pain, Horner's syndrome (first order neuron)

Table 3–2
Location of lesions and clinical signs (continued)

Location of lesion	Clinical signs
C6 to T2	Ataxia (thoracic limbs often worse); quadriparesis; quadriplegia; ipsilateral hemiplegia, with hopping, placing, and conscious proprioceptive deficits; depressed or absent thoracic limb spinal reflexes (with large lesion); hyperactive pelvic limb spinal reflexes; neck pain; Horner's syndrome (second order neuron)
T2 to L3	Ataxia pelvic limbs; paraparesis; paraplegia; hopping, placing, and conscious proprioceptive deficits; hyperactive pelvic limb spinal reflexes; superficial sensory level; loss of panniculus, deep pain alterations
L4 to Cd	Ataxia pelvic limbs; paraparesis; paraplegia; hopping, placing, and conscious proprioceptive deficits; depressed or absent pelvic limb spinal reflexes; superficial sensory level; deep pain alterations; distended bladder (S1–S3); dilated anus (S1–S3); atonic tail (Cd1–Cd5)
Diffuse peripheral nerve or neuromuscular junction	Ataxia all four limbs; quadriparesis; quadriplegia (rear limbs often worse); depressed or absent spinal reflexes in all four limbs; increased or decreased sensitivity (peripheral nerve only)

nerve, neuromuscular junction, or diffuse muscle lesions.

Gait deficits in the pelvic limbs only with no "head signs" are usually due to thoracolumbar spinal cord or bilateral peripheral nerve or muscle disease. The absence of "thoracic limb signs" must be confirmed. The pelvic limbs may appear more affected than the thoracic limbs, so that in comparison with the pelvic limbs, the thoracic limbs appear normal. Independent evaluation of the thoracic limbs is very important to detect minimal involvement that might alter the conclusion about the location of the lesion. An outline of the location of lesions and changes in gait is found in Table 3–2.

Evaluation of the neck and thoracic limbs

The neck and thoracic limbs are individually examined to determine whether they are affected by disease. The pelvic limbs are lifted and supported, forcing the animal to walk forward entirely on its thoracic

limbs. This is referred to as *wheelbarrowing*, and is useful to evaluate the strength and coordination of the thoracic limbs alone (Fig. 3–13). Subtle gait deficits in the thoracic limbs may become more obvious when wheelbarrowing is performed.

Postural reactions. The thoracic limb postural reactions of hopping and placing are examined. Both pelvic limbs and one thoracic limb are lifted and supported, so that the animal is relying on one thoracic limb. The animal then is hopped forward, backward, and to the side on left and right thoracic limbs separately to detect any deficit or asymmetries in initiation, strength, or coordination (Fig. 3–14).

During the placing test, the animal is lifted and supported under the abdomen and thorax and advanced toward a table. The normal response is that the animal sees the table, or feels the table edge with the dorsum of the paw if blindfolded, and advances both feet forward and places them on the table (Fig. 3–15). Left and right thoracic limbs also should be evalu-

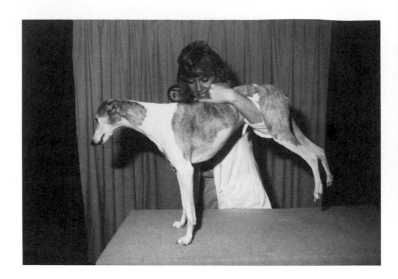

Figure 3–13. *Wheelbarrowing* and evaluating the thoracic limb function.

ated separately to detect asymmetries. Initiation of the hopping and placing responses are thought to originate in the frontal lobe cerebral cortex and basal nuclei, and may be affected by disease processes rostral to the midbrain. The strength and coordination of the hopping response is due to the proper function of motor and sensory tracts caudal to the midbrain. The animal may be suspended in the air by the pelvic region and lowered slowly to the ground (see Fig. 3–1). The normal posture is to extend the neck and

thoracic limbs, which support weight as the feet touch the ground. Hopping and placing deficits are usually ipsilateral with lesions below the midbrain, but contralateral with lesions of the rostral midbrain, diencephalon, and cerebral cortex.

Proprioception. Proprioceptive position testing is performed by standing the forelimb knuckled over at the paw and observing the ability of the animal to correct this abnormal position (Fig. 3–16). The limb also may be adducted or ab-

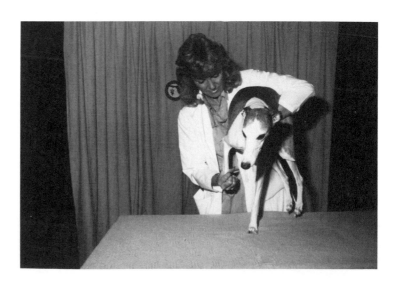

Figure 3–14. Individual thoracic limb function is evaluated by *hopping* on each limb.

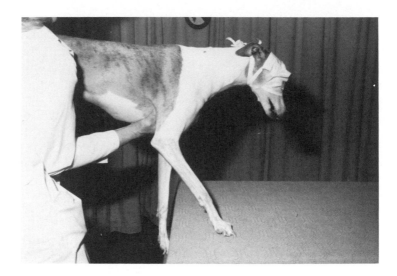

Figure 3–15. The *placing response* is used to evaluate for subtle dysfunction of the thoracic limbs.

ducted into abnormal postures, which the animal with normal proprioceptive sense should correct. Proprioception is a function of peripheral sensory nerves and sensory tracts from the spinal cord through the thalamus to the parietal lobe cerebral cortex. Proprioceptive deficits are usually ipsilateral with lesions below the diencephalon, but contralateral with lesions of the diencephalon and cerebral cortex.

Extensor strength. With the animal standing, the strength of the forelimbs may be examined by pressing down on the withers and noting the strength and symmetry of the extension of the limbs combating the downward pressure. The animal also may be suspended by its pelvis and lowered to the ground to observe the extension of the forelimbs and their ability to support weight. This also is an excellent test of vestibular function.

Spinal reflexes of the thoracic limbs. Examination of the spinal reflexes of the thoracic limbs specifically tests certain cer-

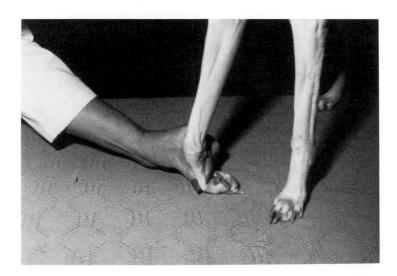

Figure 3–16. Testing *proprioception* of the thoracic limbs by standing the paw knuckled over and observing correction for this abnormal position.

vical spinal cord segments and nerves of the brachial plexus. The response of the spinal reflexes may be graded with the following scale: 0 = absent, 1+(+) = depressed, 2+(++) = normal, 3+(+++) = hyperactive, and 4+(++++) = hyperactive with clonus. The animal is held in lateral recumbency so the limbs relax as much as possible. A tense, stiff limb can override the reflex activity. If a normal animal is extremely nervous, the spinal reflexes may appear exaggerated. A percussion hammer or pleximeter is used to tap the tendon or muscle to ellicit a response.

A depressed or absent spinal reflex is produced by a lesion of the sensory peripheral nerve, dorsal roots, spinal cord segments, ventral roots, motor peripheral nerves, neuromuscular junctions, or muscles of the specific reflex arc (see Fig. 1–3). An absent spinal reflex often is an indicator of lower motor neuron (LMN) disease, and results in a flaccid type of paresis or paralysis. If the spinal cord segments and nerves of a particular reflex are known, then a depressed or absent spinal reflex can be used to localize the lesion to that specific segment, nerve root, or nerve (see Table 3–2).

Hyperactive spinal reflexes are associated with upper motor neuron (UMN) lesions anywhere rostral to the reflex arc in the spinal cord, brain stem, and the frontal lobe cerebral cortex (see Fig. 1–4). If an animal is paralyzed and the spinal reflexes are hyperactive, this is referred to as a spastic type of paralysis. The limbs may not be rigid, so spastic paralysis should not be confused with extensor rigidity (Chap. 14).

The biceps reflex (Fig. 3–17) is elicited by holding a relaxed thoracic limb with the elbow slightly flexed, placing the forefinger on the biceps tendon on the proximal medial aspect of the elbow, and tapping the finger with a percussion hammer. Although this reflex is sometimes difficult to elicit, a slight shortening of the tendon usually can be palpated in the normal animal. The left and right sides should be compared. If the reflex is present, spinal cord segments and nerve roots C6 to 7 and the musculocutaneous nerve are intact. The biceps reflex can become hyperactive in lesions above C6.

The triceps reflex (Fig. 3–18) is elicited by holding a relaxed thoracic limb with the elbow slightly flexed and tapping the triceps tendon with a percussion hammer, or by placing the forefinger or thumb on the tendon and tapping the finger or thumb

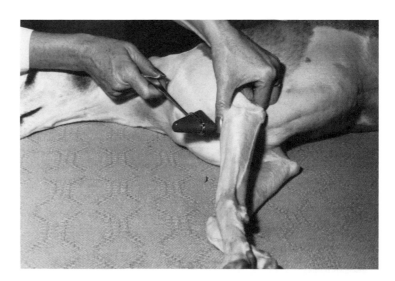

Figure 3–17. Testing the *biceps tendon reflex* by tapping with the pleximeter and observing a slight flexion of the elbow.

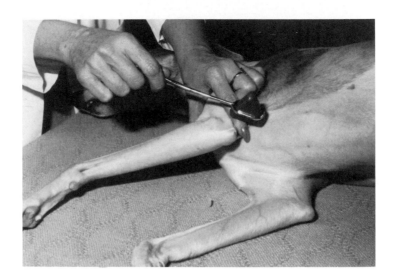

Figure 3–18. Testing the *triceps tendon reflex* by tapping with the pleximeter and observing a slight extension of the elbow.

with the hammer. Although the response is often small, in normal animals, a slight extension of the elbow may be visualized or palpated. The left and right sides should be compared. If the reflex is present, then spinal cord segments and nerve roots C7 to T2 and the radial nerve are intact. The triceps reflex may become exaggerated in lesions above C7.

The extensor carpi radialis muscle reflex (Fig. 3–19) is elicited by tapping the muscle with the percussion hammer (pleximeter), and a slight extension of the carpus is seen

in the normal animal. This response becomes diminished or absent in lesions of C7 to T2 spinal cord segments and nerve roots and the radial nerve. The response can also become hyperactive in lesions above C7.

The flexor, toe pinch, or withdrawal reflex (Fig. 3–20) is tested by pinching the animal's toe either with the fingers or a pair of hemostatic forceps and observing a withdrawal or flexion of the limb away from the stimulus. The presence of this reflex does not mean that the animal con-

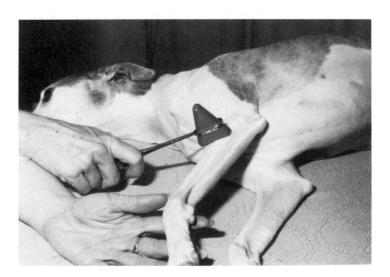

Figure 3–19. Testing the *extensor carpi radialis muscle reflex* by tapping with the pleximeter and observing a slight extension of the carpus.

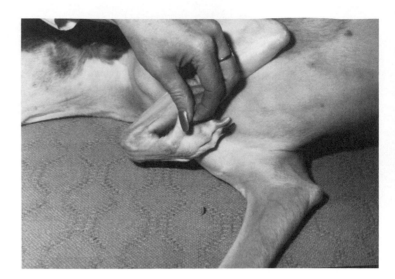

Figure 3–20. Testing the *toe pinch, withdrawal,* or *flexor reflex* of the thoracic limb by pinching the toe and observing a withdrawal response of the limb.

sciously feels the pinching. It only indicates that spinal cord and nerve root segments C6 to T2 and the musculocutaneous (flexion of the elbow) and median and ulnar (flexion of the carpus and digits) nerves are intact. When testing the flexor reflex of the left thoracic limb, the right thoracic limb should be observed for extension. If the opposite limb extends as the one tested flexes, this is called the crossed extensor reflex and indicates a lesion above the level of C6, usually on the side of the extended limb. When observed in acute injuries, crossed extensor reflex may indicate severe spinal cord damage, but this exaggerated reflex is often observed in chronic lesions above the C6 spinal cord segment and is not necessarily a grave sign. A further discussion of the use of spinal reflexes to localize lesions is found in Chapter 16.

Deep pain. During testing of the withdrawal reflex, evaluation of peripheral nerve and spinal cord integrity can be performed by increasing the stimulus strength and observing a behavioral response, such as the animal's crying in pain or trying to bite the examiner. This is the deep pain response, and is carried by small nonmyelinated axons, which are the most resistant to the effects of compression. The loss of

deep pain and the withdrawal reflex is usually due to damage to the sensory portion of the radial, median, and ulnar nerves or spinal cord segments C6 to T2. Damaged peripheral nerves potentially can regenerate and recover unless the nerve roots have been torn from the spinal cord (Chap. 18). The loss of deep pain with an intact flexor reflex indicates damage to ascending spinal cord tracts. Because these tracts are multiple and bilateral in animals, deep pain is usually lost only in severe injuries, and its continued absence 72 hours after an injury often means a grave prognosis. If the animal is already in extreme pain or very anxious from its injury, the response to the deep pain test may be minimal to absent, even when peripheral nerves or spinal cord tracts are actually intact. Loss of deep pain from severe cervical spinal cord lesions is rare, as such animals die from damage to upper motor neurons necessary for respiration. Damage to descending sympathetic pathways may produce loss of temperature regulation. Ascending degeneration into vital centers in the nearby medulla oblongata also may result in death in high cervical spinal cord injuries.

Babinski sign. The Babinski sign is best elicited in animals by a medial to lateral upward stroking of the metacarpal bones with the metal end of a percussion hammer. In normal animals, the toes flex slightly in response to this stroking. With a positive Babinski sign, the toes extend. The presence of a Babinski sign in man indicates corticospinal tract damage. In dogs, the Babinski sign is often seen with UMN lesions in general and is not related to disease in a specific motor system. A Babinski sign is more common in UMN lesions to the pelvic limbs than in UMN lesions to the thoracic limbs.

Superficial sensation. Superficial sensation, sharp localizing pain is carried by large diameter axons, which are more susceptible to compression than deep pain axons. Superficial sensation can be tested by light pin-pricking or pinching of the skin with hemostatic forceps. The light pin-pricking is most helpful in detecting hyperesthesia, and pinching of the skin is most useful in detecting anesthesia. Various segments of the skin, referred to as dermatomes, are innervated by specific nerve roots. There is much duplication of innervation in the cervical dermatomes as compared with thoracolumbar dermatomes, and lesions are not as easily localized in the cervical region as in the thora-

columbar region. The presence of neck pain or muscle spasms on manipulation of the neck is a more reliable indicator of a cervical lesion than superficial sensation alterations. Below the elbow on the thoracic limb, the dermatomes are well defined for the radial, median, ulnar, and musculocutaneous nerves, and can easily be tested for anesthesia (Chap. 18).

Neck pain. If the animal cries out or tries to bite, or if the muscles become rigid when the neck is manipulated, focal cervical nerve root or meningeal irritation is probably present (Fig. 3–21). The neck should be manipulated only if a cervical vertebral fracture or luxation is unlikely.

Muscle atrophy. Severe localized muscle atrophy of the thoracic limb indicates damage to the particular nerve root or peripheral nerve that innervates that muscle, and can be very helpful in localizing the lesion (Chap. 18).

Localization of lesions. Lesions above the level of the midbrain rarely produce gait deficits, but do produce deficits in hopping, placing, and proprioceptive positioning in the limbs. Unilateral lesions produce contralateral deficits, i.e., the le-

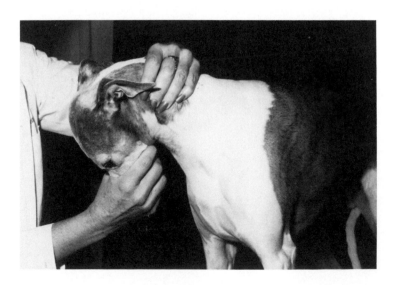

Figure 3–21. Manipulation and palpation of the neck to examine for pain and muscle spasms.

sion is on the opposite side of the deficit. Spinal reflexes are normal to hyperactive ($++$, $+++$, or $++++$).

Lesions below the level of the midbrain through the cervical spinal cord produce gait deficits in the limbs and deficits in hopping, placing, and proprioception. Unilateral lesions of the rostral midbrain usually produce contralateral deficits. Unilateral lesions of the caudal midbrain and below produce ipsilateral deficits. Spinal reflexes are normal or hyperactive unless the specific spinal cord segments or peripheral nerves to the reflex arc are involved. A lesion is probably located in the cervical spinal cord if there are no "head signs," but an abnormal gait in all four limbs, abnormal postural reactions, and decreased or increased spinal reflexes of the thoracic limbs, and abnormal postural reactions and increased spinal reflexes of the pelvic limbs are present.

If there are no "head signs" or thoracic limb signs, and abnormalities of the pelvic limbs were observed during gaiting, then the lesion is located below T2 in the thoracolumbar spinal cord or in nerves and muscles associated with the lumbosacral plexus. A summary of the changes in forelimb responses at various anatomic sites is found in Table 3–2 and further discussed in Chapter 16.

Evaluation of the pelvic limbs, anus, and tail

Examination of the pelvic limbs is carried out in a similar manner to that of the thoracic limbs. The thoracic limbs are gently lifted and the animal is forced to walk (wheelbarrow) on the pelvic limbs alone, to evaluate strength and coordination of limb movements (Fig. 3–22). Animals are reluctant to perform this on a slippery surface, so a carpeted surface or grass should be used.

Postural reactions. The thoracic limbs and one pelvic limb may be lifted, supporting and balancing the animal, so that hopping on the remaining pelvic limb may be evaluated for initiation, strength, and coordination of movement (Fig. 3–23). The hopping responses of the pelvic limbs should be compared for symmetry.

A small dog or cat may be lifted to a table edge, and when the pelvic limb paws touch the edge of the table the animal should place them on the table top. The animal can be lifted off the ground by the

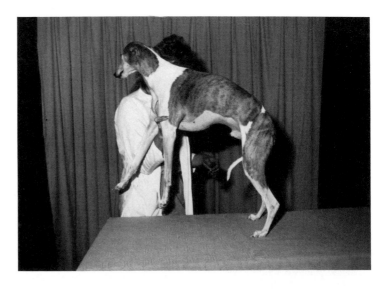

Figure 3–22. The *wheelbarrowing* maneuver of the pelvic limbs.

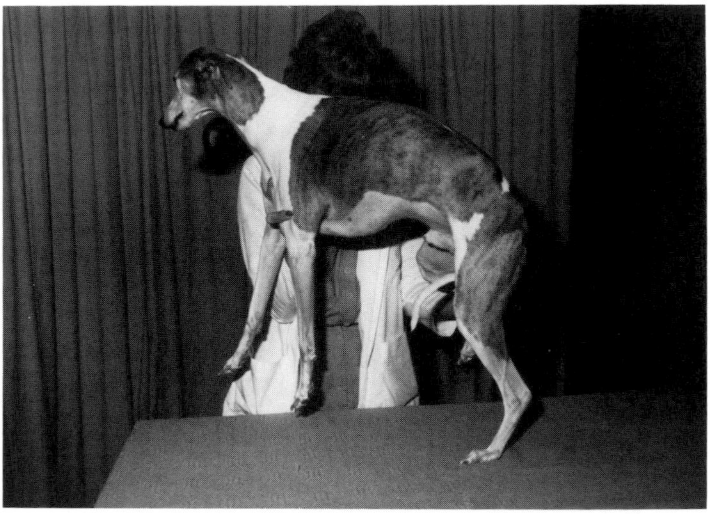

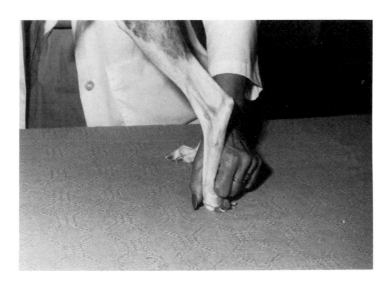

Figure 3–23. *Hopping* on each pelvic limb to detect subtle dysfunction.

chest and axillary region, and then slowly lowered to see if both pelvic limbs will extend and support weight.

Proprioception. The pelvic limb paw may be knuckled onto its dorsal surface or severely adducted or abducted, to see if the animal can replace it to its proper position, testing proprioceptive sense (Fig. 3–24).

Extensor strength. Pressure may be applied downward to the pelvic limbs, with the animal standing, to observe extensor strength as the animal pushes upward against the pressure. Some animals may sit, if they have been taught in this manner.

Spinal reflexes of the pelvic limbs, anus, tail, and bladder. Spinal reflexes of the pelvic limbs are more easily elicited and often more obviously affected by a lesion than those of the thoracic limbs. It is easier to get the limbs to relax if the animal is held in lateral recumbency, rather than suspended by the chest and

Figure 3–24. Testing *proprioception* of the pelvic limb by standing the paw knuckled onto the dorsum and observing correction for this abnormal position.

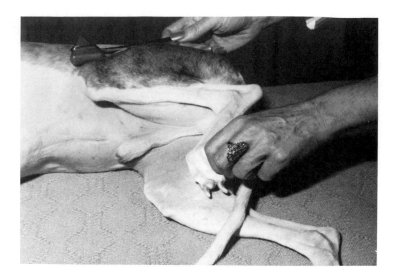

Figure 3–28. Testing the *toe pinch, withdrawal, or flexor reflex* of the pelvic limb by pinching the toe and observing a withdrawal response.

a large overflow bladder that drips urine and is easily expressed. Lesions above S1 to S3 can produce a small bladder that may be difficult to express and reflexively spurts out urine. Lesions are discussed further in Chapter 19.

When attempting to localize spinal cord and nerve root signs with the vertebral site of involvement, the anatomic relationships in the lumbar vertebrae and spinal cord must be considered (Figs. 3–30, 3–31). This is often more critical in the lumbar than in the cervical region. The spinal cord ends at vertebra L6 in the dog and the sacrum in the cat, but the nerve roots continue inside the canal and exit behind the vertebrae they are numbered after. Because a spinal reflex can be diminished by affecting the spinal cord segment or the nerve roots, they are vulnerable over several vertebrae. The lumbar spinal reflex changes associated with disease in various vertebrae are outlined in Table 3–2 and further discussed in Chapter 17.

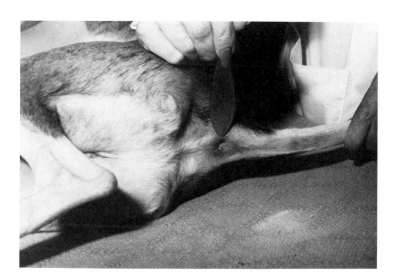

Figure 3–29. Testing the *anal reflex* by touching the perineal region and observing anal contracture.

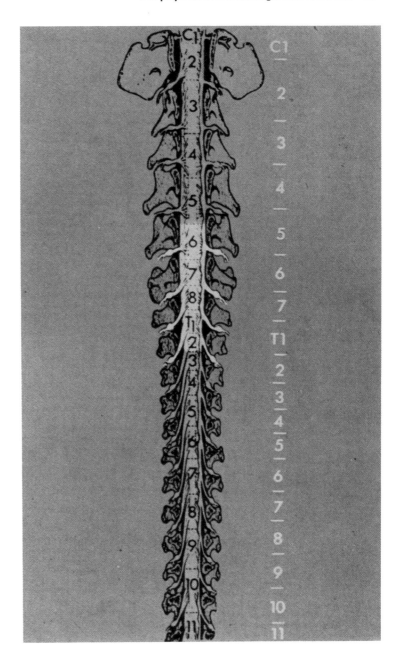

Figure 3–30. The relationship of spinal cord segments and nerve roots to vertebrae in the cervical region. C6 to T2 spinal cord segments are displayed in white and are the main contributions to the brachial plexus (after Miller, 1964).

Deep pain. A stimulus stronger than the toe pinch is applied to the toe, and the animal is observed for a behavioral response such as crying out or turning to bite the examiner, indicating that deep pain is intact. As was discussed with the thoracic limbs, a loss of deep pain and loss of flexor reflex could be due to disease of peripheral nerves, which are capable of regeneration. An intact withdrawal reflex, with crossed extension and no deep pain 72 hours after an acute injury, can indicate extensive spinal cord damage and a guarded prognosis for the animal's recov-

Table 5–1
Cerebrospinal fluid parameters and normal values

Parameter	Normal values
Pressure	Less than 100 mm CSF (cats)
	Less than 170 mm CSF (dogs)
Color	Transparent
Clarity	Clear
Refractive index	1.3347 to 1.3350
Urinary reagent strips	pH 8 ± 1
	Glucose—trace to +
	Protein—trace to 30
	Blood—negative
Pandy's test	No turbulence
Spectrophotometer protein	10 to 25 mg/dl (cisterna magna)
Total cell count	Less than 8/microliter
Cell type	Small lymphocytes and a few monocytes

particularly bacterial infections, with an increased number of neutrophils. Pink or red CSF usually is due to contamination with blood during the collection procedure.

Refractive index

The refractive index may be determined with a refractometer. The normal value is a refraction between 17 and 20 or a refractive index between 1.3347 and 1.3350. The refractive index is often elevated when either the cells or protein in the CSF are increased.

Urinary reagent strips

The CSF can be dropped on urinary reagent strips to estimate pH, glucose, protein, and blood. The normal value for pH is 8 ± 1; for glucose, trace to +; protein, trace to 30; and blood, negative. If the protein content of CSF is markedly elevated, the elevation produces an appropriate color change on the dip stick. Mild elevations in CSF protein, however, are not seen by this method, and other tests for the evaluation of protein content are indicated.

Pandy's test

Another simple qualitative measure of protein is the Pandy's test. Pandy's solution is made by mixing 10 mg carbolic acid crystals in 100 ml distilled water. A few drops of CSF and 1 ml of Pandy's solution are mixed in a test tube. The CSF protein content is increased if the mixture becomes turbid after shaking the test tube. The Pandy test should be negative and no turbidity should be seen in normal CSF.

Spectrophotometer protein determination

The most accurate and reliable measure of protein is that taken with a spectrophotometer. CSF may be frozen and sent out to a private laboratory equipped to measure CSF protein if a spectrophotometer is not available in the individual veterinary hospital. Normal values should be established for each laboratory. If protein content is elevated, a CSF protein electrophoresis may give more insight into the type of disease process involved.[63,64] An increase in CSF gammaglobulin may occur in canine distemper virus infections.

Total cell count

Undiluted CSF is applied to one side of a standard dual-chambered hemocytometer for total cell counts. The other side of the chamber is filled with CSF mixed with a diluting fluid. The diluting fluid is composed of 0.2 g crystal or methyl violet dissolved in 10 ml of glacial acetic acid brought to a 100 ml volume with distilled water. In a 1:10 WBC diluting pipet, the diluting fluid is drawn to the 1 mark and CSF drawn to the 11 mark. The fluids are gently mixed. The diluting fluid lyses RBCs and stains WBC nuclei in approximately 2 minutes. Counting all cells in 5 of the 9-mm^2 areas and multiplying by 2 on the undiluted side and by 2.2 on the diluted side equals the total number of cells per microliter of fluid. The number of cells on the undiluted side equals WBCs and RBCs, and the number of cells on the diluted side are WBCs alone. Normal CSF contains no RBCs. Recent hemorrhage or peripheral blood contamination results in RBCs. Less than 8 WBCs per microliter is normal. A differential cell count should be performed even if white cells are not increased, as an abnormal distribution of cell types may be found.[11] If the cell count is elevated, the percentage of each cell type should be calculated.

Elevated cell counts may occur in inflammations, neoplasia, trauma, or spinal cord compression. Cell counts over 300 WBC per microliter are most commonly associated with an inflammatory process.

Differential cell counts

One milliliter of fresh-mixed CSF is placed in a sedimentation chamber to prepare a slide for a differential cell count. The sedimentation chamber is made from a test tube that is cut to form a double open-ended glass cylinder. The smooth end of the cylinder is sealed to a standard glass microscope slide with paraffin wax to form a chamber to hold the CSF (Fig. 5–2). After 25 minutes, the cells settle to the bottom of the chamber onto the glass slide. The supernate is gently aspirated, the chamber is removed by breaking the paraffin seal, and a small amount of CSF remains inside the paraffin ring. The slide is air dried and sprayed with a cell fixative.* Excess paraffin is removed with a razor blade. A Wright's stain or any other commercial WBC stain is applied to the slide. A cover slip can be applied with mounting media. Normal CSF has a cellular population of a few mononuclear cells, mostly small lymphocytes and a few monocytes. The presence of neutrophils when there has been no blood contamination is considered abnormal. Monocytes exhibiting phagocytic activity are found in many nervous system disorders.

A membrane filtration technique also may be used to collect cells in a 13-mm-diameter millipore filter for a differential cell count (Fig. 5–3).[49,66]† Ten drops to 1 ml of CSF is mixed with 2 ml of 40% ethanol. Once mixed with the ethanol, the cells are preserved and will not degenerate if immediate examination is not possible. A Swinny-type hypodermic adapter‡ contains the millipore filter. The CSF and alcohol mixture is placed in a syringe attached to the adapter and then passed

---

* Profixx, Scientific Products, McGraw Park, Illinois.
† Millipore Corporation, SMWP—01300, HAWP—01300, Bedford, Massachusetts.
‡ Gelman Instrument Company, Ann Arbor, Michigan.

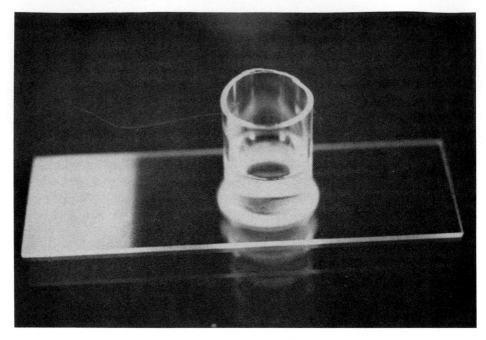

Figure 5–2. Sedimentation chamber containing cerebrospinal fluid (CSF).

through the millipore filter. The filter and collection of cells are removed again, fixed in 95% ethanol, and rinsed in distilled water. The filter is placed in Harris' hematoxylin for 3 to 4 minutes and then in distilled water and 95% ethanol for 30 seconds each. It then is placed in absolute alcohol and xylene for 1 minute each, and the filter becomes transparent and can be placed on a slide. The filter technique requires more specific equipment than the sedimentation technique. The examiner also must adjust to viewing the cells at several angles in the filter technique, as they are rounded and not flattened as in the sedimenting technique. Either technique, however, can be employed in veterinary practice.

Cells from CSF may also be collected on a slide using a cytocentrifuge; however, this equipment is not available in many private veterinary hospitals. Most commercial diagnostic laboratories with a cytocentrifuge cannot process the CSF within 20 to 30 minutes after collection unless some special arrangements can be made. Elevated WBC counts that are primarily neutrophils have been reported with bacterial infections, steroid-responsive meningitis, acute viral encephalitis, and some meningiomas.[5,37,70,76]

Elevated WBC counts that are primarily lymphocytes have been reported with chronic viral infections and steroid-responsive meningitis.[37,70,76]

Mixed populations of small and large lymphocytes, monocytes, macrophages, and neutrophils have been reported with granulomatous meningoencephalitis, distemper virus encephalitis, steroid-responsive meningoencephalitis, and neoplasia (Fig. 5–4).[4,5,70]

Miscellaneous tests

Fluorescent antibody tests for distemper virus may be performed on the CSF cell preparations in some special laboratories.

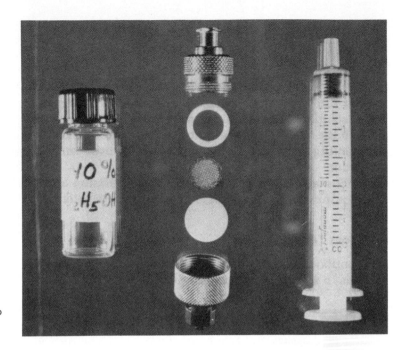

Figure 5-3. Equipment needed to collect CSF cells on a millipore filter for cytologic examination.

In CNS necrosis, certain enzyme levels in CSF may be elevated. CPK, LDH, and ALT determinations may be performed in commercial laboratories. Elevated levels may support a diagnosis of active necrosis in the CNS.

If bacterial or fungal disorders are suspected, CSF may be cultured. Several milliliters of fluid are needed for the best results. Gram stains and india ink preparations of CSF cytology may demonstrate bacterial or fungal organisms, respectively.

CSF titers for canine distemper virus, feline infectious peritonitis virus, and other agents confirm the diagnosis of meningoencephalomyelitis produced by these organisms. A negative CSF titer does not

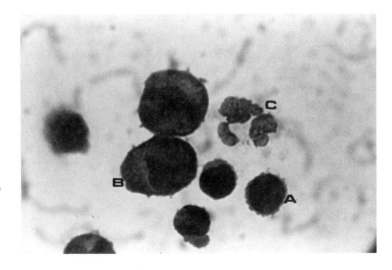

Figure 5-4. Cerebrospinal fluid from a dog with steroid-responsive meningoencephalitis. There is a mixed population of cells. A = small lymphocytes, B = macrophages, and C = neutrophil (Courtesy of Dr. Dennis Myer, University of Florida).

rule out infections. A further discussion of serum and CSF titers is found in Chapter 7. A list of titers is found in Table 7–8. Virus isolation from CSF also may be attempted if the facilities are available.

CSF electrolytes may be evaluated in electrolyte disturbances. CSF osmolality and pH may be used to support the diagnosis of osmolality and acid-base imbalances.

CSF analysis is an invaluable diagnostic aid for the evaluation of the neurologic patient. The mechanisms of disease, specific disorders, and CSF changes are listed in Table 5–2.

Electroencephalography

The electroencephalogram (EEG) is a recording of the electrical activity of the cerebral cortex. The normal EEG is a summation of subthreshold electrical alterations of cortical neuronal membranes. Cerebral electrical activity is influenced by that of subcortical structures, particularly the diencephalon and midbrain. Disease processes of the cerebral cortex, diencephalon, and midbrain produce the greatest alterations in the EEG. There are several techniques and electrode placements used to obtain EEGs in animals. One technique uses five electrodes and eight leads.[45,47] The electrode and lead arrangement are demonstrated in Figure 5–5. The skin and underlying muscle are infiltrated with local anesthetic. Alligator clips are fastened to the scalp with contact paste or subdermal needle electrodes are inserted. Cotton is placed in the animal's ears to decrease auditory input and a mask is placed over the animal's eyes to decrease visual input. Then the animal is held gently on its side by an assistant. The environment should be quiet, at a comfortable temperature, and dimly lit.

The normal, alert EEG has an asynchronous wave form with a frequency ranging from 15 to 30 hertz (Hz) and an amplitude from 5 to 15 microvolts (μV) (Fig. 5–6). As the animal relaxes, superimposed synchronous slow-wave activity is seen (Fig. 5–7). As relaxation continues and sleep occurs, the frequency slows to 1 to 3 Hz and the amplitude increases to 150 to 300 μV. The state of consciousness of the animal during the EEG recording must be considered for proper interpretation of any changes in the wave forms.

The EEG reaches maturity at approximately 6 months of age in most dogs and cats. Prior to this time, some slow-wave activity may be seen in the normal animal. In aged dogs, the EEG amplitude may decrease to less than 5 μV. The age of the animal must therefore be considered for an accurate interpretation of the EEG.

Sedation and anesthesia produce synchronous slowing and increasing amplitude of the EEG. Spindle formations in the EEG are commonly seen in barbiturate anesthesia. The EEG pattern varies with the depth of anesthesia. The examiner must have experience with effects of various drugs to correctly interpret the EEG during anesthesia. The EEG may be recorded as the animal awakens from anesthesia and then is reexamined in the awake state if abnormalities are suspected.

Phenothiazine-derivative tranquilizers such as acepromazine produce slow-wave activity, but also may produce seizure discharges from epileptic foci. Phenothiazine tranquilizers may be used as an activating agent to study epilepsy in some special cases. Short-acting barbiturates also have been used to activate epileptic foci. In some research laboratories, pentylenetetrazole has been used to activate seizure discharges on the EEG, but this technique is not used in many neurology practices. Photostimulation and hyperventilation are two techniques for activating seizure discharges used in man, but are not particularly applicable to unanesthetized animals.

Routine anticonvulsant therapy does

not alter the alert EEG of the dog or cat unless the animal is overdosed or sedated. For most routine EEG examinations, the animal is maintained on the daily anticonvulsant therapy.

A routine EEG recording is obtained with the animal in an awake, nonsedated state if the animal is cooperative. When the animal is awake, various artifacts can occur, but with a little experience these artifacts are easily recognized and do not interfere with the interpretation of EEG activity. Electrodes are placed over the temporalis muscles, and spike discharges from these muscles are commonly seen in a tense animal. The electrical activity of the muscle can be decreased or eliminated with infiltration of a local anesthetic. Eye blinks, ear twitches, body tremors, and head movement will cause the baseline to shift and produce a movement artifact. Panting will produce a rhythmic bobbing of the head and rhythmic waving of the baseline that corresponds with each breath. Occasionally, the ECG will be seen on the EEG and can be correlated with the heart rate. With a quiet environment, a little reassurance to the animal, and a patient technician, an accurate, artifact-free EEG tracing may be obtained on most pet animals.

Disease processes may affect the EEG in several ways. There is no specific EEG change for a certain disease. The significance of any EEG changes can only be interpreted properly in light of the history, physical and neurologic examinations, and basic clinicopathologic test results on the animal. The EEG is a method of obtaining another objective bit of information on cerebral cortex function. Without a complete data base, this information is of little use in solving the animal's problem.

A disease process may alter the normal, alert EEG waveforms by producing an increase in amplitude with little or mild slowing (Fig. 5–8), an increase in amplitude with greater slowing (Fig. 5–9), a decrease in amplitude with little or no slowing (Fig. 5–10), or a decrease in amplitude with slowing (Fig. 5–11). Also, fast-activity and slow-activity mixtures with spindles and spike discharges may be seen. The activity may be asynchronous or synchronous. Abnormal activity may be continuous in the alert state, may occur during relaxation only, or occur in bursts or paroxysms. The activity may be asymmetric, affecting one hemisphere or one electrode area.

The EEG changes seen in different disease processes are described in detail elsewhere.[45] Those disease processes that produce abnormal EEGs are listed in Table 5–3.

A few disorders of the brain do not alter the normal EEG. A normal EEG can also be useful information to support a certain diagnosis. Those neurologic disorders that might have a normal EEG associated with them are listed in Table 5–4.

Electromyography

The electromyogram (EMG) is a recording of the electrical activity of muscle. Any disease process affecting the ventral horn cell within the gray matter of the spinal cord, the ventral root within the spinal canal, the peripheral nerve, the neuromuscular junction, or muscle can produce changes in the muscle that are detected by EMG. The EMG is used as an extension of the neurologic examination to evaluate the electrical activity of the neuromuscular system.[7,9]

The EMG equipment consists of an oscilloscope, which displays the waveforms, and an auditory amplifier, which projects sound for each waveform.

The two basic types of studies performed during the EMG examination are needle EMG and nerve stimulation studies. Needle EMG examination is performed by inserting an exploring needle

Table 5–2
Diseases and typical cerebrospinal fluid changes

Disorder	Pressure	Appearance	Protein	Cell count	Primary cell type
Congenital and familial disorders					
Hydrocephalus (congenital)	N	Clear	N	N	N
Hydrocephalus (postnatal)	N	Turbid	↑	↑	Neutrophils or *mononuclear cells
Globoid leukodystrophy	N	Turbid	↑	↑	Globoid cells, macrophages
Infections and Inflammations					
Canine distemper virus	N or ↑	Clear or turbid	N or ↑	N or ↑↑	*Mononuclear cells, neutrophils
Feline infectious peritonitis	N or ↑	Clear or turbid	N or ↑	N or ↑↑	*Mononuclear cells
Cryptococcosis	↑ or viscous	Turbid, xanthochromic	↑	↑↑	Neutrophils, *mononuclear cells, and eosinophils
Toxoplasmosis	N or ↑	Xanthochromic	↑	↑↑	Neutrophils, *mononuclear cells, and eosinophils

Bacterial	N or ↑	Turbid	↑	↑↑	Neutrophils
Granulomatous meningoencephalitis	N	Clear or turbid	↑	↑↑	*Mononuclear cells, neutrophils
Steroid-responsive meningoencephalitis	N	Clear or turbid	↑ or ↑↑	↑↑	*Mononuclear cells, neutrophils, eosinophils
Trauma					
Intervertebral disc protrusion	N	Clear, xanthochromic	↑	N or ↑	*Mononuclear cells
Vascular					
Fibrocartilaginous infarct	N	Clear	↑	N	N
Degeneration					
Degenerative myelopathy	N	Clear	↑ (lumbar)	N	N
Neoplasia					
Cerebral	↑ or N	Clear	↑	N or ↑	N or *mononuclear cells, neutrophils
Spinal cord	N	Clear	↑	N or ↑	N or *mononuclear cells, neutrophils

N = normal; ↑ = mildly increased; ↑↑ = greatly increased.
* mononuclear cells = lymphocytes, monocytes, and macrophages.

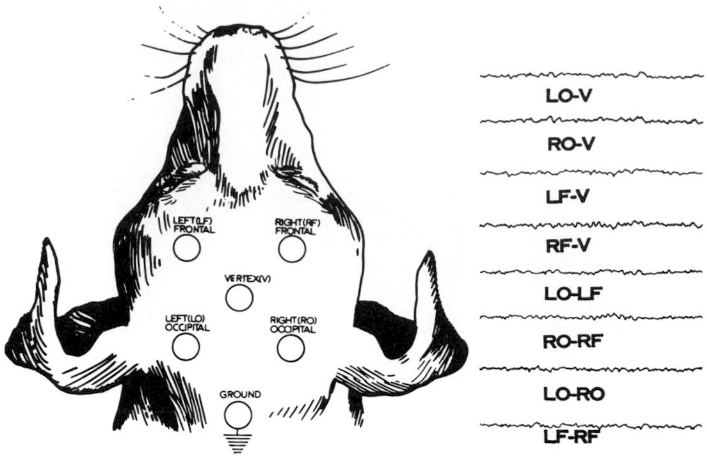

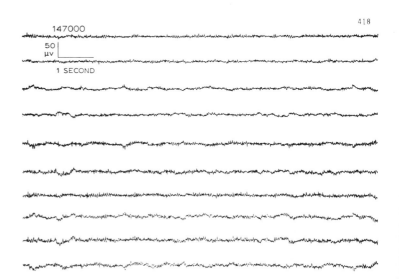

Figure 5–5. The electrode arrangement used to record the EEG, and the electrode combinations used for each lead. (From Redding, R.: Anatomy and Physiology. *In* Canine Neurology. Edited by B.F. Hoerlein. Philadelphia, W.B. Saunders, 1978.)

electrode into a muscle to examine its intrinsic electrical activity.

Three sources of electrical activity are recorded from the muscle during needle EMG examination. If the animal is awake or only lightly anesthetized, voluntary muscle contractions, referred to as *motor unit action potentials* (MUAP), may be seen (Fig. 5–12). These are biphasic or triphasic potentials that vary in amplitude depending on their distance from the recording needle electrode. MUAPs have a sharp, popping sound. In man, muscle diseases often produce a decrease in amplitude and

an increase in number of MUAPs for a given muscle contraction, whereas neuropathies produce an increase in amplitude and a decrease in number of MUAPs. These changes often are difficult to evaluate in animals. Polyphasic MUAPs may suggest a disease process in an animal (Fig. 5–13). In a tense animal, the MUAPs can make examination for any other electrical activity impossible, so the animals often are anesthetized for the rest of the examination. Routine general anesthetic agents have little effect on the needle EMG.

The second source of electrical activity

Figure 5–6. The alert normal EEG. Note some muscle artifact in each lead. Last two leads are between left occipital and right frontal electrodes and right occipital and left frontal electrodes, respectively. Others are the lead arrangement described in Fig. 5–5.

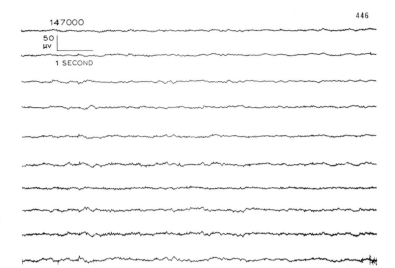

Figure 5–7. Relaxed normal EEG. Note the lack of muscle artifact as compared with Fig. 5–6. Last two leads are between left occipital and right frontal electrodes and right occipital and left frontal electrodes, respectively. Others are the lead arrangement described in Fig. 5–5.

seen during the needle EMG examination is produced by the mechanical irritation of the needle electrode as it is inserted into the muscle, and is referred to as *insertional activity*. In normal muscle, which is properly innervated, the insertional activity is a brief burst, which has a crisp sound that ceases as soon as movement is discontinued. In denervated, inflamed, or degenerating muscle, insertional activity is prolonged, and *positive sharp waves* and *bizarre high-frequency discharges* may be seen. Positive sharp waves can be few, many, or long trains of 50 to 100/sec discharges, with a

characteristic waveform that has an initial large deflection in the downward, or positive, direction on the oscilloscope, followed by a smaller upward, or negative, deflection (Fig. 5–14). Trains of positive waves sound like a race car speeding by. Bizarre high-frequency (BHF) discharges may also be seen in insertion, and have a variety of bizarre forms or sounds, which are repetitive at over 200/sec (Fig. 5–15). These potentials are sometimes referred to as pseudomyotonia.

Myotonic discharges are bizarre high-frequency discharges that wax and wane

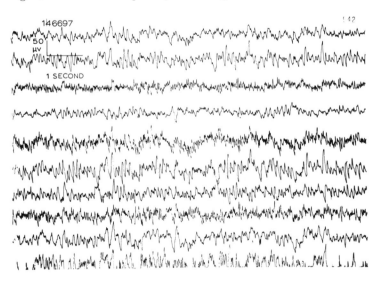

Figure 5–8. Increased amplitude and mild slowing of the EEG associated with hydrocephalus in a 7-month-old Pomeranian dog. Lead arrangement as in Fig. 5–5. Last two leads are between left occipital and right frontal electrodes and right occipital and left frontal electrodes, respectively.

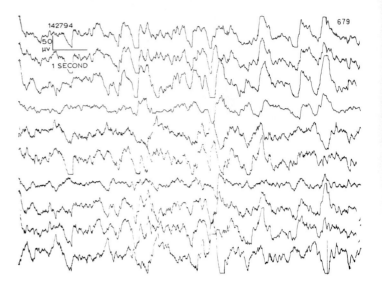

Figure 5–9. Increased amplitude and moderate slowing of the EEG following a cranial trauma in a 9-month-old Beagle dog. Lead arrangement as in Fig. 5–5. Last two leads are between left occipital and right frontal electrodes and right occipital and left frontal electrodes, respectively.

spontaneously in shape and sound like a dive bomber. These potentials are only found in the muscle membrane defect of myotonia.

Generally, when the needle electrode is held quietly in a relaxed muscle, no electrical alterations are visualized on the oscilloscope or heard through the speakers. In denervated or severely inflamed muscle, spontaneous discharges called fibrillation and fasciculation potentials occur.

These spontaneous discharges are a third source of electrical activity. Fibrillation potentials are small, biphasic potentials that sound like eggs frying, and although they occur spontaneously, they may also occur during insertional activity (Fig. 5–16). Although fibrillation potentials usually are associated with denervated muscle fibers, they may be present in muscle inflammation.

Fasciculation potentials are irregular

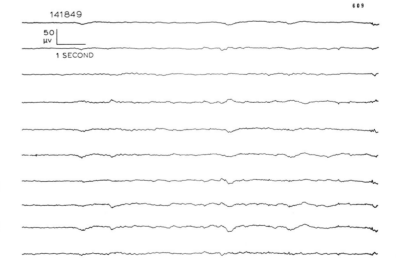

Figure 5–10. Decreased amplitude and mild slowing of the EEG associated with a relaxed tracing of a 2-year-old Doberman Pinscher with hypothyroidism. Lead arrangement as in Fig. 5–5. Last two leads are between left occipital and right frontal occipital and left frontal electrodes, respectively.

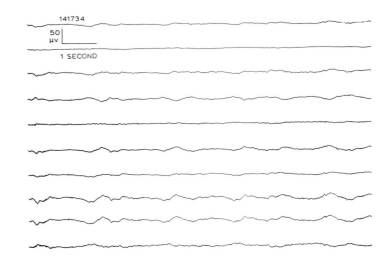

141734

50 μv

1 SECOND

Figure 5–11. Decreased amplitude and slowing of the EEG associated with severe cerebral edema secondary to cerebral neoplasia in a 3-year-old Schnauzer. The animal died shortly after this recording was made. Lead arrangement as in Fig. 5–5. Last two leads are between left occipital and right frontal electrodes and right occipital and left frontal electrodes, respectively.

Table 5–3
Diseases with abnormal electroencephalograms

Congenital and familial disorders
  Hydrocephalus
  Lissencephaly
  Lysosomal storage diseases

Infections and other inflammations
  Viral encephalitis
  Bacterial meningitis
  Rickettsial encephalitis
  Steroid-responsive meningoencephalitis
  Granulomatous meningoencephalitis
  Other types of encephalitis

  Mycotic encephalitis
  Toxoplasmosis encephalitis
  Postencephalitis acquired epilepsy

Metabolic disturbances
  Chronic hypoglycemia
  Chronic hypoxia
  Hypothyroidism
  Hepatic encephalopathy

  Uremic encephalopathy
  Osmolality disturbances
  Postmetabolic acquired epilepsy

Toxicity
  Lead
  Organophosphate

Nutritional deficiency
  Thiamine

Trauma and vascular
  Cerebral edema
  Cerebral hemorrhage
  Concussion

  Infarct
  Post-traumatic acquired epilepsy

Neoplasia
  Cerebral, diencephalon, and midbrain

Table 5–4
Diseases of the brain that may have normal electroencephalograms

Congenital and familial disorders
  True epilepsy
Metabolic disturbances
  Hypoglycemia
  Hepatic encephalopathy (at certain times)
Neoplasia
  Pituitary tumor (if small)

in shape, form, and rate of firing. Fasciculations may be grossly visible through the skin, but are not always a sign of neuromuscular disease, as they may also be seen in extreme nervousness, exhaustion, or acid-base imbalances.

During the needle EMG examination, the major muscles of the pelvic and thoracic limbs are each tested, along with individual paravertebral muscles from the tail to the rostral cervical region. Skeletal muscles innervated by cranial nerves, such as the tongue, larynx, facial, temporalis, masseter, and extraocular muscles, also may be examined. It may take 5 to 7 days after an insult to a nerve before abnormal EMG findings can be detected in the muscle. The distribution of the disease process can be outlined by knowing the specific innervation to each abnormal muscle tested, and it can be determined whether a focal, multifocal, or diffuse disease is present. Table 5–5 lists the distribution of EMG abnormalities and possible diseases.

If the EMG is normal in a paralyzed animal, then the lesions probably involve mainly white matter tracts rather than gray matter lower motor neurons. If a focal nerve root lesion is found and an intervertebral disc herniation or tumor is in the differential, the needle EMG findings can support the need to do a myelogram when plain radiographs are normal.

If a multifocal or diffuse neuromus-

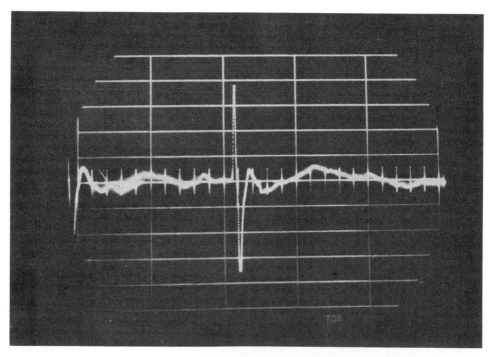

Figure 5–12. A single motor unit action potential. 100 μv/cm, 30 msec/ major division.

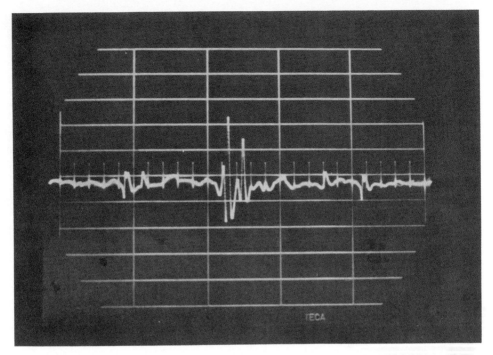

Figure 5–13. A polyphasic motor unit action potential. 100 μv/cm, 30 msec/ major division.

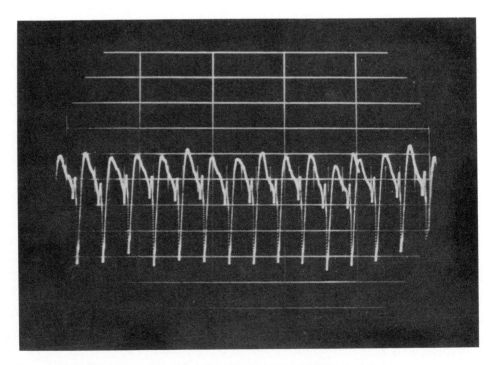

Figure 5–14. Positive sharp waves. 100 μv/cm, 30 msec/ major division.

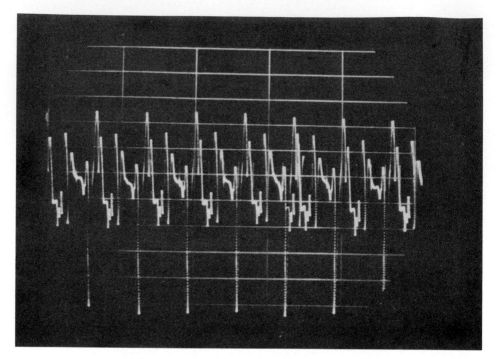

Figure 5–15. Bizarre high-frequency discharges. 100 μv/cm, 30 msec/ major division.

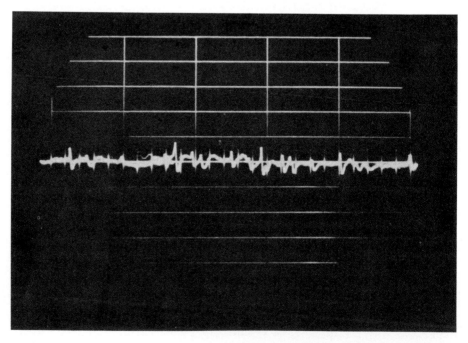

Figure 5–16. Fibrillation potentials. 100 μv/cm, 30 msec/ major division.

Table 5–5
Distribution of EMG abnormalities and possible diseases

Focal nerve root lesions
   Intervertebral disc protrusion or
   herniation
   Cervical vertebral malformations
   Vertebral fractures
   Discospondylitis
   Fibrocartilaginous infarct
   Spinal cord or nerve root neoplasia
Focal peripheral nerve lesions
   Brachial plexus trauma
   Other cranial and spinal nerve trauma or
   neoplasia
Diffuse neuromuscular lesions
   Polyradiculitis
   Polyradiculoneuritis
   Polyneuritis
   Polymyositis

cular disease process is suspected from the needle EMG examination, then nerve stimulation studies are indicated.[9,34,40] A supramaximal electrical stimulation is applied to the nerve. This is a level of stimulation that evokes the highest amplitude response from the muscle called an M wave. A normal muscle response is biphasic or triphasic, with an amplitude of 15,000 μV or greater (Fig. 5–17). In severe nerve or muscle disease, the M wave may be polyphasic or small. If the nerve has been severed or completely degenerated, there will be no response to electrical stimulation 72 hours after the insult. In neuromuscular junction blockade, as with tick paralysis or botulism, there may be a depressed or absent response. A 5/sec series of repeated stimulations will not alter the normal response in shape or amplitude (Fig. 5–18). In myasthenia gravis, organophosphate toxicity, and distal axonopathies, a decremental response is seen as a decrease in amplitude of the first three evoked M waves (Fig. 5–19). An intravenous injection of edrophonium chloride (Tensilon) will abolish this response in myasthenia gravis and distal axonopathies but worsen the response in organophosphate toxicity.

The F wave is a low-amplitude wave seen several milliseconds after the M wave.[26,27,46] The F wave is thought to be produced by an electrical impulse traveling to the cell body of the motor nerve and then back down the motor nerve to elicit a small response in the muscle.

The H wave or H reflex is another low-amplitude wave seen several milliseconds after the F wave, but only if the stimulus voltage is low.[25–27,54,55] The H wave is thought to be produced by the electrical impulse traveling up the sensory nerve to reflexively stimulate the motor nerve and elicit a response in the muscle.

F and H waves and latencies have been studied in normal and in a few abnormal dogs and cats following stimulation of the ulnar and tibial nerves. The F wave may be inconsistent in normal animals, but the H wave may be useful to localize diseases to the proximal portion of the nerve.[26]

By stimulating the nerve at two different sites, a nerve conduction velocity can be calculated (Fig. 5–20).[7,9,34] The normal motor nerve conduction velocity in an adult animal is usually 50 m/sec or greater in dogs, and generally faster in cats.[53,67,72] A value of less than 50 m/sec supports a diagnosis of peripheral neuropathy. If multiple peripheral nerves are tested in all limbs and are slow, then a diagnosis of polyneuropathy can be made. Table 5–6 outlines typical needle EMG, nerve stimulation, and motor nerve conduction velocity changes found in various neuromuscular diseases.

If a sensory neuropathy is suspected from the data base and the needle EMG is normal, sensory nerve conduction velocity studies are needed to confirm the diagnosis.[19,42,44,46] The electrode arrangement for sensory nerve conduction velocity studies is outlined in Figure 5–21. A signal

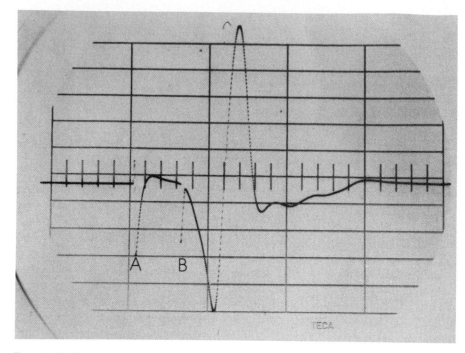

Figure 5–17. The evoked response recorded from the muscle following stimulation of a nerve. *(A)* the shock artifact, *(B)* the onset of the evoked response. The time between *A* and *B* is the nerve latency. 200 μv/cm, 5 msec/ division.

averager is often used to enhance visualization of the evoked response. Note that there are two recording sites instead of two stimulating sites as in motor nerve conduction velocity studies. Detailed descriptions of both motor and sensory nerve conduction velocity studies are found elsewhere.[19,42]

Cortical evoked responses

Brain stem auditory evoked responses

Brain stem auditory evoked responses (BAER) can be recorded using electrodiagnostic equipment* with a signal averager

─────────
* Neurostar, Teca Corporation, Pleasantville, New York.

and a click stimulus generator.[46,56,57] The animal may be anesthetized with a short-acting barbiturate and halothane gas. A recording electrode is placed on the head in the area of the vertex electrode on the EEG recording (Fig. 5–5). Seven sequential waveforms are produced, but only the first five are evaluated. The five waveforms correspond to potentials in the vestibulocochlear nerve, cochlear nucleus, nucleus of the trapezoid body, the lemniscal nuclei, and caudal colliculus, respectively (Fig. 5–22). The BAER is useful to evaluate animals for vestibulocochlear nerve disease as well as brain stem problems.[24,35,38,58]

Somatosensory evoked responses

Somatosensory evoked responses or potentials (SSEP) are tested by stimulation of a peripheral nerve such as the sciatic nerve

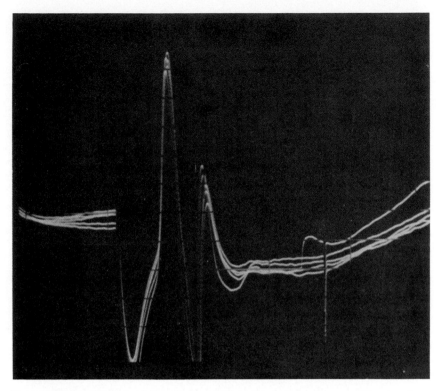

Figure 5–18. Repetitive stimulation of a nerve with no decremental response. 100 μv/cm, 5 msec/ division. (From Chrisman, C.L.: Electromyography in Animals. *In* Pathophysiology in Small Animal Surgery. Edited by M.J. Bojrab. Philadelphia, Lea & Febiger, 1981.)

and recording from an electrode on the scalp over the somatosensory cortex of the parietal lobe cerebral cortex. The animal is anesthetized with sodium pentobarbital or a short-activating barbiturate and halothane gas. Electrodiagnostic equipment with a nerve stimulator and signal averager can be used for the study.* The presence of this response suggests integrity of the sensory peripheral nerve, spinal cord, and brain stem pathways through the internal capsule to the parietal lobe cortex. Somatosensory evoked responses are useful to demonstrate pathway integrity in spinal cord and brain stem trauma to determine a prognosis.

---

* Neurostar, Teca Corporation, Pleasantville, New York.

Visual evoked responses

Visual evoked responses or potentials (VEP) are tested by applying a series of photic flashes into the retina and recording the response from the scalp over the visual region of the occipital lobe cortex.[21,59] Animals are anesthetized with thiopental and halothane. Red light flashes produce a VEP with less electroretinogram (ERG) artifact than white light.[6] The test is useful to demonstrate the integrity of the visual pathway.

Spinal cord evoked responses

A needle recording electrode placed on the dorsal lamina of cervical or lumbar

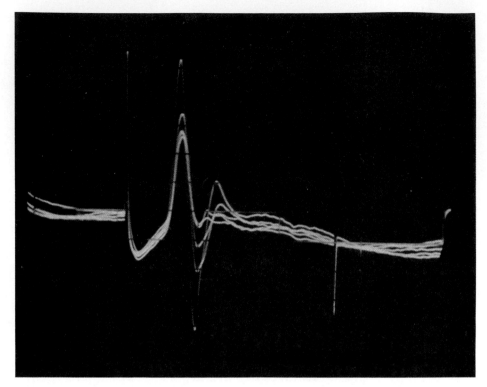

Figure 5–19. Repetitive stimulation of a nerve with a decremental response in a 2½-year-old Cairn Terrier with myasthenia gravis. 200 μv/cm, 5 msec/ division. (From Chrisman, C.L.: Electromyography in Animals. *In* Pathophysiology in Small Animal Surgery. Edited by M.J. Bojrab. Philadephia, Lea & Febiger, 1981.)

vertebrae can be used to detect an electrical response in the spinal cord following stimulation of a peripheral sensory nerve.[20,43,46,62] Animals are anesthetized with thiopental and halothane. Electrodiagnostic equipment with a nerve stimulator and signal averager can be used for the study.* The amplitude, shape, and latency of the evoked response can be examined and can be useful to further study spinal cord function. This test may be used to evaluate the integrity of the spinal cord white matter in spinal cord injury.[51]

---

*Neurostar, Teca Corporation, Pleasantville, New York.

Neuroradiography

Plain radiographs of the vertebral column

Plain radiographs of the vertebral column are usually indicated when focal or multifocal spinal cord and nerve root disease are suspected (Chap. 4).

Special techniques used to improve radiographs of the vertebral column are described elsewhere.[50,69] However, if the clinician follows a few simple rules, the diagnostic quality of any radiographs can be greatly improved. The animal should be anesthetized so that the vertebral column may be stretched and held straight. Only a few vertebrae at a time should be

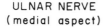

ULNAR NERVE
(medial aspect)

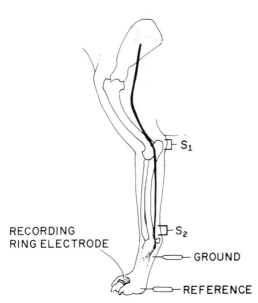

RECORDING
RING ELECTRODE

GROUND

REFERENCE

S₁

S₂

Figure 5–20. The electrode placement for ulnar nerve stimulation. (S1) the proximal simulation site, (S2) the distal stimulation site. The time from S1 to the recording ring electrode is latency 1. The time from S2 to the recording ring electrode is latency 2.

$$\text{Motor nerve conduction velocity} = \frac{\text{Distance between S1 and S2}}{\text{latency 1} - \text{latency 2}} = \text{m/sec}$$

(From Chrisman, C.L.: Electromyography in Animals. *In* Pathophysiology in Small Animal Surgery. Edited by M.J. Bojrab. Philadephia, Lea & Febiger, 1981.)

radiographed. If the lesion can be localized by the neurologic and EMG examinations to a specific vertebral region, then these vertebrae should be in the center of the x-ray beam. A complete spinal series usually consists of five to six lateral and five to six ventrodorsal views, which include cranial cervical to midcervical, midcervical to cranial thoracic, midthoracic, thoracolumbar junction, lumbar, and often lumbosacral junction radiographs.

Radiographs may aid greatly in diagnosing many vertebral column disorders that secondarily affect the spinal cord (Table 5–7).[33,39] If there are no lesions found on the plain radiographs, other differential diagnoses may be considered (Table 5–8). Any lesions seen on the radiographs must be evaluated in light of the neurologic examination findings to make sure a lesion at that site would produce the neurologic deficit the animal shows. It is not uncommon to have multiple fractured vertebrae, intervertebral disc herniations, or discospondylitis lesions.

Plain radiographs of the skull

Plain radiographs of the skull are often in the diagnostic plan when a lesion above the level of the foramen magnum is suspected[50,69] (Chap. 4).

Radiographic study of the skull may vary depending on the location of the lesion. If vestibular signs are compatible with inner ear disease, then ventrodorsal, left and right lateral oblique, and open mouth views are all used to study the osseous bullae and the petrous temporal bone.

If cerebral and cerebellar lesions are suspected, generally ventrodorsal and straight lateral views are used. Occasionally rostral-caudal views through the frontal sinus regions may be useful to further demonstrate tumors and fractures involving the frontal sinus.

Of the number of cerebral disorders, those with lesions that can be seen with routine skull radiographs are few (Tables 5–9, 5–10).

Myelography

Myelography may be indicated when a focal spinal cord lesion is suspected, plain radiographs show a questionable lesion or are negative, and no inflammatory response is seen on CSF analysis (Tables 5–11, 5–12). Contrast media may be injected into the cerebellomedullary cistern or in the subarachnoid space at L4 to L5. The

Table 5–6
Needle EMG and nerve stimulation studies in neuromuscular disorders

Disorder	Needle EMG findings	Nerve stimulation	Nerve conduction velocity
Polyradiculopathy	Trains of positive waves and fibrillation potentials; bizarre high-frequency discharges; decreased number MUAP; polyphasic MUAP	Evoked response normal or polyphasic	Normal
Polyradiculoneuropathy or polyneuropathy	Trains of positive waves and fibrillation potentials; bizarre high-frequency discharges; decreased number MUAP; polyphasic MUAP	Evoked response normal or polyphasic	Decreased
Neuromuscular junction (NMJ)	Normal insertion; decreased or no MUAP (NMJ blockade)	Decreased or no evoked response (NMJ blockade); decremental response on repetitive stimulation (myasthenia gravis)	Normal (if can be recorded)
Polymyopathy	May be normal insertion or trains of positive waves and fibrillation potentials; increased number but decreased amplitude of MUAP	Evoked response normal or low amplitude and polyphasic	Normal

contrast media and CSF mixture surround the spinal cord and demonstrate focal spinal cord compression or expansion (Fig. 5–23).[18] Myelography can be risky, and the animal must be carefully evaluated prior to, during, and following the procedure. Convulsions, hyperthermia, and death are still the main complications, and the risk of these must be carefully weighed against the necessity of getting an accurate diagnosis. Iohexol (180)* is currently the safest, most diagnostic myelographic agent available. There are less side effects than previously described for metrizamide.[1,14,68,73,74,77] A dose of 0.33 ml/kg is

injected in the subarachnoid space in the cerebellomedullary cistern for cervical myelography or the lumbar region for thoracolumbar myelography. A dose of 0.45 ml/kg is used for cervical myelography injected at the lumbar site.

Both Iohexol and metrizamide produce a transient hemorrhagic leptomeningitis that produces no longterm complications.[8,65] However, neither substance should be used in the presence of meningomyelitis. CSF analysis is therefore performed prior to myelography.

Cerebral angiography

When cerebral neoplasia is high on the list of differential diagnoses, a cerebral angio-

___

* Omnipaque 180, Winthrop Pharmaceuticals, New York, New York.

SUPERFICIAL RADIAL NERVE
(lateral aspect)

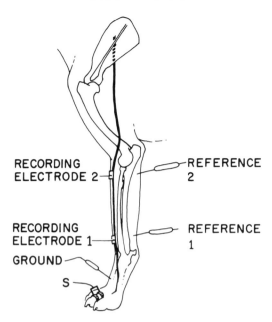

Figure 5–21. Electrode arrangement for sensory nerve conduction velocity. (S) site of stimulation of sensory nerves of the toes. An action potential may be recorded from the nerve at recording electrode 1 and 2. The sensory nerve conduction velocity (SNCV) can be calculated in two ways:

$$SNCV = \frac{\text{Distance from S to recording electrode 1 (or 2)}}{\text{Time from S to recording electrode 1 (or 2)}} = m/sec$$

$$SNCV = \frac{\text{Distance between recording electrode 1 and 2}}{\text{Latency 2 - Latency 1}} = m/sec$$

Latency 1 is the time from S to recording electrode 1. Latency 2 is the time from S to recording electrode 2. (From Chrisman, C.L.: Electromyography in Animals. *In* Pathophysiology in Small Animal Surgery. Edited by M.J. Bojrab. Philadephia, Lea & Febiger, 1981.)

gram may aid in outlining the area of involvement.[15,31,48] Contrast media is injected into either the carotid artery or the vertebral artery to outline the major arterial and venous supply of the brain (Fig. 5–24). Space-occupying lesions may displace blood vessels from their normal position, or be highly vascular themselves. Radiographic fluoroscopic equipment, ar-

terial catheters, and technical skill are required to perform cerebral angiography successfully, and its use has been mainly limited to institutions. As other noninvasive types of imaging such as computerized axial tomography (CT) scans and magnetic resonance imaging (MRI) scans become available for animals, the need for cerebral angiography has decreased at many institutions.

Ventriculography

Ventriculography can be used to demonstrate ventricular size and position when hydrocephalus or any disorder producing a midline shift is suspected. Specific details on the technique or ventriculography are described elsewhere.[69] After removal of some CSF, air is introduced into the ventricular system and dorsoventral, ventrodorsal, and rostral-caudal skull radiographs are taken. The air rises to the top of each position and outlines the extent of the ventricular system. Normal ventricles can be difficult to inject with air (Fig. 5–25A,B), but enlarged ventricles are easily injected. Contrast media can cause complications such as seizures or apnea, which makes them riskier to use than air. Pneumoventriculography (air injected into the ventricles) is a safe and useful method of confirming the extent of hydrocephalus. Other noninvasive types of imaging have become available, and the need for ventriculography has decreased, as the ventricular system is readily demonstrated on ultrasound, CT, and MRI scans.

Radioisotope scanning

Radioisotope or nuclear scanning has been used to diagnose space-occupying lesions such as neoplasia, hematomas, and abscesses in animals.[23] Radioactive isotopes are injected intravenously into the animals, and the isotope distribution in the brain is recorded with a special gamma camera.

Table 5–11
Disorders with lesions seen on the myelogram

Congenital and familial disorders
  Spinal dysraphia
  Meningocele, myelocele
Trauma and vascular
  Intervertebral disc herniation
  Spinal cord edema
  Spinal cord compression
Neoplasia
  Intramedullary spinal cord tumors
  Extramedullary spinal cord tumors

mals.[29,75] The procedures are safe, non-invasive, and have better diagnostic capabilities than the other radiographic techniques for the brain and spinal cord. All animals are anesthetized to prevent movement artifact.

Figure 5–26 shows a scanner used to obtain computerized axial tomograms of the brain. During the CT scan an x-ray beam is transmitted through a cross-sectional slice of the animal's brain or spinal cord. The CT image is reconstructed by computer analysis of the transmitted x-ray data from multiple exposures. Ventrodorsal and occasionally lateral views are taken,

and reproduce the brain images as transverse (coronal) and dorsal (horizontal) sections, respectively (Fig. 5–27A and C). An organic iodide contrast medium containing 400 mg of iodide per milliliter is injected intravenously into the cephalic vein. Neoplastic processes will often be enhanced by the use of the iodide contrast medium (Fig. 5–27B and C). Figure 5–27D shows the transverse brain section at necropsy. Cerebral neoplasia, hydrocephalus, cerebral hemorrhage, and abscesses may be diagnosed using CT scans of the brain.[16,17,30,32] The computerized pictures appear as the slices of brain would be seen at necropsy.

MRI uses the animal's own body proton reactions in the presence of a strong magnetic field. Energy changes in proton spins produce a signal that can be reconstructed by computer analysis to create an image. Gadolinium can be injected intravenously and is absorbed by tissue where the blood-brain barrier is no longer intact and brain and spinal cord lesions can be further delineated. Soft tissue contrast is often superior in MRI as compared with CT scans (Fig. 5–28).

Both CT and MRI scans are available through centers providing diagnostic services for humans and some veterinary teaching hospitals.

Table 5–12
Disorders with no lesions seen on the myelogram

Congenital and familial disorders
  Spinal dysraphia
  Afghan myelopathy
  Lysosomal storage diseases
  Dysmyelinogenesis
Infections and other inflammations
  Myelitis—viral, bacterial, fungal, protozoal
  Meningitis—myelography may aggravate
  Granulomatous meningoencephalitis
Degenerations
  Degenerative myelopathy (German Shepherds)

Miscellaneous neuroradiographic techniques

Several neuroradiographic techniques may occasionally be used to study a particular problem. Vertebral sinus venography may be performed by the injection of an aqueous contrast media into a vertebral body. The contrast media then drains into the vertebral sinuses and their integrity can be studied.[69]

Injection of contrast media into the angularis oculi veins fills the cavernous sinus at the base of the brain, and may aid in

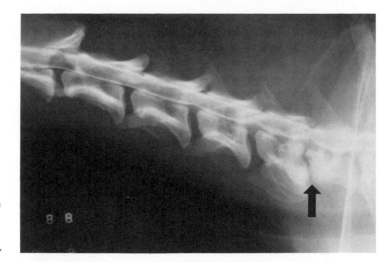

Figure 5–23. A cervical myelogram on a dog using iohexal. There is an intervertebral disc protrusion and discospondylitis at the C6–7 intervertebral space (arrow) (Courtesy of Dr. Norman Ackerman, University of Florida).

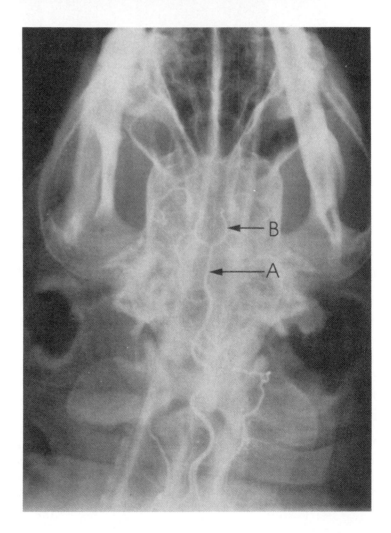

Figure 5–24. Ventrodorsal view of a cerebral angiogram after injection of contrast media in the vertebral artery of a normal dog. (A) basilar artery, (B) circle of Willis.

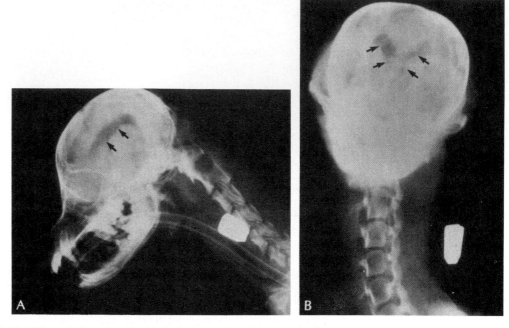

Figure 5–25. *(A)* Lateral view of a pneumoventriculogram in a dog. Lateral ventricles indicated by arrows. *(B)* Frontal view of a pneumoventriculogram in a dog. Lateral ventricles indicated by arrows.

the diagnosis of hemorrhage and tumors in this region.[31]

Occasionally, contrast media may be injected into spinal arteries to outline the vascular integrity of the spinal cord.

Simple tomography blurs the images of all structures not in a predetermined plane, so various planes of a structure may be visualized. This can be useful in studying vertebral and petrous temporal bone changes associated with infections or tumors. Tomography may be used with pneumoventriculography.

Biopsy of the nervous system and muscle

Histologic examination of tissue from a biopsy specimen can further characterize lesions. If a nonresectable lesion is identified in the cerebral cortex or diencephalon by the MRI or CT scan, then a biopsy may be taken on selected patients to attempt a tissue diagnosis. With the advent of new drugs and techniques in chemotherapy and radiation, biopsy of nervous system tissue may increase. Lesions of the brain stem below the diencephalon and the spinal cord are usually not biopsied, as the manipulation would result in further neurologic deficit.

In cases of chronic progressive cerebellar dysfunction, a biopsy of the cerebellum may be performed (Chap. 15). Biopsy of the cerebellum rarely produces any detectable change in the neurologic status of the patient.

A biopsy of a peripheral nerve may be obtained by removing only a few fascicles of the involved nerve while keeping the main portion of the nerve intact. This results in little additional neurologic dysfunction (Chap. 16).

A biopsy of muscle tissue is useful to characterized polymyopathies of dogs and

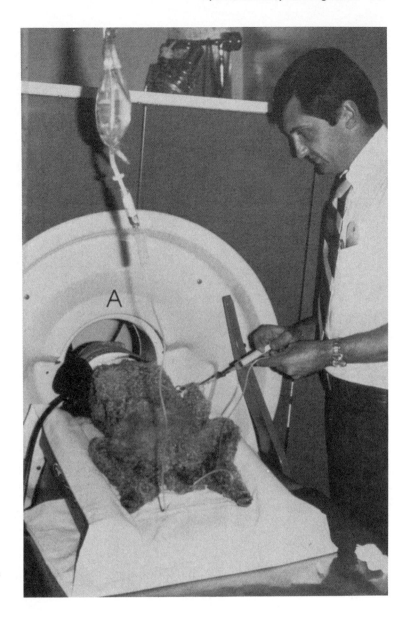

Figure 5–26. Computerized axial tomography of a 10-year-old Poodle thought to have cerebral neoplasia. The animal is anesthetized, placed on his back, and his head is inserted into the gantry of the scanner *(A)*. The radiologist is injecting an organic iodide contrast media into the cephalic vein catheter.

cats. Histochemical evaluation of the muscle can determine which fiber types are most involved (Chap. 16).

Miscellaneous ancillary aids

Ultrasonography

A-mode echoencephalography is performed by sending ultrasonic waves through the brain from the left to the right side. Deflections of the sound waves occur at all interfaces and can be demonstrated on an oscilloscope.[61] The main usefulness of the echoencephalogram has been to detect midline shifts due to hemorrhage, brain swelling and neoplastic processes.[60] It is a safe, simple procedure. However, it requires special equipment, and its use has been limited.

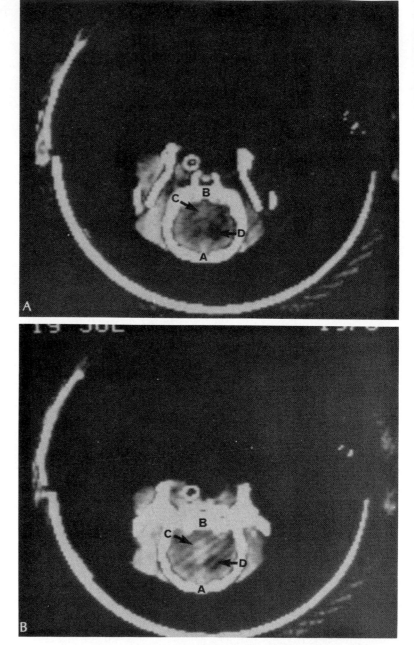

Figure 5–27. A, CT scan of a 13-year-old Boston terrier thought to have cerebral neoplasia. *(A)* dorsal cranial vault, *(B)* floor of the cranial vault, *(C)* suspected site of the tumor, *(D)* enlarged right lateral ventricle. **B,** CT scan of same Boston terrier after injection of organic iodide showing enhancement of neoplasm. *(A)* dorsal cranial vault, *(B)* floor of the cranial vault, *(C)* the enhanced tumor in the left subcortical region, *(D)* enlarged right lateral ventricle.

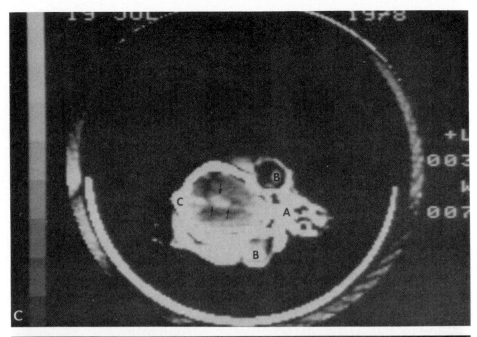

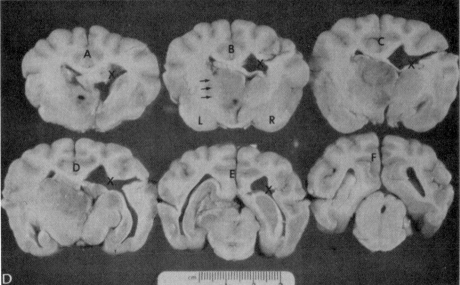

Figure 5–27. C, Head placed in lateral recumbency to produce a dorsal (horizontal) brain section. *(A)* dog's nose, *(B)* dog's eyes, *(C)* occipital protuberance. Neoplastic process has been enhanced by organic iodide contrast media and is indicated by the arrows. CT scan of same dog as in Figs. A and B. **D,** Views of the caudal surfaces of the transverse brain sections at necropsy of case in Figs. A through C. *(A)* through *(F)* indicate rostral to caudal sections. Section *(B)* corresponds best to the CT scan in Figs. A and B. The neoplasm is indicated by arrows and was an astrocytoma; (L) left side and (R) right side. Note the right lateral ventricle enlargement (X).

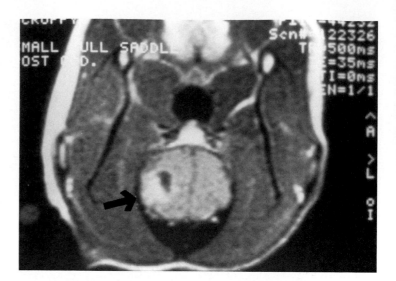

Figure 5–28. A magnetic resonance imaging (MRI) scan of a dog with seizures and a suspected brain tumor in the right frontal cerebral cortex (arrow) (Courtesy of Dr. Norman Ackerman, University of Florida).

Real time ultrasound has been used in diagnostics, but has limited application to study brain diseases if the calvarium is intact. The ultrasound anatomy of the canine brain has been experimentally studied through burr holes in the calvarium.[22] Dogs with an open fontanelle can be studied with ultrasound, and ventricular size can be assessed. In these dogs, ultrasound can replace invasive techniques like ventriculography.

Cystometry

Cystometry is a technique used to study the intravesical pressure in the bladder during the detrusor reflex in animals. It is a simple, safe technique, but does require some special equipment. Fluid is introduced into the bladder, and when a certain capacity is reached, the detrusor reflex is initiated. The cystometrogram (CMG) is recorded with a pressure transducer and physiograph. The CMG measures bladder-wall elasticity, detects uninhibited bladder contractions as seen during denervation, and demonstrates the integrity of the detrusor reflex (Chap. 19).

Audiometry

Deafness may be tested using electroencephalography and the alerting response to sound.[47] The animal is allowed to fall into a light sleep, which results in a slow-wave activity on the EEG. Then various frequency sound stimulations are given to the animal. An alerting response, or disappearance of the slow-wave activity, is observed if the animal can hear and respond to the sound. However, the BAER discussed earlier is a more objective and specific way to study deafness than EEG audiometry (Chap. 13).

References

1. Adams, W.M. and Stowater, J.L.: Complications of metrizamide myelography in the dog: A summary of 107 clinical case histories. Vet. Radiol., *22*:27, 1981.
2. Adams, W.M.: Myelography. Vet. Clin. North Am. (Small Anim. Pract.), *12*: 295, 1982.
3. Bailey, C.S. and Higgins, R.J.: Comparison of total white blood cell count and total

protein content of lumbar and cisternal cerebrospinal fluid of healthy dogs. Am. J. Vet. Res., *46*:1162, 1985.

4. Bailey, C.S. and Higgins, R.J.: Characteristics of cerebrospinal fluid associated with canine granulomatous meningoencephalitis: A retrospective study. J. Am. Vet. Med. Assoc., *188*:418, 1986.

5. Bailey, C.S. and Higgins, R.J.: Characteristics of cisternal cerebrospinal fluid associated with primary brain tumors in the dog: A retrospective study. J. Am. Vet. Med. Assoc., *188*:414, 1986.

6. Bichsel, P., et al.: Recording of visual evoked potentials in dogs with scalp electrodes. J. Vet. Intern. Med., *2*:145, 1988.

7. Bowen, J.M.: Electrophysiologic diagnosis: Electromyography. *In* Veterinary Neurology. Edited by J.E. Oliver, B.F. Hoerlein, and I.G. Mayhew. Philadelphia, W.B. Saunders, 1987.

8. Carakostas, M.C., et al.: Effects of metrizamide myelography on cerebrospinal fluid analysis in the dog. Vet. Radiol., *24*:267, 1983.

9. Chrisman, C.L.: Diseases of peripheral nerves. *In* Textbook and Veterinary Internal Medicine. Vol. I. Edited by S.J. Ettinger. Philadelphia, W.B. Saunders, 1989.

10. Chrisman, C.L.: Cerebrospinal fluid evaluation. *In* Current Veterinary Therapy VIII. Edited by R.W. Kirk. Philadelphia, W.B. Saunders, 1983.

11. Christopher, M.M., Perman, V., and Hardy, R.: Reassessment of cytologic values in canine cerebrospinal fluid used by cytocentrifugation. J. Am. Vet. Med. Assoc., *192*:1726, 1988.

12. Cook, J.R. and DeNicola, D.B.: Cerebrospinal fluid in common neurologic problems. Vet. Clin. North Am. *18*:475, 1988.

13. DeLahunta, A.: Cerebrospinal fluid and hydrocephalus. *In* Veterinary Neuroanatomy and Clinical Neurology. Philadelphia, W.B. Saunders, 1983.

14. Drayer, B., et al.: Iopamidol vs metrizamide: A double blind study for cervical myelography. Neuroradiology, *24*:77, 1982.

15. Dorn, A.S.: A standard technique for canine cerebral angiography. J. Am. Vet. Med. Assoc., *161*(12):1669, 1972.

16. Fike, J.R., et al.: Computerized tomography of brain tumors of the rostral and middle fossa in the dog. Am. J. Vet. Res., *42*:275, 1981.

17. Fike, J.R., et al.: Differentiation of neoplastic from nonneoplastic lesions in dog brain using quantitative CT. Vet. Radiol., *27*:121, 1986.

18. Funkquist, B.: Myelographic localization of spinal cord compression in dogs. Acta Vet. Scand., *16*:269, 1975.

19. Holliday, T.A., Ealand, B.G., and Weldon, B.G.: Sensory nerve conduction velocity. Am. J. Vet. Res., *38*:1543, 1977.

20. Holliday, T.A., Weldon, W.E., and Ealand, B.G.: Percutaneous recording of evoked spinal cord potentials of dogs. Am. J. Vet. Res., *40*(3):326, 1979.

21. Howard, D.R. and Breazile, J.E.: Normal visual cortical evoked response in the dog. Am. J. Vet. Res., *33*:2155, 1972.

22. Hudson, J.A., et al.: Ultrasonographic anatomy of the canine brain. Vet. Radiol., *30*:13, 1989.

23. Kallfelz, F.A., et al.: Scintigraphic diagnosis of brain lesions in the dog and cat. J. Am. Vet. Med. Assoc., *172*:589, 1978.

24. Kay, P., Palmer, A.C., and Taylor, P.M.: Hearing in the dog as assessed by auditory brain stem evoked potentials. Vet. Rec., *114*:81, 1984.

25. Knecht, C.D. and Redding, R.W.: Monosynaptic reflex (H wave) in clinically normal and abnormal dog. Am. J. Vet. Res., *42*:1586, 1981.

26. Knecht, C.D., Redding, R., and Hyams, D.: Stimulation techniques and response characteristics of the M and F waves and H reflex in dogs. Vet. Res. Commun., *6*:123, 1983.

27. Knecht, C.D., Redding, R.W., and Wilson, S.: Characteristics of F and H waves of ulnar and tibial nerves in cats: Reference values. Am. J. Vet. Res., *46*:977, 1985.

28. Kornegay, J.N., et al.: Somatosensory evoked potentials in clinically normal dogs. Am. J. Vet. Res., *42*:70, 1981.

29. Kraft, S. L., et al.: Canine brain anatomy on magnetic resonance images. Vet. Radiol., *30*:147, 1989.

30. LeCouteur, R., et al.: Computed tomography of brain tumors in the caudal fossa of the dog. Vet. Radiol., *22*:244, 1981.

31. Lee, R. and Griffiths, I.R.: A comparison of cerebral arteriography and cavernous sinus venography in the dog. J. Sm. Anim. Pract., *13*:225, 1972.

32. Loden, D., et al.: Diagnosis of intracranial lesions by computerized tomography in three dogs. J. Am. Anim. Hosp. Assoc., *19*:303, 1983.

33. Luttgen, P.J., et al.: Neuroradiology in common neurologic problems. Vet. Clin. North Am., *18*:501, 1988.

34. Malik, S.H. and Church, D.B.: A new method for recording and analysing evoked motor potentials from dogs. J. Sm. Anim. Pract., *30*:13, 1989.

35. Marshall, A.E.: Use of brain stem auditory evoked response to evaluate deafness in a group of Dalmatian dogs. J. Am. Vet. Med. Assoc., *188*:718, 1986.

36. Mayhew, I.G. and Beal, C.R.: Techniques of analysis of cerebrospinal fluid. Vet. Clin. North Am., *10*:155, 1980.

37. Meric, S.M.: Canine meningitis. J. Vet. Intern. Med., *2*:26, 1988.

38. Morgan, J.L., et al.: Effects of neomycin on the waveform of auditory evoked brain stem potentials in dogs. Am. J. Vet. Res., *41*:1077, 1980.

39. Morgan, J.P. and Takayoshi, M.: Degenerative changes in the vertebral column of the dog: A review of radiographic findings. Vet. Radiol., *29*:72, 1988.

40. Nafe, L.A. and Lee, A.E.: Evaluation of evoked muscle potentials from stimulation of ulnar nerves of the dog. Am. J. Vet. Res., *44*:669, 1983.

41. Parker, A.J., Marshall, A.E., and Sharp, J.G.: Study of the use of evoked cortical activity for clinical evaluation for spinal cord sensory transmission. Am. J. Vet. Res., *35*:673, 1974.

42. Redding, R.W., Ingram, J.T., and Colter, S.B.: Sensory nerve conduction velocity of cutaneous afferents of the radial, ulnar, peroneal and tibial nerves of the dog. Am. J. Vet. Res., *43*:517, 1982.

43. Redding, R.W., Lee, A.H., and Wilson, S.G.: Spinal evoked potentials and spinal conduction velocity of the cat: Reference values. Am. J. Vet. Res., *45*:2175, 1984.

44. Redding, R.W. and Ingram, J.T.: Sensory nerve conduction velocity of cutaneous afferents of the radial, ulnar, peroneal and tibial nerves of the cat. Am. J. Vet. Res., *45*:1042, 1984.

45. Redding, R.W. and Knecht, C.D.: Atlas of electroencephalography in the dog and cat. New York, Prager Scientific, 1984.

46. Redding, R.W. and Myers, L.J.: Electrophysiologic diagnosis: Evoked response. *In* Veterinary Neurology. Edited by J.E. Oliver, B.F. Hoerlein, and I.G. Mayhew. Philadelphia, W.B. Saunders, 1987.

47. Redding, R.W.: Electrophysiologic diagnosis: Electroencephalography. *In* Veterinary Neurology. Edited by J.E. Oliver, B.F. Hoerlein, and I.G. Mayhew. Philadelphia, W.B. Saunders, 1987.

48. Rising, J.L. and Lewis, R.E.: Femorovertebral cerebral angiography in the dog. Am. J. Vet. Res., *33*:665, 1972.

49. Roszel, J.F.: Membrane filtration of canine and feline cerebrospinal fluid for cytologic evaluation. J. Am. Vet. Med. Assoc., *160*:720, 1972.

50. Shebitz, H. and Wilkens, H.: Atlas of Radiographic Anatomy of the Dog and Cat, 3rd ed. Philadelphia, W.B. Saunders, 1978.

51. Shores, A., Redding, R.E., and Knecht, C.D.: Spinal evoked potentials in dogs with acute compressive thoracolumbar spinal cord disease. Am. J. Vet. Res., *48*:1525, 1987.

52. Simpson, S.T. and Reed, R.B.: Manometric values for normal cerebrospinal fluid pressure in dogs. J. Am. Anim. Hosp. Assoc., *23*:629, 1987.

53. Sims, M.H. and Redding, R.W.: Maturation of nerve conduction velocity and evoked muscle potential in the dog. Am. J. Vet. Res., *41*:1247, 1980.

54. Sims, M.H. and Selcer, R.R.: Occurrence and evaluation of a reflex evoked muscle potential (H reflex) in the normal dog. Am. J. Vet. Res., *42*:975, 1981.

55. Sims, M.H.: Recovery cycle of the reflex evoked muscle potential (H reflex): Excitability of spinal motor neurons in the healthy dog. Am. J. Vet. Res., *43*:89, 1982.

56. Sims, M.H. and Moore, R.E.: Auditory evoked response in the clinically normal dog: Early latency components. Am. J. Vet. Res., *45*:2019, 1984.

57. Sims, M.H. and Moore, R.E.: Auditory

evoked response in the clinically normal dog: Middle latency components. Am. J. Vet. Res., *45*:2028, 1984.

58. Sims, M.H. and Shull-Selcer, E.: Electrodiagnostic evaluation of deafness in two English Setter littermates. J. Am. Vet. Med. Assoc., *4*:398, 1985.

59. Sims, M.H. and Laratta, L.J.: Visual evoked potentials in cats using a light-emitting diode stimulator. Am. J. Vet. Res., *49*:1876, 1988.

60. Smith, C.W., et al.: Detection of artificially produced intracranial midline shifts of the brain in the dog with A-mode echoencephalography. Am. J. Vet. Res., *33*:2423, 1972.

61. Smith, C.W., et al.: Use of A-mode echoencephalography in the dog. Am. J. Vet. Res., *33*:2415, 1972.

62. Snyder, B.G. and Holliday, T.A.: Pathways of ascending evoked spinal cord potentials of dogs. EEG and Clin. Neurophysiol., *58*:140, 1984.

63. Sorjonen, D.C., Warren, J.N., and Schultz, R.D.: Qualitative and quantitative determination of albumin IgG, IgM, and IgA in normal cerebrospinal fluid of dogs. J. Am. Anim. Hosp. Assoc., *17*:833, 1981.

64. Sorjonen, D.C.: Total protein, albumin quota and electrophoretic patterns in cerebrospinal fluid of dogs with central nervous system disorders. Am. J. Vet. Res., *48*:301, 1987.

65. Spencer, C.P., et al.: Neurotoxicologic effects of the nonionic contrast agent iopamidol on the leptomeninges of the dog. Am. J. Vet. Res., *43*:1958, 1982.

66. Steinberg, S.A. and Vandervelde, M.: A comparative study of two methods of cytological evaluation of spinal fluid in domestic animals. Folia Vet. Latina, *20*:235, 1974.

67. Steiss, J.E. and Marshall, A.E.: Electromyographic evaluation of conduction time and velocity of the recurrent laryngeal nerves of clinically normal dogs. Am. J. Vet. Res., *49*:1533, 1988.

68. Stowater, J.L. and Kneller, S.K.: Clinical evaluation of metrizamide as a myelographic agent in the dog. J. Am. Vet. Assoc., *175*:191, 1979.

69. Ticer, J.W.: Radiographic Techniques in Veterinary Practice. 2nd ed. Philadelphia, W.B. Saunders, 1984.

70. Vandervelde, M. and Spano, J.S.: Cerebrospinal fluid cytology in canine neurologic disease. Am. J. Vet. Res., *38*:1827, 1977.

71. Vaughn, et al.: A rostrocaudal gradient for neurotransmitter metabolites and a caudorostral gradient for protein in canine cerebrospinal fluid. Am. J. Vet. Res., *49*:2134, 1988.

72. Walker, T.L., Redding, R.W., and Braund, K.G.: Motor nerve conduction velocity and latency in the dog. Am. J. Vet. Res., *40*:1433, 1979.

73. Wheeler, S.J. and Davies, J.V.: Iohexol myelography in the dog and cat: A series of one hundred cases, and a comparison with metrizamide and iopamidol. J. Small Anim. Pract., *26*:247, 1985.

74. Widmer, W.R., et al.: A comparison of iopamidol and metrizamide for cervical myelography in the dog. Vet. Radiol., *29*:108, 1988.

75. Wortman, J.A.: Principles of x-ray computed tomography and magnetic resonance imaging. Semin. Vet. Med. Surg., *1*:176, 1986.

76. Wright, J.A.: Evaluation of cerebrospinal fluid in the dog. Vet. Rec., *103*:48, 1978.

77. Wright, J.A. and Clayton-Jones, D.C.: Metrizamide myelography in sixty eight dogs. J. Small Anim. Pract., *22*:415, 1981.

Chapter 6

Medical management of the neurologic patient

The therapy for a neurologic patient may be medical, surgical, or both. The techniques used in neurosurgery for the cranium, vertebral column, and peripheral nerves are well described elsewhere and will not be discussed here.[11,18,19] Table 6–1 reviews the most commonly used neurosurgery techniques and some of their indications. The medical management of the neurologic patient is discussed in this chapter. Seizures, muscle spasms, nervous system inflammation, edema, and infection are problems that may require medical management. Although the cause and prognosis of these problems may vary greatly, many of the principles of the symptomatic therapy are the same.

Acute management of seizures

Seizures may be a sign of such disorders as encephalitis, intoxication, hypoglycemia, epilepsy, and cerebral neoplasia (Chap. 8). If the animal is presented in multiple or continual seizures (status epilepticus), the seizure must be stopped, regardless of the cause, before further evaluation can be performed.

Table 6–2 outlines the basic steps in managing status epilepticus of unknown cause.

Table 6–1
Neurosurgical Techniques and Indications

Techniques	Indications
Cranial vault surgery	
Lateral rostral tentorial craniotomy Bilateral rostral tentorial craniotomy Transfrontal craniotomy Caudal suboccipital or caudotentorial craniectomy Ventral craniectomy	All techniques are used to explore various regions of the brain to arrest hemorrhage, remove hematomas, decompress cerebral edema, remove brain tumors, remove epileptic foci, and perform a biopsy of the brain.
Paracranial surgery	
Bulla osteotomy	Used to explore the middle ear, to drain infection, or to remove tumors.
Vertebral column surgery	
Ventral fenestration (cervical)	Removal of degenerated or protruding intervertebral disc material.
Ventral slot (cervical)	Removal of herniated intervertebral disc material, and ventral decompression.
Dorsal laminectomy	Dorsal decompression and exploration of the spinal cord, removal of exposed intervertebral disc material, or neoplasia.
Dorsal hemilaminectomy (thoracolumbar)	Removal of herniated intervertebral disc material or neoplasia, decompression, and exploration of the spinal cord.
Dorsolateral fenestration (thoracolumbar)	Removal of degenerated or protruding intervertebral disc material to prevent future herniations.
Vertebral body plating, pinning, and screwing Vertebral body fusion Vertebral articular facet screwing and wiring Vertebral spinous process plating or wiring	All techniques used to repair and stabilize fractured, luxated, and subluxated vertebrae.

Anticonvulsant drugs

The drugs most commonly used to stop seizures are intravenous injections of diazepam and sodium pentobarbital (Na pentobarbital). Intravenous diazepam stops the seizure discharge without heavily sedating the animal.[1,6] Immediate evaluation of the animal's neurologic status may be made if the animal is not heavily sedated or anesthetized. Diazepam has a wide margin of safety. However, it is more expensive than Na pentobarbital, and as diazepam is a drug which is often abused,

many veterinarians may not want the responsibility of having it in their hospitals. Although diazepam may not be as effective as Na pentobarbital in controlling seizures from chemical intoxication, it is often the first drug of choice in stopping seizures of unknown cause. The dosage is listed in Table 6–2. The initial dose may be repeated 2–3 times over several minutes for continuing seizures.

Sodium pentobarbital is readily available in most practices, and is relatively inexpensive compared with diazepam. If diazepam has already been given, then Na

Table 6–2
Management of status epilepticus

1. Immediate anticonvulsant therapy
   a. Diazepam   2 mg intravenously to a 5-kg dog or cat
                         5 mg intravenously to a 10-kg dog
                         10 mg intravenously to a 20-kg dog
       Each dose can be repeated 2 or 3 times over several
       minutes in an attempt to stop the seizures.
   b. Sodium pentobarbital—intravenously to effect, usually not
       to exceed 3–15 mg/kg
2. Evaluate respirations, establish a patent airway, and give
   oxygen if needed.
3. Place intravenous catheter and flush with heparinized saline
   to keep patent.
4. Evaluate for hypoglycemia, draw a blood sample, analyze,
   and if low, administer 50% dextrose intravenously or orally
   as needed to control hypoglycemia.
5. Monitor vital signs
   a. If temperature elevated over 105° F after 10 minutes, give
       cool water bath until temperature is 102° F.
   b. If cerebral edema is suspected, give oxygen, mannitol, and
       glucocorticoids.
6. Maintenance anticonvulsant therapy
   a. Phenobarbital intravenously or intramuscularly 1–2 mg/kg
       every 6 hours for 24 hours if seizures are persistent, to
       produce anticonvulsant levels more rapidly
   b. Resume or initiate oral anticonvulsants every 8–12 hours
       if indicated as soon as the animal can swallow.
7. Collect data base (history, physical examination, neurologic
   examination, complete blood count, serum chemistry profile,
   and urinalysis).

pentobarbital is given slowly intravenously to effect, but usually 1–2 ml (65 mg/ml) will stop the seizures. The effective dosage of Na pentobarbital alone is less than the anesthetic dosage, and usually between 3 and 15 mg/kg will stop the seizure, but at that point the animal is heavily sedated. This sedation may be desired in cases of known chemical intoxications until the chemical is cleared from the body. The sedation of the animal makes it difficult to evaluate its neurologic status. Respiration should be monitored closely if diazepam and Na pentobarbital are mixed, as they produce respiratory depression in combination. If Na pentobarbital injections do not stop the seizures, then gas anesthesia may be used, and the anesthetic periodically discontinued to see whether the seizures have stopped. Recovery from Na pentobarbital anesthesia can produce a hyperexcitable state of paddling and thrashing, and this should be differentiated from continued seizure activity.

Intravenous phenobarbital is not as useful in stopping seizures, as it can take up to 15 or 20 minutes for a complete effect. Injectable phenobarbital given intravenously or intramuscularly may be more useful after the seizure has been stopped to provide a prolonged anticonvulsant effect.

Injectable phenothiazine-derivative tranquilizers such as acepromazine or disassociative anesthetic agents such as ketamine hydrochloride are contraindicated in the management of any seizure disorder. These drugs actually reduce the seizure threshold and can potentiate the seizures.

Evaluate respiration

Status epilepticus results in hypoxia because of the difficulty of proper respiration produced by the severe muscle contractions. Mucous membranes may appear cyanotic during the seizure. In most cases, once the seizure is stopped the airway becomes patent and mucous membrane color and respiratory function return to normal. Hypoxia or anoxia from prolonged status epilepticus can lead to cerebral edema. Oxygen may be administered through a face mask or endotracheal tube to combat the cerebral edema. Elevate the head to facilitate blood flow.

Serum glucose determination

Hypoglycemia may cause seizures. Prolonged seizure activity also may cause hypoglycemia, which complicates the seizure control and can cause brain damage. Seizures from hypoglycemia are difficult to control with anticonvulsant therapy alone. Therefore, an immediate serum glucose determination should be made if hypoglycemia is suspected. If seizures are due to hypoglycemia, no anticonvulsant may be needed and an injection of 50% dextrose will stop further seizures in most cases. A quick Dextrostix (Ames Company, Elkhart, Indiana) examination using 1 drop of whole blood may be performed. If the Dextrostix reaction indicates hypoglycemia, administration of 50% dextrose may be tried. The Dextrostix may not be as reliable for hypoglycemia as it is for hyperglycemia, and therefore, serum glucose determinations should also be per-

formed as soon as possible by other standard laboratory methods.

In many dogs and cats, the serum glucose value is elevated because of the stress of the seizure releasing epinephrine and glucose stores into the blood stream. If the serum glucose determination is low (below 60 mg/dl), it must be decided whether this is a primary sign of the underlying disease process or a complication of the prolonged seizure. Fifty percent dextrose may be given intravenously to effect, at a dose from 2 to 25 ml or approximately 1–4 mg/kg, depending on the size of the animal and its response to therapy. If an insulinoma is the suspected cause of hypoglycemia, the animal should be maintained on a constant 10% or more dextrose intravenous infusion until further studies or surgery can be performed. Otherwise, 2–3 hours after 50% dextrose injection, the serum glucose level may fall severely because of the outpouring of insulin from the tumor (Chap. 8).

A serum calcium determination can be performed; however, hypocalcemia with no history of recent whelping or lactation is rare. Prophylactic injections of calcium are not recommended. Determination of the serum calcium is part of the routine clinical pathologic evaluation of a seizure patient (Chap. 8).

Management of complications

The vital signs of the animal should be closely monitored. The body temperature elevates during status epilepticus, but should return to normal once the seizure is stopped. Cool water baths may be given to reduce body temperature if greater than 105° F, but discontinue bath once the body temperature reaches 102° F. Do not do this routinely as hypothermia may result and slow recovery from the seizure.

Complications of status epilepticus are anoxia or hypoxia, hypoglycemia, lactic acidosis, and pulmonary edema. Anoxia or hypoxia produces cerebral edema. If hypoxic brain swelling is suspected from the length of the seizure and the animal is semicomatose or comatose, a patent airway should be established with an endotracheal tube and oxygen given. Agents to reduce acute cerebral edema, such as intravenous administration of mannitol, may be given followed by repeated injections of glucocorticoids. See Nervous System Edema treatment below.

Hypoglycemia should be corrected as described in the discussion on serum glucose determination, then monitored, as chronic hypoglycemia can produce permanent brain damage or an epileptic focus.

Lactic acidosis is due to the excessive muscle activity, and generally corrects itself once the seizures stop. Rapid correction of systemic acidosis may actually worsen the CNS acidosis (Chap. 1).

In cases of recurrent seizures, chronic oral anticonvulsant therapy may be necessary. Drugs, dosages, and indications of chronic anticonvulsant therapy are discussed in Chapter 8.

Maintenance anticonvulsant therapy

Once seizures have been stopped, maintenance anticonvulsant therapy should be continued on those animals that have a history of seizures or have been on oral anticonvulsants. Oral anticonvulsants may be given as soon as the animal can swallow. The effectiveness of the previous anticonvulsant regimen should be evaluated, and either continued or changed (Chap. 8).

Intramuscular injections of diazepam are of little use for maintenance anticonvulsant therapy in dogs, but may be useful in cats.

Intravenous injections of 1–2 mg/kg phenobarbital every 6–12 hours over the next 24 hours may be useful to facilitate anticonvulsant levels in dogs and cats; however, often this is not necessary, and oral medication is resumed.

Muscle spasms

Muscle spasms can be a painful complication of nerve root compression or irritation from intervertebral disc material, neoplasia, fractured vertebrae, or meningitis. Several drugs may be used to provide relief to the animal.

Diazepam (Valium) is a potent central-acting muscle relaxant. Administation of 1–2 mg diazepam intravenously may be given to a 5 kg dog or cat for acute muscle spasms. A dose of 2–5 mg diazepam may be given to a 10–20 kg dog intravenously. Diazepam (1–5 mg) can be given orally every 6–8 hours for maintenance. Diazepam therapy can provide great relief to dogs with protruded or herniated intervertebral disc material. In dogs and cats with spastic paraplegia and spasms of the external urethral sphincter, the use of diazepam may allow the bladder to be more easily expressed.

Methocarbamol (Robaxin) is another useful antispasmodic drug for the dog. Intravenous injections of 40 mg/kg of methocarbamol relieve acute muscle spasms. Oral methocarbamol may be administered as maintenance therapy at 20–40 mg/kg every 8 hours, once spasms are under control.

Pain control

Pain commonly is associated with vertebral osteomyelitis, fractures, neoplasms, discospondylitis, and nerve root and meningeal neoplasms, as well as some neurosurgical procedures. The pain associated with intervertebral disc disease is usually controlled with diazepam and glucocorticoid therapy. For 12–48 hours after a ventral cervical vertebral slot, fenestration, laminectomy, or vertebral fracture repair, additional pain control may be needed.

Buprenorphine hydrochloride (Buprenex) 0.1–0.3 mg/kg or butorphanol (Torbutrol) 0.1–0.4 mg/kg may be given subcutaneously (SC) to dogs and cats repeated every 4–8 hours if needed for 12–48 hours to control pain during the immediate postoperative period.[14,16,23] Buprenorphine and butorphanol are longer acting than the narcotics, but like narcotics are contraindicated in head injury patients as they increase intracranial pressure.

Narcotics such as oxymorphone (Numorphan), morphine sulfate (Morphine), and meperidine (Demerol) are very short acting in dogs and cats. Morphine may be given SC or intramuscularly (IM) to dogs at 0.1–1 mg/kg and cats at 0.05–0.1 mg/kg. To avoid hyperexcitability, the lowest effective dose should be administered to cats. Meperidine may be given IM to dogs at 5–10 mg/kg and cats at 1–4 mg/kg. If postoperative sedation is desired, acepromazine may be combined with either morphine or meperidine. For dogs, 0.05 mg/kg acepromazine and 0.1 mg/kg morphine are given SC or 1 mg/kg meperidine mixed with the above dose of acepromazine is given IM.[23] For cats, 0.01 mg/kg acepromazine and 0.1 mg/kg meperidine mixed with acepromazine is given IM.[23] If narcotics have been given, do not use buprenorphine or butorphanol, as they are narcotic antagonists and will reverse any existing narcotic effect.

Pain associated with discospondylitis and vertebral osteomyelitis may be controlled by nonsteroidal anti-inflammatory drugs piroxicam, phenylbutazone, buffered acetylsalicylic acid (aspirin), or acetaminophen (Tylenol). Phenylbutazone can be used in cats, but acetylsalicylic acid must be used only once every 3 days. Acetamin-

ophen cannot be used in cats, as it produces methemoglobinemia. All the nonsteroidal anti-inflammatory drugs produce gastrointestinal irritation, which can lead to gastric, duodenal, or colonic ulcers. Nonsteroidal anti-inflammatory drugs should never be used in combination with each other or glucocorticoids, as gastrointestinal ulceration may result in perforation and death.

Piroxicam (Feldene) may be given to dogs over 25 kg at a dosage of 10 mg once daily. A 10-mg capsule is currently the smallest size produced. Piroxicam alters platelet function and may cause nose bleeds and produces gastrointestinal disturbances, so overdosing small dogs could be harmful. Piroxicam should not be used before surgery.

Phenylbutazone (Butazolidin) may be given to dogs at 8–10 mg/kg (not to exceed 800 mg/day) orally every 8–12 hours for 5–7 days.[14] A dose of 6–12 mg/kg of phenylbutazone may be given to cats orally every 12–24 hours for 5–7 days. Phenylbutazone may produce bone marrow suppression, so a complete blood count (CBC) should be monitored with prolonged usage.

Buffered acetylsalicylic acid (aspirin) may be given to dogs in a dosage not to exceed 10 mg/kg every 8 hours orally.[14] Prolonged daily administration should be avoided, as gastrointestinal disturbances and bleeding disorders are common. Acetylsalicylic acid should not be administered for 5–7 days prior to any surgery. Acetylsalicylic acid may be given to adult cats once every 3 days orally, at a dosage not to exceed 6 mg/kg.

Acetaminophen (Tylenol) may be given to dogs (not cats) at 5 mg/kg orally daily in divided doses. Signs of toxicity include anorexia, vomiting, and hemoglobinuria.

There are no good longterm analgesic drugs for pain from nerve root and men-

ingeal neoplasia. Surgical excision is recommended if possible. If surgical excision
is impossible, euthanasia is the most humane alternative.

Nervous system and muscle inflammation

Inflammation of the nervous system or
muscle may lead to excessive scarring and
disruption of function. An attempt should
be made to control the inflammatory response with glucocorticoids unless a bacterial, protozoal, or fungal infection is
present.

The glucocorticoids are the most
potent anti-inflammatory drugs for nervous tissue.[6] A comparison of the relative
glucocorticoid potency of commonly used
corticosteroids is listed in Table 6–3. Methylprednisolone, prednisolone, or prednisone are the most frequently used by the
author. Other authors use dexamethasone.[5,7,15]

For acute or severe nervous system inflammation, methylprednisolone sodium
succinate (Solu-Medrol) 30 mg/kg is administered intravenously and then reduced to 15 mg/kg every 6–8 hours for 24
hours. Dexamethasone at 2 mg/kg intravenously may also be given instead, but

may be less effective acutely. Dexamethasone has a longer effect than methylprednisolone sodium succinate.

Prednisolone or prednisone then can
be administered orally on a daily or alternate-day therapy regimen to correct or
control chronic inflammation of the nervous system. A dosage of 1–2 mg/kg daily,
divided into 12-hour doses, is recommended for a few days, then a decreasing
dosage plan such as 1 mg/kg for 3–5 days,
then 0.5 mg/kg for 3–5 days, then 0.25 mg/
kg for 3–5 days, then 0.12 mg/kg for 3–5
days, then 0.12 mg/kg every other day can
be followed over the next 2 weeks or
month, depending on the individual patient's needs. To control immune-mediated disorders or the signs of neoplastic
disease after the acute phase, alternate-day
therapy is suggested to prevent complete
suppression of the adrenal gland, as therapy may have to be continued over several
months. The dosage must be adjusted according to individual needs to control the
neurologic signs. Dexamethasone 0.1 mg/
kg may be substituted for prednisone orally and used with decreasing doses, but
lasts longer than 24 hours and so is not
good for alternate-day therapy. The author uses prednisolone or prednisone primarily, so these are suggested in this book.
Hemorrhagic gastroenteritis, pancreatitis,

Table 6–3
Comparison of glucocorticoids

Generic name	Relative anti-inflammatory potency	Relative sodium-retaining potency
Hydrocortisone	1	1
Prednisolone	4	0.8
Prednisone	4	0.8
Methylprednisolone	5	0.5
Triamcinolone	5	0
Betamethasone	25	0
Dexamethasone	25	0

hepatopathy, and duodenal and colonic ulcers also may be a complication at higher dosages especially in paraplegic dogs and cats.[17,20] Gastrointestinal complications may be less with prednisone or prednisolone than with dexamethasone in the author's experience. A combination of cimetidine (Tagamet) 4 mg/kg orally every 6–8 hours followed in 2 hours by sucralfate (Carafate) 250 mg to 1 g orally is recommended. Polyuria, polydipsia, polyphagia, and excessive panting are almost always present at higher dosages, and are more evident with prednisolone and prednisone therapy than with dexamethasone therapy.

Immune-mediated muscle inflammation such as polymyositis and masseter and temporalis myositis responds well to glucocorticoid therapy.

Prednisone and prednisolone are often preferred over dexamethasone for longterm control, as alternate-day therapy is often effective and less stressful on the adrenal glands.

Nonsuppurative inflammations of the CNS associated with viral infections, or granulomatous meningoencephalitis (reticulosis) and steroid-responsive meningoencephalomyelitis frequently respond to glucocorticoid therapy. Longterm alternate-day prednisone therapy may be necessary to control clinical signs (Chap. 8).

Phenylbutazone (Butazolidin), acetylsalicylic acid (aspirin), and flunixine meglumine (Banamine) have little anti-inflammatory effect on nervous tissue, but affect bone and joint inflammation, and therefore, relieve some discomfort. However, these nonsteroidal anti-inflammatory drugs should not be used in place of a glucocorticoid if nervous system inflammation and edema are to be treated. Nonsteroidal anti-inflammatory drugs should never be used in conjunction with glucocorticoids, as gastrointestinal ulceration is more likely than with either drug alone.

Nervous system edema

Edema of nervous tissue may be due to infections, trauma, neoplasia, hypoxia, and other metabolic disturbances, or may occur as a result of manipulation during surgery. The edema may lead to further compromise of the intrinsic vascular system and neuronal damage.

Oral glycerol or 50% glucose, and intravenous mannitol, urea, and 50% glucose are osmotic diuretics that have an effect on nervous system edema. Mannitol (20%) is currently the most commonly used drug for the treatment of nervous system edema.[6] Because mannitol is a large molecule that stays in the vascular compartment, it elevates the osmolality of plasma and draws fluids from the nervous tissue into the plasma.

In acute cerebral edema, 0.5–2.0 g/kg of 20% mannitol solution is given intravenously very slowly or in a drip over a 10–15-minute period and methylprednisolone sodium succinate (Solu-Medrol) 30 mg/kg is administered intravenously at the same time.[6,8] Mannitol may be repeated once in 30 minutes to 1 hour, depending on the condition of the animal. Mannitol decreases the immediate cerebral edema and methylprednisolone sodium succinate supplies protection in a few hours. Continued therapy with dexamethasone or prednisolone may prevent recurrence of edema.[5,15] Mannitol should not be given if the animal is dehydrated, in congestive heart failure, shock, or if there is known cerebral hemorrhage. Chronic nervous system edema can be controlled with daily, then alternate-day, prednisolone or prednisone.

In acute spinal cord injuries from trauma or intervertebral disc herniation, Mannitol (20%) is contraindicated. Methylprednisolone sodium succinate (Solu-Medrol) 30 mg/kg is administered intravenously to cats and dogs initially and then reduced to 15 mg/kg every 6–8 hours. Decreasing doses may be given over the next 5–7 days or prednisone or prednisolone at 1 mg/kg orally may be begun and then reduced every 3 days for 7–10 days (See Nervous System and Muscle Inflammation).

Infections of the nervous system

If the blood–brain barrier is intact, few antibiotics will cross it to develop significant levels in nervous tissue.[4] When possible, cerebrospinal fluid (CSF) culture and sensitivity should be used to guide the treatment of CNS infections.

Chloramphenicol, trimethoprim, metronidazole, sulfonamides, moxalactam, minocycline, and rifampin all penetrate the blood–brain barrier. Chloramphenicol has a wide spectrum of antibacterial activity, but is mainly bacteriostatic in action, which may be a problem when trying to control chronic infections. The usual dose is 50 mg/kg given every 6–8 hours orally. Few problems with asplastic anemia associated with the use of chloramphenicol have been encountered in dogs and cats as compared with humans.[21,22] Chloramphenicol produces anorexia in cats. Chloramphenicol may increase blood levels of phenobarbital and phenytoin and produce signs of toxicity in dogs.[9]

Sulfonamides may reach effective concentrations in cerebrospinal fluid. Sulfonamides are usually protein-bound in serum, and because there is little protein to bind to in the CSF, more of the drug is available. Sulfonamides have a wide range of antimicrobial activity, and are bacteriostatic in action. Sulfadiazine is most commonly used for the CNS. Trimethoprim also can enter CSF, and may be indicated from culture and sensitivity studies. Trimethoprim sulfadiazine (Tribrissen) 15 mg/kg every 12 hours orally is often used to treat CNS infections. Drug reactions producing polyarthritis, keratitis sicca, skin rashes, and bleeding problems have been reported, especially in Doberman Pinschers. Trimethoprim sulfadiazine administration is very effective and safe in most dogs and cats.

Ampicillin and penicillin G do not enter the CNS under normal conditions. In cases of bacterial meningitis, however, levels reached are adequate to be effective for therapy. Ampicillin is given at a dose of 22 mg/kg orally every 8 hours or 11–22 mg/kg intravenously, subcutaneously, or intramuscularly every 6–8 hours. Penicillin G may be given at a dose of 10,000–20,000 units/kg intravenously every 4–6 hours in bacterial meningitis.

Metronidazole 25–50 mg/kg orally every 12 hours may be given to dogs with an anaerobic meningitis. Side effects of metronidazole include vestibular dysfunction (Chap. 12).

In general, cephalosporins have relatively poor penetration into brain tissue and CSF. Cephradine (Velosef) 20 mg/kg orally every 8 hours may be useful for treating bacterial infections of bone. A combination of trimethoprim sulfadiazine (Tribrissen) and cephradine (Velosef) for 6–8 weeks may be useful to treat many cases of inner and middle ear infections and discospondylitis or osteomyelitis from bacterial infections.

Amphotericin B (Fungizone) is fungistatic or fungicidal for many of the systemic mycotic infections. With an intact blood–brain barrier, little amphotericin B is absorbed into the cerebrospinal fluid. Intrathecal infusions of amphotericin B have been advocated for treatment of fungal meningitis in man, but few reports are available in veterinary literature. Amphotericin B (Fungizone) is given at 0.25–0.50 mg/kg in 0.5–0.1 liter 5% dextrose in water intravenously over 6–8 hours every other day to a total dosage of 8–10 mg/kg unless the blood urea nitrogen (BUN) and creatinine rise. Therapy is discontinued if the latter occurs. Rifampin (Rifamate) 10–20 mg/kg orally every 8 hours and flucytosine (Ancobon) 100–175 mg/kg orally divided every 6–8 hours are added to amphotericin B to treat CNS histoplasmosis and aspergillosis.

Amphotericin B and flucytosine are combined to treat cryptococcosis. Ketoconazole (Nizoral) 15 mg/kg orally every 12 hours may be used to treat cryptococcal infections. New azole antifungal drugs such as fluconazole have good penetration in CSF and may be available for use in the future.[3]

Controversial medical therapies

Several medical therapy regimens have been evaluated for use in the treatment of acute spinal cord injuries. Spinal cord trauma research has shown that, after the initial injury, secondary reactions in the blood vessels of the spinal cord result in severe hemorrhagic necrosis and spinal cord destruction with 24–48 hours. Some experimental data suggest that the hemorrhagic necrosis is due in part to an excessive local release of catecholamines (epinephrine, norepinephrine, and dopamine). Anticatecholamine therapy given within the first 24 hours should theoretically diminish the hemorrhagic necrosis and improve the changes of recovery from spinal cord trauma. Several anticatecholamine therapies have been tested experimentally, but as yet are not widely advocated because nothing conclusive has been established.

In spinal cord hemorrhage, plasminogen is activated to break down blood clots. Antifibrinolytic therapy has been suggested to stabilize clot formation and reduce hemorrhagic necrosis. Epsilon amino caproic acid (EACA) is a fibrinolytic inhibitor, and has been suggested for use in spinal cord trauma. A dosage of 330 mg/kg was given to dogs in one study.[10] In another study, there was no improvement seen.[13]

Dimethyl sulfoxide (DMSO) has been used in experimental spinal cord and brain trauma because of its anti-inflammatory and diuretic properties. Some experimentors have injected 2.2–3.0 g/kg of a 20 g/dl solution of DMSO intravenously and improved the clinical recovery of animals with experimental spinal cord trauma.[2] Other studies have shown little recovery with this method.[13]

Naloxone, crocetin, thyrotropin-releasing hormone, and solcoseryl are other drugs that have been studied in experimental spinal cord injuries and produced no difference in recovery rates between treated and control groups.[7,8]

Perhaps in the next few years, enough experimental data may be acquired that new recommendations may be made concerning the treatment of humans and animals with CNS trauma. As a better understanding of the neurochemical basis of disease processes is developed, new, rational, and effective neuropharmacologic therapies may be advocated.

Medical and surgical therapies are discussed further with the individual problems of the nervous system.

References

1. Averill, D.R.: Treatment of status epilepticus in dogs with diazepam sodium. J. Am. Vet. Med. Assoc., *156*:432, 1970.
2. DelaTorre, J.C. et al.: Modification of experimental head and spinal cord injuries using dimethylsulfoxide. Trans. Am. Neurol. Assoc., *97*:230, 1972.
3. Dismukes, W.E.: Azole antifungal drugs: Old and new. Ann. Intern. Med., *109*:177, 1988.

4. Fenner, W.R.: Treatment of central nervous system infections in small animals. J. Am. Vet. Med. Assoc., *185*:1176, 1984.
5. Franklin, R.T.: The use of glucocorticoids in treating cerebral edema. Compend. Contin. Ed., *6*:442, 1984.
6. Greene, C.E.: Principles of medical therapy. *In* Veterinary Neurology. Edited by J.E. Oliver, B.F. Hoerlein, and I.G. Mayhew. Philadelphia, W.B. Saunders, 1987.
7. Hoerlein, et al.: Evaluation of dexamethasone, DMSO, mannitol and solcoseryl in acute spinal cord trauma. J. Am. Anim. Hosp. Assoc., *19*:216, 1983.
8. Hoerlein, et al.: Evaluation of naloxone, crocetin, thyrotropin releasing hormone, methylprednisolone, partial myelotomy, and hemilaminectomy in the treatment of acute spinal cord trauma. J. Am. Anim. Hosp. Assoc., *21*:67, 1985.
9. Koup, J.R., et al.: Interaction of chloramphenicol with phenytoin and phenobarbital. Clin. Pharmacol. Ther., *24*:372, 1978.
10. Mendenhall, H.V., et al.: Aggressive pharmacologic and surgical treatment of spinal cord injuries in dogs and cats. J. Am. Vet. Med. Assoc., *168*:1026, 1976.
11. Oliver, J.E. and Hoerlein, B.F.: Cranial surgery. *In* Veterinary Neurology. Edited by J.E. Oliver, B.F. Hoerlein, and I.G. Mayhew. Philadelphia, W.B. Saunders, 1987.
12. Parent, J.: Effects of dexamethasone on pancreatic tissue and on serum amylase and lipase activities in dogs. J. Am. Vet. Med. Assoc., *180*:743, 1982.
13. Parker, A.J.: Lack of functional recovery from spinal cord trauma following dimethylsulfoxide and epsilon amino caproic acid therapy in dogs. Res. Vet. Sci., *27*:253, 1979.
14. Potthoff, A. and Carithers, R.W.: Pain and analgesia in dogs and cats. Compend. Contin. Ed., *11*:887, 1989.
15. Sims, M.H. and Redding, R.W.: The use of dexamethasone in the prevention of cerebral edema in dogs. J. Am. Anim. Hosp. Assoc., *11*:439, 1975.
16. Sawyer, D.C. and Rech, R.H.: Analgesia and behavioral effects of butorphenol, nalbuphine, and pentazocine in the cat. J. Am. Anim. Hosp. Assoc., *23*:438, 1987.
17. Sorjonen, D.C., et al.: Effects of dexamethasone and surgical hypotension on the stomach of dogs: Clinical endoscopic and pathologic evaluations. Am J. Vet. Res., *44*:1233, 1983.
18. Sorjonen, D.C.: Small animal cervical surgery. *In* Veterinary Neurology. Edited by J.E. Oliver, B.F. Hoerlein, and I.G. Mayhew. Philadelphia, W.B. Saunders, 1987.
19. Swaim, S.F.: Small animal thoracolumbar, lumbosacral and sacrocaudal surgery. *In* Veterinary Neurology. Edited by J.E. Oliver, B.F. Hoerlein, and I.G. Mayhew. Philadelphia, W.B. Saunders, 1987.
20. Toombs, J.P., et al.: Colonic perforation following neurosurgical procedures and corticosteroid therapy in four dogs. J. Am. Vet. Med. Assoc., *177*:68. 1980.
21. Watson, A.D.J. and Middleton, D.J.: Chloramphenicol toxicosis in cats. Am. J. Vet. Res., *39*:1199, 1978.
22. Watson, A.D.J.: Further observations on chloramphenicol toxicosis in cats. Am. J. Vet. Res., *41*:293, 1980.
23. Webb, Alistair: Dept. Anesthesiology, University of Florida, personal communication.

Part II

Problems
in clinical
neurology

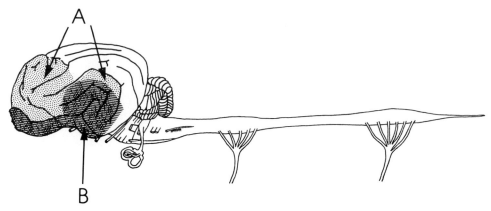

Figure 7–1. Location of lesions producing behavior and personality disorders. (*A*) cerebrum—frontal and temporal lobes (dots), (*B*) limbic system and hypothalamus (horizontal lines) beneath the cerebrum.

Location of the lesion (Figure 7–1): *cerebrum and diencephalon (limbic system, hypothalamus)*

Mechanisms of disease and differential diagnosis

Congenital and familial disorders

Hydrocephalus
Lissencephaly
Lysosomal storage disease

Infections and other inflammations

Distemper virus
Granulomatous meningoencephalitis (reticulosis) (Chap. 12)
Steroid-responsive meningoencephalitis
Feline infectious peritonitis virus
Rabies virus
Toxoplasmosis
Pug encephalitis
Mycosis
Miscellaneous encephalitis

Metabolic disorders

Hepatic encephalopathy
Uremic encephalopathy
Hypoglycemia (Chap. 8)
Hyperglycemia
Other hyperosmolar disturbances (Chap. 10)
Acid-base imbalances
Hypoxia (Chap. 9)

Toxicity

Lead
Miscellaneous toxicities

Nutritional Disorders

Thiamine deficiency

Trauma and vascular disorders

Hemorrhage, edema, and infarcts (Chap. 10)
Feline cerebral infarct

Degeneration

Neuronal degeneration of cocker spaniels

Neoplasia

Astrocytoma
Oligodendroglioma
Ependymoma
Choroid plexus papilloma
Glioblastoma
Spongioblastoma
Meningioma
Chromophobe adenoma
Metastatic tumors

Chapter 7

Behavior and personality disorders

Behavior and personality changes due to organic brain diseases are usually produced by lesions in the telencephalon or diencephalon (Fig. 7–1). Table 7–1 gives examples of changes in behavior and location of the lesion. There is an overlap in function between various areas of the telencephalon and diencephalon, so similar behavior changes can be produced by lesions in different anatomic regions.

Animals may have seizures along with their behavior abnormalities (Chap. 8). Lesions in the hypothalamus also may produce endocrinopathies. If the olfactory bulbs or connections into the hypothalamus are diseased, olfactory disturbances can occur, and are most commonly manifested by difficulty in finding food. Lesions in the midbrain and other areas of the ascending reticular activating system produce sleepiness, semicoma, or coma. These are discussed in Chapter 10.

Patient evaluation

The clinician must first decide if the behavior abnormality of an animal is neurologic or psychologic in origin. Early stages of a neurologic disorder may be difficult to differentiate from psychologic disturbances when the neurologic examination is normal. The development of further

Table 7–1
Behavior changes and locations of lesions

Behavior changes	Possible location of lesions
Loss of recognition of owner	Frontal lobe, internal capsule
Dementia	Frontal lobe, internal capsule
Inability to learn	Frontal lobe
Aggressiveness, irritability, passiveness, hypersexuality	Temporal lobe, limbic system, hypothalamus
Compulsive pacing or circling	Frontal lobe, internal capsule, basal nuclei (caudate nucleus)
Polyuria, polydipsia, polyphagia, aphagia, pica	Hypothalamus
Sleepiness, semicoma, coma	Frontal lobe, thalamus, subthalamus, midbrain
Inability to find food	Olfactory system

neurologic deficits on serial patient evaluations can help support the suspicion of an underlying neurologic disease. Further diagnostic tests then can be used to decide the mechanism of the disease process.

Signalment and history

As discussed in Chapter 2, the age, breed, and sex of the animal presented with behavior disorders can influence the type of diseases included in the differential diagnosis. Table 7–2 is an outline of the most common diseases in the differential diagnosis of certain age groups with behavior disorders due to neurologic disease. Congenital abnormalities are considered in animals under 1 year of age. Neoplastic processes are more commonly seen after 5 years of age. Other mechanisms can be included in the differential diagnosis at any age, but young animals may be more susceptible than adults to infections and automobile accidents, and be more inclined to chew on foreign objects and thus risk developing a toxic disorder.

A complete description of the type of behavior abnormality and the onset, course, and duration of the problem can further aid in differentiating the possible cause of the underlying disease process. If the abnormal behavior is a paroxysmal event, it could be a type of seizure (Chap. 8).

Physical and neurologic examinations

The physical and neurologic examination findings that support neurologic disease are discussed in Chapter 3.

In small, frontal lobe cortex, limbic system, or hypothalamic lesions, the neurologic examination may be normal other than the reported or observed behavior abnormalities. Lesions above the midbrain rarely produce obvious changes in strength and coordination of the gait unless they are acute (trauma and vascular lesions).

Unilateral lesions of the frontal lobe cerebral cortex and internal capsule may produce hopping and placing deficits in the contralateral thoracic and pelvic limbs.

Table 7–2
Differential diagnosis of behavior disorders and age groups

Young dogs and cats (under 1 yr of age)

Hydrocephalus (congenital)
Lissencephaly
Lysosomal storage diseases
Meningoencephalitis
Trauma
Lead poisoning
Thiamine deficiency
Hypoglycemia
Hepatic disorders—portacaval shunt
Metabolic disorders secondary to other congenital diseases

Older dogs and cats (over 5 yrs of age)

Cerebral neoplasia
Hypoglycemia—insulinoma
Hepatic disorders—acquired cirrhosis
Metabolic disorders secondary to acquired diseases
Thiamine deficiency
Meningoencephalitis
Trauma—infarcts
Lead poisoning (rare)

Unilateral lesions of the parietal lobe cerebral cortex, internal capsule, and thalamus may produce conscious proprioceptive deficits in the contralateral thoracic and pelvic limbs (see Table 3–2). Animals with asymmetric neurologic deficits most likely have encephalitis or neoplasia if the signs have been progressive over a few days or more. Traumatic and vascular disorders may produce asymmetric neurologic deficits, but rarely progress after 72 hours.

Ancillary diagnostic investigations

A complete blood count (CBC) and chemistry profile can support a diagnosis of infectious, metabolic, or toxic disease (Chap.

4). Special clinicopathologic investigations may be needed to further evaluate these disorders (Chap. 5).

The electroencephalogram (EEG) is an important ancillary aid in evaluating an animal with a behavior problem. If the EEG is abnormal, it supports the suspicion that a behavior disorder is due to neurologic disease rather than to a psychologic problem (see Table 5–3). However, a normal EEG does not rule out the possibility of a neurologic disorder (see Table 5–4).

The diagnosis of an infection or neoplasm may be supported by the findings of cerebrospinal fluid (CSF) analysis (see Table 5–2).

Plain, routine skull radiographs may show skull fractures and neoplasms, secondary bone changes due to hydrocephalus, and, rarely, calcified tumors (see Table 5–9).

Specialized radiographic studies such as pneumoventriculography and cerebral angiography may aid in the diagnosis of hydrocephalus. Magnetic resonance imaging (MRI) scans and computerized axial tomography (CT scan) are the most useful to diagnose hydrocephalus, hemorrhage, infarcts, and neoplasia. The diagnostic approach for animals with behavior disorders is outlined in Table 7–3.

Behavior disorders due to environmental or genetic problems with no known neurologic disease process will not be discussed here. Disorders in which seizures are a primary sign are discussed in Chapter 8.

Congenital and familial disorders

Hydrocephalus

Incidence: frequent

Hydrocephalus in animals is usually associated with an enlargement of all or part of the ventricular system and either hypoplasia or atrophy of surrounding nervous tissue. Hydrocephalus may be a congenital disorder in dogs and cats, resulting from a teratogen or a genetic disturbance. It is probably the most common congenital nervous system disorder in dogs. An abnormality in CSF flow and/or absorption in the developing brain is suspected of producing the deformity. Postnatal infections primarily involving the choroid plexus and periventricular structures can produce an acquired hydrocephalus in young dogs 6 to 8 weeks of age.[33] The causative agent is yet unknown.

Hydrocephalus may be produced in adult animals by neoplasms occluding CSF flow or by infections, such as toxoplasmosis, which might also occlude CSF flow or prevent reabsorption.

Feline infectious peritonitis virus infections can produce meningitis and ependymitis and obstruct CSF flow and absorption, and produce hydrocephalus in cats.

This discussion is limited to congenital hydrocephalus and acquired hydrocephalus of young animals.

Signalment and history. Congenital hydrocephalus is commonly seen in toy breeds of dogs, such as Chihuahuas and Poodles, and the brachycephalic breeds, such as Boston terriers and Pekingese. It can occur sporadically in any breed dog or cat. Affected animals are usually the smallest in the litter. Abnormality in behavior is generally noticed by 4 to 5 months of age, but depends on the degree of hydrocephalus. The complaints may be dementia, inability to be "house trained" or taught tricks, aggressive, irritable or irrational behavior, or seizures. Some animals only have seizures and the owners are unwilling to admit to any behavior disturbances. Often, there is little progression of the signs, and the neurologic deficit remains unchanged.

Acquired hydrocephalus secondary to infection in young puppies has an acute onset of neurologic signs at 6 to 8 weeks of age, and has been seen in several breeds. The animals are normal, then suddenly become irritable and hyperexcitable when handled, cry excessively, circle compulsively, and act blind. The skull may rapidly enlarge.

Physical and neurologic examinations. The skull may appear enlarged with open skull sutures or fontanelles. Some toy breeds commonly have skull sutures that never completely close, and are considered to have normal behavior. Some hydrocephalic dogs have normal-appearing skulls and closed skull sutures.

The findings of the neurologic examination may vary with the degree of hydrocephalus, the portions of the ventricular system involved, and the areas of

Table 7–3
Diagnostic approach for the evaluation of behavior disorders of neurologic origin

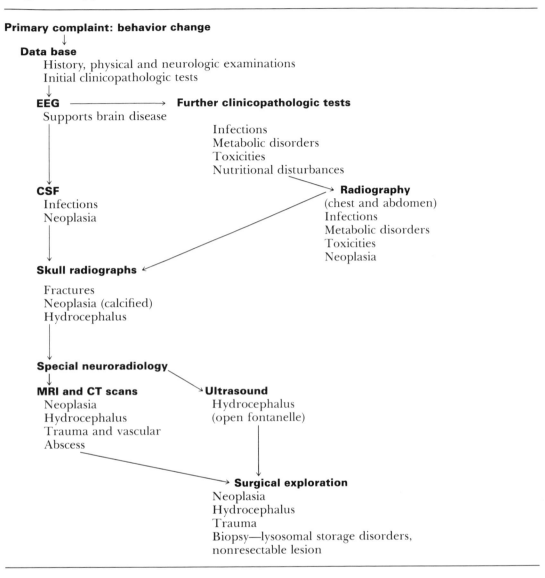

Primary complaint: behavior change

Data base
    History, physical and neurologic examinations
    Initial clinicopathologic tests

EEG ⟶ **Further clinicopathologic tests**
Supports brain disease
        Infections
        Metabolic disorders
        Toxicities
        Nutritional disturbances

CSF   **Radiography**
Infections   (chest and abdomen)
Neoplasia   Infections
                 Metabolic disorders
                 Toxicities
                 Neoplasia

Skull radiographs

    Fractures
    Neoplasia (calcified)
    Hydrocephalus

Special neuroradiology

MRI and CT scans   **Ultrasound**
    Neoplasia   Hydrocephalus
    Hydrocephalus   (open fontanelle)
    Trauma and vascular
    Abscess

                   Surgical exploration
                   Neoplasia
                   Hydrocephalus
                   Trauma
                   Biopsy—lysosomal storage disorders,
                   nonresectable lesion

nervous tissue affected. If the lateral and third ventricles are involved, irritability, aggressiveness, dementia, and seizures may be seen. The animal may be blind and have difficulty localizing sounds. If the ventricular size is asymmetric, the animal may circle to one side. If the aqueduct through the brain stem, the fourth ventricle, and the central canal of the spinal cord are dilated, the animal may be ataxic and have hypermetria. Delayed hopping, placing, and proprioceptive responses also may be present.

The eyeballs may appear to have divergent strabismus, but this is usually not caused by oculomotor nerve (cranial nerve III) paresis. Instead, it is usually associated with skull and orbit deformities.

Ancillary diagnostic investigations.
The EEG changes associated with congenital hydrocephalus may vary somewhat, but often have a high amplitude, 100 to 200 μv, and mixtures of frequencies varying from 2 to 5 Hz and 6 to 12 Hz (see Fig. 5–6). The EEG changes associated with acute encephalitis can be similar to those produced by hydrocephalus. Therefore, EEG findings must be interpreted with regard to the history and the physical and neurologic examinations, and can be used only to further support a diagnosis of hydrocephalus.

CSF collected either from the lateral ventricle or cisterna magna should be analyzed. CSF pressure is normal in congenital hydrocephalus. CSF cells and protein can be normal in congenital hydrocephalus, unless the animal has received a recent head injury and has cerebral hemorrhage. CSF analysis is the best way to confirm an infection producing hydrocephalus. Xanthochromia, neutrophils, macrophages, and some mononuclear cells may be seen in the CSF.

On routine skull radiographs, a loss of convolutional markings from the internal surface of the calvarium may give a "ground glass" appearance to the cranial vault. The calvarium may also appear thin, with open skull sutures.

The extent of the ventricular enlargement can be visualized with the aid of a pneumoventriculogram. The normal pneomoventriculogram is pictured in Figure 5–22A,B. Figure 7–2A,B,C shows a pneumoventriculogram of an animal with hydrocephalus. Noninvasive techniques are replacing the use of pneumoventriculography in most hospitals.

If the fontanelle is open, real-time ultrasonography can be used to demonstrate the ventricular enlargement. CT and MRI scans can also demonstrate the extent of dilated ventricles (Figs. 5–24, 7–6A).

Therapy and prognosis. No therapy is required for congenital hydrocephalus in an animl that has had a stable neurologic status over several months. If its behavior is acceptable, the animal may continue as a pet. If seizures occur frequently, anticonvulsant therapy can be administered to control the seizure activity (Chap. 8). The prognosis for the animal that is not deteriorating further is good, but the owner should understand that the animal will never be normal. The thin calvarium and thin cerebral cortex make the animal especially susceptible to head injury and cerebral hemorrhage.

If the animal is severely affected and the course is progressive, shunting of CSF from the lateral ventricle to the jugular vein or peritoneal cavity may be attempted.[43] Often the neurologic damage is severe by the time the diagnosis is made. Progressive neurologic signs frequently will respond to glucocorticoids as described in Chapter 6. Prednisone at a dose of 1–2 mg/kg orally divided every 12 hours may improve neurologic status. The dose can be decreased every 3–5 days and discontinued after 3–4 weeks if improvement continues.

An animal with acute, progressive neurologic signs owing to an inflammatory process may benefit from glucocorticoids (Chap. 6). A ventricular shunt also may be of some benefit in a few cases. The prognosis for young animals with progressive, acquired hydrocephalus is poor. Even if the infection is eradicated, the hydrocephalus and resulting neurologic deficit are often permanent sequelae.

Lissencephaly

Incidence: Rare

Lissencephaly is a decrease or absence of gyri and sulci resulting in a smooth cerebral cortex (Fig. 7–3). Behavior abnormalities and seizures are the common presenting complaint.[31] Lissencephaly is rare, but has been described in Lhasa Apsos, Beagles, Irish Setters, and cats. The signs may be subtle when the animal is very young, but in the case of the Lhasa Apso, behavior abnormalities usually become apparent by 3 months of age. The animals are difficult or impossible to housetrain and can be irritable and aggressive. At other times they may be demented and depressed. Visual and olfactory impairment may be present. Generalized seizures are usually seen before 1 year of age (Chap. 8).

An abnormal mental attitude and bilateral menace-response deficits are often present on the neurologic examination. Other cranial nerves are normal. The gait is normal. Postural reactions are usually present but are slow. Conscious proprioception may be absent in the pelvic limbs.

Clinicopathologic tests, including CSF analysis, are normal in animals affected by lissencephaly. EEG activity is slowed and increased in amplitude, with frequencies ranging from 4 to 10 Hz and amplitude varying from 24 to 100 μv. Paroxysmal wave forms are also seen. Plain skull radiographs may be normal or show a decrease in convolutional markings of the calvarium. Cerebral angiography has been reported to be normal.

The presence of lissencephaly may be suspected from the signalment, history, neurologic deficit, and EEG results. Lack of convolutional markings may be apparent on an MRI scan.

Anticonvulsant therapy may be used to attempt control of the seizures, but the behavior abnormalities and other neurologic deficits are permanent. The animals are often not acceptable pets. The diagnosis of lissencephaly is confirmed by exploratory craniotomy or necropsy. It is not known at present whether this is an inherited problem in the Lhasa Apso breed.

Lysosomal storage disorders

Incidence: Rare

Lysosomal storage disorders are produced by enzyme defects within the lysosomes of the cells of the nervous system. The enzyme deficiency disrupts the normal metabolic degradation process of lipids, glycoproteins, glycogen, or mucopolysaccharides. Undigestible material accumulates within the affected lysosomes, disrupts cellular function, and produces cellular death. Although the enzyme defect may be present in many cells of the body, the clinical signs are most frequently associated with changes in the cells of the nervous system. Lysosomal storage disorders are relatively rare in small animals, and are outlined as a group here, even though not all affected animals have behavior changes. Table 7–4 lists the lysosomal storage diseases described in dogs and cats, the enzyme defect, the material that accumulates in the lysosomes, the main cells of the nervous system affected, the signalment, and the presenting clinical signs.

Lysosomal storage diseases are most often seen in animals under 1 year of age. The neurologic status of the affected animals progressively deteriorates and the animals die.

Animals suffering from GM_2 gangliosidosis, ceroid lipofuscinosis, neuronal glycoproteinosis, and fucosidosis may present initially with behavior changes, dementia, blindness, and seizures.[3,22] These disorders may be included in the differential diagnosis, particularly in German Shorthaired Pointers, English Setters, Springer Spaniels, and some other dogs and cats. The signs progress over a few months until the animals become ataxic, paralyzed, and eventually die. GM_1 gangliosidosis, sphingomyelinosis, glucocerebrosidosis and alpha mannosidosis all begin with ataxia and head tremors (Chap. 15).[21,53]

Animals with globoid cell leukodystrophy commonly display paraparesis or pelvic limb ataxia (Chap. 17).

A lysosomal storage disorder may be suspected from the signalment, history, and physical and neurologic examinations.

An antemortem diagnosis of some of

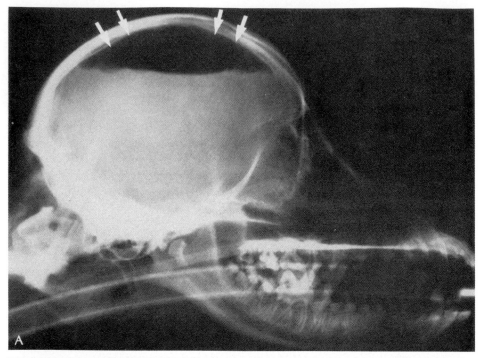

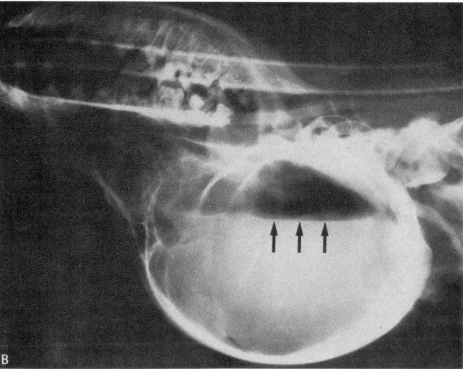

Figure 7–2. Pneumoventriculogram of a dog with hydrocephalus. The air bubble rises to the top of the ventricular system. The ventricle extends to the surface of the calvarium with only a thin rim of cerebral cortex (arrows). (*B*) Pneumoventriculogram of same dog as in *A*, with the air bubble rising to the top (arrows) and outlining the ventral aspect of the enlarged ventricles.

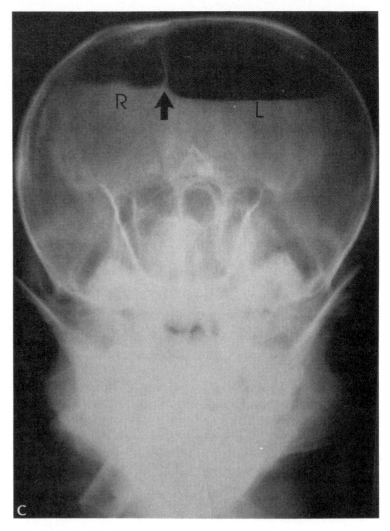

Figure 7-2. (*C*) Frontal view of the pneumoventriculogram of the same dog in Figures *A* and *B*. The air bubble has risen to the surface and outlines asymmetry of the left (L) and right (R) ventricular enlargement. Arrow indicates the medial surface of left and right ventricles.

the lysosomal storage disorders may be made by analysis of the deficient enzyme in leukocytes.[29] Performing a biopsy of affected tissues, including parts of the nervous system, and histologic examination can also aid in the diagnosis. Table 7–5 outlines some of these antemortum diagnostic tests.

Most lysosomal storage disorders have an autosomal recessive inheritance. Par-

ents of affected dogs are, therefore, both carriers. Carrier and normal animals in a kennel may be detected by the level of the specific enzyme in their leukocytes or urine (Table 7–5). The carrier animal has an enzyme level that is intermediate between the normal and affected animals. By breeding only animals with a known normal enzyme level, the problem can be eradicated from a kennel.

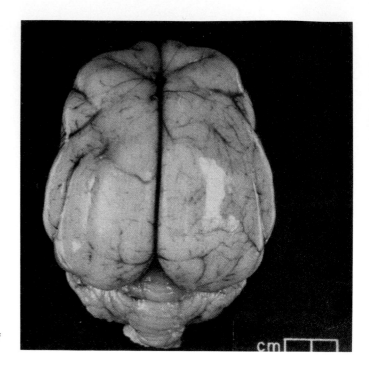

Figure 7–3. Lissencephaly in a 9-month-old female Lhasa Apso with uncontrollable seizures. Note the loss of convolutional markings on the surface of the brain.

Infections and other inflammations

There are many causes of meningoencephalitis in dogs and cats and an overview of these is found in Tables 7–6 & 7–7. Serum and CSF titers for some of the organisms producing meningoencephalitis are listed in Table 7–8.

Distemper virus

Incidence: Frequent

The distemper virus, a paramyxovirus, is a common cause of neurologic disease in dogs.[12,30,51,73] The virus affects many tissues, including those in the respiratory, gastrointestinal, integumentary, and nervous systems, producing pneumonia, gastroenteritis, hyperkeratosis, and nonsuppurative meningoencephalomyelitis, respectively. The nervous system involvement has different clinical manifestations, and distemper virus infection may be listed in the differential diagnosis of many of the neurologic problems dealt with in this book.

Signalment and history. Any age, breed, or sex of dog can become infected with the distemper virus. In young, unvaccinated dogs, a respiratory or gastrointestinal disorder commonly precedes the development of neurologic signs. The neurologic signs may become apparent while disease in the other systems is still present, or as long as several months after recovery from the initial systemic disease. Mature or vaccinated dogs often have only those signs associated with the nervous system involvement.

Occasionally, neurologic signs may develop in 1 to 2 weeks after vaccination with modified live virus, because of a vaccine-induced encephalomyelitis.[7,19]

The course of distemper virus infection can be as variable as its clinical manifestations. The infection may be fatal within a few days, progress over several weeks and then become fatal or stabilize with no further deterioration, or be slowly progressive over several months.

Physical and neurologic examinations. The physical examination can be normal or any or all of the following signs may be observed. The animal may have an elevated temperature, a serous or mucopurulent nasal and ocular discharge, bronchopneumonia, with coughing and difficulty breathing, vomiting, diarrhea, and dehydration. A pustular dermatitis may be observed on the abdomen. The foot pads and nasal epithelium may be hyperkeratotic. An active chorioretinitis may be seen on examination of the ocular fundus. Pitting of the enamel of the teeth indicates a high fever during the development of the enamel, which may have been associated with distemper infection.

The findings of the neurologic examination can be extremely variable, depending on the neuroanatomic site most involved with the infection. If the frontal lobe of the cerebral cortex is involved, the animal will be demented, may pace or circle compulsively, and may act blind. Seizures are common if the cerebral cortex is affected. During the typical "chewing gum" convulsion of distemper encephalitis, the animal stares blankly off into space and then begins chomping the jaws, twitching several muscle groups and salivating, without falling onto its side. This is a type of mild, generalized seizure (Chap. 8). Severe generalized and partial seizures and partial seizures that secondarily generalize may occur with distemper encephalitis. The animal may have only seizures and no other neurologic deficit. It may be blind due to optic neuritis (Chap. 9). Generalized ataxia, hypermetria, and head tremors associated with involvement of the cerebellum are commonly seen (Chap. 15).

Other common signs are ataxia and paresis of the pelvic limbs (Chap. 17) due to thoracolumbar spinal cord involvement, which can progress to quadriplegia if the cervical spinal cord becomes involved (Chap. 16).

Brain stem and multiple cranial nerve involvement are less common, but they can occur (Chap. 11).

An animal may develop myoclonus in the temporalis and masseter muscles or limb muscles (Chap. 14). Myoclonus, sometimes referred to as chorea, is a rhythmic contraction of a group of muscles, which is continual even during sleep. The origin of the rhythmic discharge producing the muscle contraction is suspected of being located in the gray matter of the spinal cord in cases of myoclonus of the neck, trunk, and limbs, and in the gray matter of the brain stem in cases of myoclonus in the muscles of the head.

Severe self-mutilation leading to the destruction of the limbs or tail may be associated with distemper virus infections (Chap. 20). Whether the self-mutilation is due to a peripheral sensory neuritis or to involvement of the parietal lobe cerebral cortex or sensory pathways through the brain stem or spinal cord is unknown. Occasionally, peripheral neuritis is seen with flaccid paralysis of a limb, but this is rare. The presence of signs from multiple anatomic sites confirms a multifocal disease process.

Ancillary diagnostic investigations. Although distemper virus infections are common and may be strongly suspected from the history and physical and neurologic examinations, the diagnosis can be difficult to prove antemortem. Leukopenia, seen on a peripheral blood smear, may support the diagnosis, but is not always present at the time of the evaluation.

Conjunctival, prepucial, and vulvar skin scrapings and tracheal washings can be applied to a microscope slide, stained with Wright's stain, and the cells examined for intracytoplasmic eosinophilic inclusion bodies characteristic of distemper virus.

Table 7-4
Lysosomal Storage Disorders of Dogs and Cats

Disorder	Enzyme defect	Material accumulating	Nervous system cells involved	Signalment	Presenting clinical signs
GM$_1$ gangliosidosis	Beta-galactosidase	GM$_1$ ganglioside	Neurons	Siamese and Korat cats, Beagles, other cats and dogs 3–6 mos	Ataxia, head tremors, spastic quadriparesis
GM$_2$ gangliosidosis	Hexosaminidase A and B	GM$_2$ ganglioside	Neurons	German Shorthaired Pointers—males, other cats and dogs 6–12 mos	Dementia, blindness, seizures
Sphingomyelinosis (Niemann-Pick disease)	Sphingomyelinase (phosphocholine hydrolase)	Sphingomyelin	Neurons	Siamese and DSH cats; Poodles 4–6 mos	Ataxia, head tremors, hypermetria
Glucocerebrosidosis (Gaucher's disease)	Glucocerebrosidase	Glucocerebroside	Neurons and many reticuloendothelial cells	Silky terriers 6–8 mos	Ataxia, tremors
Ceroid lipofuscinosis (amaurotic familial idiocy)	P-phenylenediamine-mediated peroxidase	Ceroid and lipofuscin	Neurons	English Setters 1–2 yrs; Salukis 1–2 yrs; Siamese cats 6–12 mos; Border Collies 1–2 yrs; Chihuahuas 6–12 mos; Cocker Spaniels 1–2 yrs; Dachshunds 1–2 yrs	Dementia, blindness, seizures
Globoid cell leukodystrophy (Krabbe's disease)	Beta-galacto-cerebrosidase	Galactocerebroside	Macrophages (globoid cells) in white matter	West Highland White terriers, Hounds, Cairn terriers, Beagles, Poodles, Pomeranians, cats 6–12 mos	Rear limb ataxia or paresis, quadriparesis
Neuronal glycoproteinosis (Lafora's disease)	Unclassified	Glycoprotein	Neurons	Poodles, Beagles, Bassetts, mixed breeds, 5–12 mos	Dementia, seizures
Glycogen storage disease (type II) (Pompe's disease)	Alpha glucosidase	Type II glycogen	Neurons, neuroglia	Cats, dogs 12 mos; German Shepherds 2–6 mos	Generalized muscle weakness, seizures
Alpha mannosidosis	Alpha mannosidase	Oligosaccharides	Neurons, neuroglia	Persian cats 2–4 mos; DLH cats 6 mos—1 yr; DSH cats 6 mos—1 yr	Generalized tremors, ataxia, head tremors, spastic paraplegia, opisthotonus
Fucosidosis	Alpha-L-fucosidase	Alpha-L-fucose	Neurons, neuroglia	English Springer Spaniels 1–3 yrs	Ataxia, incoordination, change in temperament, head pressing

Table 7-5
Antemortem diagnosis of lysosomal storage diseases

Disorder	Clinicopathologic tests	Biopsy
GM$_1$ gangliosidosis	Assay for beta-galactosidase in leukocytes and skin fibroblast cultures. Can detect heterozygote carriers	Lymph node—stored material in lymphocytes and macrophages Cerebellum—stored material in Purkinje cells
GM$_2$ gangliosidosis	Assay for hexosaminidase A and B in leukocytes. Can detect heterozygote carriers	Cerebrum—stored material in neurons
Sphingomyelinosis	Assay for sphingomyelinase in leukocytes, bone marrow, and skin fibroblast cultures. Can detect heterozygote carriers	Bone marrow—vacuolated histiocytes Cerebellum—stored material in Purkinje cells
Glucocerebrosidosis	Assay for glucocerebrosidase in leukocytes and skin fibroblast cultures	Lymph node, liver, or bone marrow—presence of large spherical cells with lacy cytoplasm (Gaucher's cells) Cerebellum—stored material in Purkinje cells
Globoid cell leukodystrophy	CSF analysis—presence of macrophages filled with myelin (globoid cells) Assay for beta-galactocerebrosidase in leukocytes. Can detect heterozygote carriers	Peripheral nerve—myelin loss Lymph nodes—globoid cells
Ceroid lipofuscinosis	—	Lymph nodes—yellow-green granular deposits Cerebellum—stored material in Purkinje cells
Neuronal glycoproteinosis	—	Lymph nodes and liver—Lafora's bodies (intracytoplasmic inclusion bodies) Cerebellum—Lafora's bodies
Alpha mannosidosis	Assay urine for elevated levels of oliogosaccharide (hexasaccharides) and bound mannose	
Fucosidosis	Measure alpha-L-fucosidase in plasma and leukocytes. May detect heterozygote carriers	

Table 7-6
Meningoencephalitis of dogs

Viruses
*1. Distemper
2. Rabies
3. Herpes
4. Parvovirus
5. Adenovirus
6. Pseudorabies

Fungi
*1. Cryptococcosis
2. Aspergillosis
3. Blastomycosis
4. Histoplasmosis
5. Coccidioidomycosis
6. Phaeohyphomycosis

Rickettsia and Spirochetes
1. Erlichiosis
2. Rocky Mountain spotted fever
3. Lyme disease (Borrelia)

Protozoa
1. Toxoplasmosis
2. Neosporidiosis
3. Acanthamoeba
4. Babesiosis
5. Encephalitozoonosis
6. Trypanosomiasis

Algae
1. Prototothecosis

Bacteria
1. Staphylococcus
2. Listeria
3. Brucella
4. Leptospira
5. Other aerobic organisms
6. Anaerobic organisms
7. Nocardia
8. Actinomyces

Unknown causes
*1. Granulomatous meningo-encephalitis (GME) reticulosis
*2. Steroid-responsive meningoencephalitis
3. Miscellaneous nonsuppurative meningoencephalitis
4. Pug encephalitis

Parasites
1. Dirofilaria immitis
2. Toxicara canis
3. Ancylostoma caninum
4. Cysticercosis
5. Cuterebriasis

* Most common causes of encephalitis in dogs. Others are sporadic or rare.

The same skin scrapings and washings may be applied to a slide and sent to a laboratory to be examined for viral antigen with fluorescent antibody techniques. These tests may support the diagnosis if they are positive, but do not rule out distemper virus disease of the nervous system if they are negative. The chances of a positive test are greater when systemic signs of disease are present. Recently vaccinated

Table 7-7
Meningoencephalitis of cats

Viruses	Fungi
*1. Feline infectious peritonitis	*1. Cryptococcosus
2. Rabies	
3. Pseudorabies	
4. Panleukopenia	
5. Rhinotracheitis	

	Protozoa
	1. Toxoplasmosis

Bacteria	Parasites
1. Pasteurella	1. Cuterebriasis
2. Staphylococcus	2. Dirofilaria immitus
3. Other aerobic organisms	
4. Anaerobic organisms	**Unknown causes**
	1. Miscellaneous nonsuppurative meningoencephalitis

* Most common causes of encephalitis in cats. Others are sporadic and rare.

animals may show inclusion bodies and have positive fluorescent antibody tests. Fluorescent antibody tests may be applied to cells collected from the CSF. If the CSF cells fluoresce, viral antigen is present in the nervous system. On rare occasions, blood smears may demonstrate characteristic inclusion bodies in lymphocytes, neutrophils, and red blood cells.

The EEG examination may help support a diagnosis of an encephalitic process involving the cerebral cortex. EEG changes vary, according to the length of time and severity of cortical and subcortical involvement. In certain acute stages, the EEG changes are similar to hydrocephalus. Later in the course of the disease, a rhythmic hypersynchronous 7- to 9-Hz, 10- to 25-μv pattern is seen, which may continue paroxysmally for several months after the apparent infection appears to have been resolved. Residual EEG changes may be apparent for several years after an infection. If only signs of spinal cord disease are present and there are no apparent cerebral signs, the EEG may be normal or abnormal, indicating subclinical cerebral involvement.

CSF analysis can help to diagnose nervous system inflammation. In distemper infections, there may be an increase in cells, which primarily consists of lymphocytes and monocytes, and rarely neutrophils. However, many other inflammatory and neoplastic conditions of the brain may produce a similar CSF pleocytosis. The protein content of the CSF is often elevated. The CSF can show only increased protein with no increase in cells, or can be normal even in active infections. A CSF cytology may be examined using fluorescent antibodies against the distemper virus. A positive test indicates the presence of viral antigen.

Table 7–8
Serum and cerebrospinal fluid titers available for the diagnosis of meningoencephalitis

Dogs	Cats
1. Distemper virus	1. Infectious peritonitis virus
2. Parvovirus	2. Leukemia virus
3. Adenovirus	3. Toxoplasmosis
4. Herpes virus	4. Cyptococcosis
5. Lyme disease	
6. Erlichiosis	
7. Rocky Mountain spotted fever	
8. Cryptococcosis	
9. Toxoplasmosis	

Evaluation of serum and CSF distemper virus titers can aid in the diagnosis (Table 7–8). If IgG levels are elevated above 1:25 in CSF with no recent vaccination or if IgM is present in CSF and serum, an active infection is likely.

Therapy and prognosis. There is presently no specific antiviral therapy for distemper virus. The main aim of therapy is to treat any secondary bacterial infections in the other systems involved, rehydrate the animal, and administer symptomatic therapy for respiratory distress, vomiting, and diarrhea.

If a dog is having frequent seizures, anticonvulsant therapy can be administered. Phenobarbital or primidone are suggested, because of the rapid onset of their clinical effect (Chap. 8).

If the animal is severely demented and depressed from cerebral involvement, and there is no severe bacterial infection in other systems, glucocorticoid therapy may improve the neurologic status (Chap. 6). The distemper virus is known to have an immunosuppressive effect on the animal.[79] Therefore, when using glucocorticoids, the positive effects produced by reducing the nervous system inflammation must be weighed against the harm of further immunosuppression. In an animal with a deteriorating neurologic status, it is generally worth the risk of further immunosuppression. Some clinicians give the animal an antibiotic along with the glucocorticoid as protection against secondary bacterial invasion due to the immunosuppression.

If there are no cerebellar, brain stem, or spinal cord signs and there is a response to the anticonvulsant, glucocorticoid, and antibiotic therapy, the prognosis may be good for eventual recovery. Glucocorticoids usually are given at decreasing doses every 5–7 days for a month (Chap. 6). An anticonvulsant may have to be given indefinitely, as the animal will most likely be an epileptic the rest of its life owing to the residual brain damage produced by the encephalitis (Chap. 8). If there is no response to therapy, the animal often deteriorates and dies, or the owner may elect euthanasia.

Cerebellar signs of generalized ataxia, hypermetria, and head tremors are usually permanent. If there is no further deterioration on glucocorticoid therapy, the animal may be able to function with the gait deficit, but it is unlikely that it will improve.

If the animal develops paralysis of the pelvic limbs or of all four limbs, the prognosis is generally hopeless, as these animals rarely recover any function. In cases where only mild ataxia and weakness are present, glucocorticoid therapy can be attempted and serial neurologic examinations can be performed to monitor the progress. The owner should be warned that the paresis may progress even on therapy. If brain stem signs appear and cranial nerves are diseased, the prognosis is poor for their return of function. The animal may compensate for a loss of vestibular function or be able to live with facial paralysis; however, if swallowing is hampered by the neurologic process, the prognosis is grave.

At present, there are no oral medications that alter the myoclonus that develops from distemper virus infections. If it is severe enough to greatly disturb the dog, euthanasia is the most humane choice, as the myoclonus may last for years.

If self-mutilation begins, the prognosis is grave, as there is no therapy that seems to alter the drive for self-mutilation.

Prevention. Modified live virus vaccinations are administered for prevention of distemper virus infections. In puppies younger than 12 weeks, the first dose should be given at weaning. Vaccinations are repeated, ending at 16 weeks of age. Maternal antibodies consumed in the colostrum block the response to the vaccine, but protect the puppy against distemper virus infections. Maternal antibodies decrease after weaning and are usually gone by 16 weeks of age. A puppy with no maternal antibodies and no vaccinations, exposed to distemper virus, will most likely get an infection. Vaccination every 2 weeks, from weaning to 16 weeks of age, is probably ideal to prevent infection, but

the cost is often prohibitive to most owners. A series of 3 or 4 vaccinations with the last injection around 16 weeks is adopted by most veterinarians. Adult animals should be given a booster injection yearly, regardless of age.

Pathology. The lesions associated with canine distemper virus infections may vary in appearance and location. Focal or disseminated demyelinating lesions may be found, particularly in the cerebellar white matter and peduncles, the optic nerves and tracts, and the spinal cord.[88]

Nonsuppurative meningoencephalitis with mononuclear perivascular cuffing is found. Lesions may be multifocal and necrotic. Intranuclear or intracytoplasmic eosinophilic inclusion bodies may or may not be present in neurons, astrocytes, and ependymal cells.

Old-dog encephalitis. Old-dog encephalitis is a subacute or chronic progressive panencephalitis commonly seen in mature dogs, which is now considered by many to be another form of distemper virus encephalitis.[12] Adult dogs are commonly presented for a progressive behavior disorder characterized by dementia, blindness, pacing, and circling. The results of ancillary diagnostic investigations may be the same as with any distemper encephalitis; however, the CSF is often normal. Because such cases appear similar to those of dogs with brain tumors, an MRI or CT scan may be helpful to differentiate between them. The main difference in this form, as compared with other adult forms of distemper virus infections, is the histologic appearance of the lesions. In old-dog encephalitis there is diffuse central nervous system (CNS) sclerosis, as compared with multifocal necrosis associated with the other forms of distemper encephalitis. Old-dog encephalitis has been proposed as an animal model for studying demyelinating diseases in man.

Feline infectious peritonitis virus

Incidence: Occasional

The noneffusive form of feline infectious peritonitis (FIP) virus infections often produces panophthalmitis and pyogranulomatous meningoencephalomyelitis and hydrocephalus.[12,30,45]

Signalment and history. Any age or breed and either sex of cat can become affected, especially those in catteries or multiple-cat households. The cat may be depressed and anorexic. It may vomit and have a persistent fever despite antibiotic therapy. The cat may be demented and have seizures (Chap. 8) or be ataxic and have signs of vestibular (Chap. 12) or cerebellar deficits (Chap. 15). The cat may be presented for pelvic limb paresis only (Chap. 17). The clinical course may be variable, but is often progressive over several weeks or several months.

Physical and neurologic examinations. Anterior uveitis is commonly associated with FIP infections. Retinal hemorrhages and choroiditis also are seen. The temperature is usually elevated from 40° to 41° C. The animal may be dehydrated, debilitated, and anemic.

The neurologic examination findings can vary greatly with the site of the lesions. Cats may be demented, irritable, and have convulsions if the major lesions affect the telencephalon and diencephalon or if hydrocephalus develops from the inflammation of ependymal and subependymal regions. Neurologic deficit associated with brain stem, cerebellar, and spinal cord involvement can be seen. Often there is evidence of multifocal neurologic disease.

Ancillary diagnostic investigations. Lymphocytopenia and eosinopenia and normocytic, normochromic anemia may be evident on the CBC. An elevated plasma fibrinogen may be seen. Total serum protein content is often elevated. Elevated beta and gamma globulin content is found on serum protein electrophoresis. Elevated serum FIP titers may support the diagnosis, but may cross-react with more benign enteric corona viruses to give false-positive results.

Slowing and increased amplitude can be observed on EEG examination, indicating cerebral involvement in some disease process.

CSF analysis often has a marked increase in cells, which consists of many mononuclear cells and some polymorphonuclear cells. The CSF protein is often greatly elevated. Creatine phosphokinase (CPK) in the CSF also may be elevated. Serum and CSF FIP titers may help differentiate FIP from other diseases producing CSF pleocytosis (Table 7-8). If the titer is negative in the serum and CSF, an FIP infection is not ruled out.

Therapy and prognosis. There is no therapy for FIP infection, and the diagnosis is often confirmed at necropsy. The prognosis for an animal with FIP meningoencephalitis as it is understood at present is grave. Perhaps with better methods of antemortem diagnosis, milder nonfatal forms of the disease may be described. Many of these cats have concurrent infections with feline leukemia virus and toxoplasmosis. It is possible that the disease may be more severe when accompanied by other viral infections.

Prevention. There are currently no vaccines available against FIP infections.

Pathology. A marked pyogranulomatous inflammatory reaction with neutrophils, lymphocytes, plasma cells, and histiocytes affecting ependymal surfaces, and meninges with extension into subependymal regions and perivascular spaces is seen on histologic examination. Lesions can produce hydrocephalus by obstructing proper CSF flow and reabsorption. Other lesions may be multifocal throughout the brain stem, cerebellum, and spinal cord.

Rabies Virus

Incidence: Rare

Rabies virus infections usually produce fatal encephalomyelitis in dogs and cats.[5,12,30] The virus is transferred through the saliva from a bite by an infected animal. Bats, skunks, foxes, and raccoons are considered the natural source of infection for domestic animals. With strictly enforced rabies vaccination programs for dogs, rabies is considered a rare disease in most areas. It is a fatal disease in man, so the diagnosis of suspected cases has great public health significance to those persons bitten by or exposed to a possibly rabid animal. Rabies can have a wide variety of clinical signs that can make it difficult in many instances to differentiate from other forms of acute encephalomyelitis.

Signalment and history. The age range of reported cases of rabies in cats and dogs has varied from 8 weeks to 8 years, but any age, breed, or sex of dog or cat may be susceptible. The primary complaint of the owner may be behavior changes of depression, dementia, or viciousness. The animal may be extremely disoriented and attack inanimate objects. Other behavioral abnormalities that have been described are pruritus, coprophagia, pica, abnormal sexual behavior, and excessive playfulness.

The animal may appear demented, have excessive salivation, difficulty swallowing, and other signs of cranial nerve

and brain stem disease (Chap. 11). Ataxia and rear limb paresis are other common complaints in naturally occurring rabies and in animals recently vaccinated with modified live virus (MLV) vaccine (Chaps. 16 and 17).

There may or may not be known contact with a rabid animal. The incubation period from the bite to onset of clinical signs can vary greatly, but the clinical course of the disease from the onset of signs until death is considered to be from 3 to 8 days. Modified Live Virus vaccine-induced rabies in dogs and cats usually is seen 10–21 days after vaccination. Pelvic limb paresis develops, with the neurologic deficit most severe in the limb in which the injection was given.

Physical and neurologic examinations. One report of 19 cases of rabies infections in dogs indicated that conjunctivitis was a common finding.[59] The animal may be febrile unless presented in the terminal stages.

The findings of the neurologic examination may vary with the location of the disease process and the course of the disease. Depression and dementia are more common than aggressiveness and viciousness, although both are reported. Brain stem cranial nerve signs such as dropped jaw, facial paralysis, difficulty swallowing, and abnormal bark are comon findings and rabies should be in the differential diagnosis when brain stem disease is suspected (Chap. 11). Pelvic limb ataxia and paresis and ataxia and paresis of all four limbs are also common findings. The paresis and paralysis may be of a flaccid nature, with depressed or absent spinal reflexes.

In some forms of vaccine-induced rabies in the dog, the quadriparesis has a progressive course over 7–10 days.[65] Spinal reflexes are depressed or absent. There are no cranial nerve abnormalities and the animal is alert. The animal then begins improving after 1–3 weeks and is normal in 1–2 months. The clinical course and recovery is more typical of vaccine-induced acute polyradiculoneuritis than vaccine-induced encephalomyelitis.

Cats with vaccine-induced rabies may have flaccid paralysis of the pelvic limbs, which over a few days progresses to rigidity in all four limbs and severe dementia.[87] Gloves, masks, and protective clothing should be worn while performing the neurologic examination on any animal suspected of having rabies. A rapid progression of the neurologic signs supports the diagnosis. Distemper virus infections in dogs and feline infectious peritonitis (FIP) virus infections in cats can have neurologic signs that appear similar to rabies, although the paralysis of the pelvic limbs usually is spastic in distemper and FIP infections rather than flaccid. Distemper virus and FIP virus infections usually are not as rapidly progressive as rabies.

Ancillary diagnostic investigations. All ancillary diagnostic investigations should be performed with great caution. Little information is available on routine clinicopathologic tests in rabies. The hemogram may be normal.

The EEG may have changes suggestive of cerebral disease, but may not be distinguishable from other forms of encephalitis. The EEG changes of rabies encephalitis in dogs and cats are not reported. Electromyogram (EMG) studies on MLV vaccine-induced paralysis of dogs support the diagnosis of polyradiculoneuritis (Chaps. 5 and 16).

CSF analysis may show increased mononuclear cells and protein, as with any viral encephalomyelitis. Little information is available on CSF changes in naturally occuring rabies infections.

Serologic, saliva, and CSF rabies antibody titers may aid in the antemortem diagnosis. Rabies fluorescent antibody tests may be performed on cytology smears from nasal mucosa and the cornea. Saliva and CSF may be injected into suckling mice for virus isolation attempts.

Therapy and prognosis. At present there is no therapy for rabies infections, and the prognosis is considered grave in most of the forms of rabies infections reported. There have been a few recoveries reported in man and some suspected recoveries in animals. As our methods of antemortem diagnosis of rabies infections improve, milder forms of the disease may be recognized.

The prognosis for MLV vaccine-induced paralysis due to encephalomyelitis in cats is grave, as the signs of disease rapidly progress and the animals die.

The prognosis for MLV vaccine-induced paralysis in the dog is good if it is due to a polyradiculoneuritis, because the peripheral nerves regenerate and recovery is complete in 1 or 2 months. If encephalomyelitis is produced in dogs by the MLV virus vaccine, the prognosis is poor. Serial neurologic examinations and electromyographic studies can support the diagnosis of polyradiculoneuritis. Trains of positive waves and fibrillation potentials are present in all trunk and body musculature, and motor nerve conduction velocity may be normal or slow (Chap. 5). The relationship of immunosuppression from canine distemper or leukemia virus infection and the susceptibility to a modified live virus infection from a vaccine is still unknown.

Prevention. Enforced vaccination programs have made rabies infection a rare disease. The MLV vaccines administered intramuscularly usually give 3-year protection to most dogs. Because of the incidence of MLV vaccine-induced rabies in cats, many veterinarians are using only killed virus vaccine until problems with the MLV vaccine are solved.

The state health laboratory should be contacted whenever a person is bitten by an animal. The animal then must be confined and observed for 10 days for the development of any signs of neurologic disease.

Pathology. When rabies is suspected of being the cause of death in any animal, half of its fresh brain should be sent without fixation to the state diagnostic laboratory to be examined. Fluorescent antibody testing for rabies is performed on the nervous tissue. Mouse inoculations of brain and spinal cord tissue are used for virus isolation.

Rabies is a multifocal polioencephalomyelitis with mononuclear perivascular infiltrates. The brain stem is a predilection site for lesions. Intracytoplasmic Negri bodies are usually found in hippocampal neurons and Purkinje cells of the cerebellum.

Toxoplasmosis

Incidence: Rare

Toxoplasmosis is a protozoal infection of dogs and cats associated with the organism Toxoplasma gondii. The organism can produce a subclinical infection with few clinical signs or pneumonia, gastroenteritis, iritis, retinitis, hepatitis, encephalomyelitis, and myositis.[12,24,30] The disease is transmitted by the ingestion of feces containing oocysts or contaminated meat. Toxoplasmosis is rarely a primary disease compared with other forms of encephalitis in dogs and cats, but can occur in cats or dogs immunosuppressed by a concurrent feline leukemia virus or distemper virus infection, respectively.

Signalment and history. Any age, breed, and sex of dog or cat may be affected. As with the other forms of encephalomyelitis, there can be a variety of primary complaints. The animals may show behavior changes of dementia, irritability, and compulsive circling. Seizures may occur. Generalized ataxia and head tremor may be present (Chap. 15). The animal may have paresis in the pelvic limbs or in all four limbs (Chaps. 16 and 17). The clinical signs can have a variable course and severity. Signs can be mild and intermittent or can be rapidly fatal. Signs may become severe following immunosuppressive drug therapy. Complaints of respiratory and gastrointestinal dysfunction may be reported.

Physical and neurologic examinations. Evidence of pneumonia or gastroenteritis may be found on physical examination. The animal may or may not be febrile. Iritis and chorioretinitis may be observed on ophthalmoscopic examination.

Findings of the neurologic examination vary with the location of the lesion. Dementia and other behavior abnormalities and seizures are associated with lesions in the telencephalon and diencephalon. Ataxia and tremors may be associated with disease in the cerebellum. Ataxia and paresis of the pelvic limbs or all four limbs is often due to radiculomyelitis. The paresis can be spastic if lesions are primarily confined to the spinal cord white matter, or flaccid if the lesions involve the spinal cord gray matter and ventral nerve roots.

A stilted, stiff gait and painful muscles may be produced by associated polymyositis.

Ancillary diagnostic investigations. Antemortem diagnosis of toxoplasmosis can be difficult. Hematologic and biochemical tests are variable. Animals may have anemia, bilirubinemia, and elevated liver enzymes. Occasionally, toxoplasma oocysts can be found in the feces.

EEG changes in toxoplasmosis encephalitis can be similar to those found with other causes of encephalitis.

EMG examination can aid in the diagnosis of polymyositis (Chaps. 5 and 16).

CSF analysis is usually abnormal, and shows xanthochromia, pleocytosis with increased lymphocytes, monocytes, and occasional neutrophils. CSF protein often is elevated. Because the CSF changes may be similar to other causes of encephalitis, serum and CSF toxoplasmosis titers should be evaluated (see Table 7–8).

A rising serum antibody titer on two samples taken 1 or 2 weeks apart also supports the diagnosis of toxoplasmosis. The presence of antibodies implies a history of infection, although the absence of antibodies does not necessarily mean an absence of infection.

Therapy and prognosis. Toxoplasmosis can be a chronic disease with intermittent signs whenever the animal is stressed or immunosuppressed. Therapy with sulfadiazine (60 mg/kg/day), possibly combined with pyrimethamine (0.5–1 mg/kg/day) and a folic acid supplement, may be used to treat active infections, but may be toxic. Clindamycin 10 to 40 mg/kg daily divided into 3 or 4 doses and given either orally or intramuscularly for 2 weeks also may be given. Therapy may limit the spread of the disease until immunity is acquired and the disease becomes dormant again. The prognosis is usually grave if the dog has a concurrent canine distemper infection and the cat has a concurrent feline leukemia virus infection.

Prevention. Toxoplasmosis may be prevented by avoiding personal and animal contact with oocysts. Cat litter pans should be cleaned daily and feces burned or flushed down the toilet. All meat eaten and fed to animals should be cooked. Flies and cockroaches should be eliminated from the environment if possible.

Toxoplasmosis may produce a mild, transient disease in adult humans, but can produce severe ocular and brain disease in the human fetus.

Pathology. Toxoplasmosis may produce focal cerebral granulomas, which behave as mass lesions and produce secondary brain swelling. Toxoplasma gondii organisms may be seen free, encysted, or within macrophages. A diffuse, necrotizing granulomatous inflammatory process may be found in cerebrum, cerebellum, spinal cord, and nerve roots. Organisms are usually visible.

Inflammatory cells and organisms are often found in skeletal and cardiac muscles. Another protozoal meningoencephalomyelitis has been described in dogs that has a similar clinical course to toxoplasmosis. The organism has been called Neospora caninum, and presently can only be confirmed by a necropsy exam.[25]

Mycosis

Incidence: Rare

Mycotic agents can sporadically produce meningoencephalomyelitis in dogs and cats. Cryptococcosis, blastomycosis, histoplasmosis, coccidioidomycosis, aspergillosis, and phaeohyphomyosis (Cladosporium trichoides) are the mycoses found in the CNS.[12,28,30,42,63,92] Mycotic agents often have a geographic distribution, and disease produced by each form is more common in certain regions of the country. The organisms are in the soil and environment. An animal susceptible to the fungal agent will become infected.

Signalment and history. Any age, breed, or sex of animal may acquire a mycotic meningoencephalomyelitis, but aspergillosis is seen especially in German Shepherds. The primary complaint can vary with the anatomic location of the lesion, as with the other forms of encephalomyelitis. Behavior changes of depression and dementia may occur. Occasionally the animals may have seizures. The animal also may have weakness of the pelvic limbs or of all four limbs as the major neurologic problem (Chaps. 16 and 17). There may be a history of having lived in a region of the United States where mycotic infections are endemic. Histoplasmosis is common in the midwestern states. Cryptococcosis and blastomycosis are common in the eastern and midwestern USA. Coccidioidomycosis is most common in western and southwestern states. There may be signs of a concurrent respiratory, gastrointestinal, or integumentary disease process.

Physical and neurologic examinations. Cryptococcus neoformans infections are a common cause of chronic rhinitis and meningoencephalomyelitis in cats, and can also occur in dogs.[57,83,90] A chronic nasal discharge can precede the signs of meningoencephalitis. The infection erodes through the cribriform plate to involve the prefrontal cortex and produce behavior and olfactory disorders. Granulomatous chorioretinitis lesions may be found on ophthalmoscopic examination.

Blastomyces dermatitidis infections often produce chronic, progressive wasting of the animal and chronic pneumonia.[13,61] The animal may be febrile. Chorioretinitis, secondary glaucoma, and skin abscesses may be present. Vertebral osteomyelitis may produce involvement of nervous tissue, and occasionally meningoencephalomyelitis will be seen.

Histoplasma capsulatum infections have a variety of clinical forms and can have a variable clinical course. Chronic pulmonary, gastrointestinal, and hepatic disease are common. The animal may be febrile. Occasionally, the CNS can be involved.

Coccidioides immitis infections often begin as pulmonary disease with an unproductive cough or dyspnea.[66] The temperature may fluctuate. The bone and nervous systems also can become affected.

The neurologic signs vary greatly, depending on the area of the nervous system involved and whether the infection is focal, multifocal, or diffuse. Behavior changes are common if the telencephalon and diencephalon are diseased. Abnormalities in gait and strength of the limbs are most often due to concomitant brain stem or spinal cord disease.

Ancillary diagnostic investigations. Persistent monocytosis may be seen on the CBC. Leukocytosis is also common. The chemistry profile may have elevated liver enzymes, creatinine, and blood urea nitrogen if the liver and kidney are involved. Aspergillosis is often seen in the urine of affected dogs.

If signs of pulmonary disease are present on the physical examination, thoracic radiographs may show mycotic pneumonia.

Material from abscesses, nasal discharges, and tracheal washings should be examined microscopically for organisms, and cultures of any material collected should also be attempted. Skin tests are available for blastomycosis, histoplasmosis, and coccidioidomycosis, but they are often unreliable.

The EEG shows changes in amplitude and frequency compatible with any encephalitis if the cerebrum is affected.

Skull and vertebral radiographs may demonstrate mycotic osteomyelitis.

CSF analysis can be the greatest aid in diagnosing the cause of encephalomyelitis. (see Table 5–2). The fluid generally shows an increase in cells and protein, and the causative organism may be found. CSF also should be cultured. The CSF may be viscous. The cell count may be over 100/microliter. The increased cells may be neutrophils, eosinophils, lymphocytes, or macrophages. The protein content is often greatly elevated. India ink preparations readily demonstrate the organism. A serum and CSF titer for cryptococcosis may be positive.

Therapy and prognosis. The therapy for systemic mycotic infections is amphotericin B, rifampin, and flucytosine. The therapeutic regimen is described in detail in Chapter 6. Ketoconazole may be used to treat some cryptococcus infections. No immunosuppressive drugs should be given. In focal lesions affecting vertebrae, surgical intervention with curettage and drainage may be indicated. Sulfonamides may be used in the therapy of nocardiosis.

The prognosis is often considered poor in systemic mycotic infections, but it depends on the severity of signs in the nervous system as well as other systems.

Prevention. The relationship of immunosuppression and susceptibility to infections from mycotic agents is unknown. The diseases are so sporadic that there is currently no vaccination program used for prevention.

Granulomatous meningoencephalitis

Incidence: Occasional

Granulomatous meningoencephalitis (GME), also called reticulosis of the central nervous system, is a proliferation of reticulohistiocytic cells originating from adventitial cells of blood vessels, leptomeninges, and microglia. The proliferation of cells occurs mainly around blood vessels. It occurs most commonly in dogs, but has been reported in cats.[1,17,20,72,73] GME can be a focal or multifocal disease process, involving brain or spinal cord.

GME can be inflammatory in nature, with the cell populations consisting of lymphocytes, plasma cells, and neutrophils. GME (reticulosis) is considered neoplastic when the reticulohistiocytic elements have a high mitotic index. GME can affect a wide range of ages of dogs and cats. It has been reported in many breeds, but terriers and miniature poodles are the most commonly affected.

Signalment and history. Lesions may involve cerebral white matter, thalamus, and midbrain, and the affected animal may have behavior abnormalities and seizures. GME also may affect the pontine-medullary brain stem and produce cranial nerve deficits (Chaps. 11 and 12). Quadriparesis and paraparesis may result from focal GME in the spinal cord (Chaps. 16 and 17).

Physical and neurologic examination. GME may affect the eye and produce blindness from choroiditis, retinal detachment, and secondary glaucoma. Neurologic signs vary with the location of the lesions, but compulsive pacing or circling, dementia, and seizures can be seen.

Ancillary diagnostic investigations. GME may be difficult to differentiate from other forms of encephalitis in dogs and cats, as the clinical course and clinical signs may be the same. CSF analysis may be normal, show elevated protein only, or show an increase in cells and protein, but these findings may be seen with many encephalitides. In neoplastic GME (reticulosis), anaplastic reticulum cells may be found.

Therapy and prognosis. Glucocorticoid therapy (Chap. 6) may delay the progression of the disease process. GME is generally considered to have a grave prognosis, but that might be a reflection of the inability to arrive at an antemortem diagnosis, with confirmation of the disease process available only at necropsy. Immunohistologic techniques may be necessary to differentiate histiocytic lymphosarcoma from reticulosarcomas and neoplastic forms of GME.[89]

Steroid-responsive meningoencephalomyelitis

Incidence: *Common*

An underlying cause may not be found for many cases of meningoencephalitis, as a positive diagnosis may only be made from the necropsy findings. Adult dogs and, on rare occasions, cats may be presented for dementia and compulsive pacing or circling and have CSF pleocytosis and increased protein. All serum and CSF titers (see Table 7-8) and cultures are negative. The CSF cytology may vary from primarily neutrophils to lymphocytes with macrophages as well. In some cases eosinophilia may be present.[76]

The causes could be undetected viral infections, granulomatous meningoencephalitis, vasculitis, or immune-mediated inflammation, but many will respond within 48 to 72 hours to glucocorticoid therapy.[56,57] If no evidence or suspicion of bacterial, fungal, or protozoal disease is present, 1 to 2 mg/kg prednisone is given orally. Trimethoprim sulfadiazine 15 mg/kg every 12 hours orally may be given for 1 to 2 weeks while the glucocorticoid dose is high.

If the animal improves after 1 to 2 weeks, the antibiotics are discontinued and the prednisone dosage decreased by 25 to 50% for another 1-to 2 weeks. The dosages then are reduced over 1 to 3 months. If signs recur, the dosage prior to the recurrance is reinstituted. Alternate-day prednisone after 1 month of therapy will help deter iatrogenic Cushing's syndrome. Some dogs can discontinue prednisone after 1 to 3 months and remain normal. Others must be maintained on alternate-day doses indefinitely to be completely free of neurologic signs. The longterm prognosis for these cases is often very good.

Pug Encephalitis

Incidence: *Rare*

A necrotizing meningoencephalitis is seen in Pug dogs between 6 months and 7 years of age.[18] Behavior changes of lethargy, headpressing, and walking in circles are seen. Affected dogs may also have seizures, blindness with normal pupillary light reflexes, coma, and opisthotonus.

The CBC and serum chemistry profile studies are normal. A CSF pleocytosis of 200 to 500 cells per microliter and elevated CSF protein are found in all cases. The predominant cell type (80–98%) is small lymphocytes. The other cells are large mononuclear cells or neutrophils.

The clinical course may be acute progressive over 2 weeks or chronic progressive over several months. No therapy is known, and the prognosis is poor. Most affected dogs die naturally or are euthanized because of the severity of their neurologic signs. The diagnosis is confirmed by a necropsy examination of the brain. No causative agent has been determined. A genetic predisposition for this infection is suspected.

Miscellaneous causes of meningoencephalitis

Many different organisms sporadically produce meningoencephalomyelitis in dogs and cats. The clinical signs may be the same, and behavior changes and seizures can be seen. The diagnostic approach is the same. CSF analysis, blood and CSF cultures, and serum and CSF viral antibody titers are the only way to differentiate them (Table 7–8). Many are confirmed only at necropsy.[4,26,34,51]

Herpesvirus can produce septicemia and encephalitis in newborn puppies.[30,57] Herpesvirus has been suspected in some adult canine forms of nonsuppurative meningoencephalomyelitis.[80] Serum and

CSF herpesvirus titers should be evaluated.

Canine parvovirus may produce acute behavior changes and other neurologic signs due to vasculitis of the meninges, brain, and spinal cord.[38,91] Serum and CSF parvovirus titers should be evaluated.

Canine adenovirus I (canine infectious hepatitis) infections in the dog can produce associated encephalopathy caused by vasculitis. Necrosis and proliferation of endothelial cells of brain capillaries can produce increased vascular permeability and hemorrhages throughout the brain. Lesions are most common in the thalamus, midbrain, and medulla. Serum and CSF adenovirus titers should be evaluated.

On rare occasions, panleukopenia and rhinotracheitis viruses can produce meningoencephalitis in cats and alterations in behavior. Prenatal infections by the panleukopenia virus damage the developing cerebellum, and are discussed in Chapter 15.

The pseudorabies virus can produce excitement, dementia, and seizures in dogs and cats, owing to an encephalitis. Most animals exhibit intense pruritis. The disease is usually rapidly fatal.[32]

Nonsuppurative meningoencephalitis may be the diagnosis at necropsy in dogs and cats whose symptoms are suggestive of viral disease, but no evidence of an organism may be found.

Bacterial meningoencephalomyelitis is relatively rare in the dog and cat.[27,46] Such infections as metritis, bacterial endocarditis, and others can result in septicemia. Septicemia can produce septic embolism and microabscesses and infarction in the brain, and produce neurologic signs related to the involved region. There is usually a fever and leukocytosis. CSF analysis will show a greatly increased number of cells, which are mainly neutrophils. CSF culture may reveal the causative agent, of which the most common bacterial organisms are Pasteurella and Staphylococcus.

Nocardia, actinomyces, brucella, and leptospira also have produced infections.[70] Anaerobic bacteria Bacteroides, Fusobacterium, Peptostreptococcus, and Eubacterium have been reported in dogs and cats.[23] If a bacterial infection is suspected, aerobic and anaerobic culture of blood and CSF should be obtained.

The rickettsial diseases Erlichiosis and Rocky Mountain spotted fever, and the spirochete Borrelia burgdorferi (Lyme disease) can produce meningoencephalitis in dogs. Serum and CSF titers should be evaluated for these diseases. Oral Tetracycline 20–22 mg/kg every 8 hours for 2-3 weeks is recommended.[30,44,57]

Prototheca spp algae may produce pyogranulomatous encephalitis in dogs. The CSF may have neutrophilic, lymphocytic, or eosinophilic pleocytosis, but the organisms may not be observed. The organism may be cultured from rectal scrapings.[86] Acanthamoeba castellani has been reported to produce meningoencephalitis in a dog.[64]

Occasionally, parasites may migrate into various regions of the nervous system and produce neurologic signs (Tables 7–6 and 7–7). Parasitic migration into the telencephalon or diencephalon produces behavior abnormalities. Dirofilaria immitis has been sporadically reported to be found intravascularly and extravascularly in the brains of dogs and cats.[12,77] The adult heartworm may produce infarction or a local inflammatory reaction, resulting in behavior changes or seizures if the cortex and diencephalon are involved.

Cuterebra larvae have been reported in cat brains, producing focal encephalitis and granulomatous inflammatory reaction and behavior abnormalities of aggressiveness, hysteria, as well as seizures.[16,52,55]

Toxocara canis can migrate aberrantly in dogs, and produce a focal granulomatous inflammation in various areas of the nervous system.

Cysticercosis in the brain of dogs has

been reported to produce neurologic signs.[37]

Metabolic disorders

Hepatic encephalopathy

Incidence: Frequent

When the liver fails to remove toxic substances from the portal blood and these substances reach the brain, hepatic encephalopathy can result.[78] The accumulation of excessive toxic substances may be due to a congenital or acquired portosystemic shunt, a severely damaged nonfunctional liver, or a congenital enzyme deficiency. The toxic substances responsible for hepatic encephalopathy are suspected of being produced in the gastrointestinal tract, and include ammonia, mercaptans, short-chain fatty acids, indoles, and biogenic amines. These substances interfere with normal energy metabolism and neurotransmission in the brain.

Signalment and history. Dogs with congenital liver enzyme deficits and dogs and cats with congenital portacaval shunts commonly develop clinical signs at a young age.[8,39,40,62,67,71,75] The breed of dogs affected by congenital disease is variable. Acquired portacaval shunts and severe liver disease may occur in any age, breed, or sex.

The primary complaint is often one of periodic behavior changes. Listlessness, depression, pacing, circling, head pressing, hysteria, and viciousness all have been reported. The animals may also have seizures (Chap. 8) or appear blind (Chap. 9). The signs may become particularly severe after a large meal of protein.

Other signs of illness may include anorexia, polyuria, polydipsia, excessive panting, vomiting, diarrhea, and weight loss. The history may include intolerance to drugs, which must be metabolized by the liver.

Physical and neurologic examinations. Animals with congenital portacaval shunts may have stunted growth or be emaciated (Fig. 7–4). Ascites may be present. The animal may have renal or cystic calculi.

The neurologic examination findings can fluctuate. The abnormalities in behavior may be most severe after eating, but may improve greatly if the animal fasts. Along with behavioral changes and seizures, the animal may have ataxia. There usually are no localizing neurologic signs, and neurologic examination findings are compatible with diffuse cerebral disease.

Ancillary diagnostic investigations. Initial clinicopathologic tests may give clues that hepatic encephalopathy is the cause of the behavior disturbance. A mild microcytic hypochromic anemia and slight neutrophilic leukocytosis may be seen on the CBC. The total protein is low because of a decreased albumin. The BUN is often low. The liver enzymes are generally normal or only slightly elevated in congenital portacaval shunts, but may be elevated in acquired liver disease if active necrosis is occurring. Ammonium biurate crystals may be present in the urine.

Further clinicopathologic tests can confirm the hepatic failure. Most of the animals with portacaval shunts have elevated bromsulphalein (BSP) retention. Less that 5% retention 30 minutes after intravenous injection of 5 mg BSP/kg is normal.

Resting blood ammonia levels greater that 120 μg/dl are commonly found with hepatic encephalopathy. In animals with mild signs and only slightly elevated resting blood ammonia levels, an ammonia tolerance test may be performed.[58,82] Thirty minutes after the oral administration of 100 mg/kg of ammonia chloride, the blood

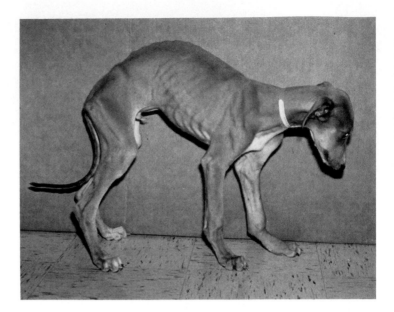

Figure 7–4. An 8-month-old greyhound presented for episodic dementia and seizures due to a portacaval shunt. Note the stunted growth and emaciation of this puppy.

ammonia level will increase 300 to 400% above fasting levels in dogs with abnormal liver function. Normal dogs will show little rise in blood ammonia.

Serum bile acids are a reliable indicator of hepatic function and easier to obtain than BSP and blood ammonia. If the animal has behavior changes or other cerebral signs, the resting bile acid level is usually elevated. If not, a fasting bile acid and 2-hour postprandial serum sample may be compared. A high protein meal such as P/D prescription diet* is given and 2 hours later a second serum sample is obtained.

EEG with hepatic encephalopathy can vary as greatly as the clinical signs. Demented and disoriented dogs have slowing and increased amplitude, similar to the changes seen in encephalitis.

CSF analysis is normal, but anesthesia is not recommended in hepatic encephalopathy.

Plain radiographs of the abdomen show a small liver in portosystemic shunts and hepatic cirrhosis. Contrast angiography of the portal system is necessary to confirm a portacaval shunt. Real time ul-trasonography may be used to locate the shunt as well.[93]

Therapy and prognosis. Partial surgical closure of the extrahepatic portacaval shunt is recommended to improve the clinical signs and prolong life.[14,54] Low-protein, low-fat, and high-carbohydrate diets reduce the amount of material catabolized into ammonia in the gut. U/D prescription diet* may be used to manage the clinical signs initially, but is too low in protein for a maintenance diet.[50] K/D prescription diet may work well in an individual dog for long term maintenance.* An enema may be given acutely to rid the colon of nitrogenous materials. The animals should be well hydrated to dilute toxins and promote diuresis through the kidney. Diuretics should be avoided; Lactulose 5–15 ml every 8 hours as needed to produce 2-3 stools per day may be used. Sedatives, anesthetics, and anticonvulsants should be

_____

* Hill's Division, Riviana Foods, Topeka, Kansas 66601.

avoided, as the animal will have little tolerance to these.

A good prognosis might be given with surgical intervention, followed by rapid improvement of the clinical signs. The longterm prognosis may still be poor in some animals. The prognosis for dogs with intrahepatic shunts is generally poor.

Uremic encephalopathy

Incidence: Frequent

Animals in renal failure may have dementia, delirium, seizures, and coma from uremic encephalopathy. Several mechanisms for the encephalopathy are proposed.[68] Uremic serum contains substances toxic to the nervous system, particularly organic acids. The organic acids are actively secreted out of the nervous system in normal dogs (see Fig. 1–5). When excessive amounts of toxin are in the serum and gain access to the nervous system, the secretion mechanism is overwhelmed. The increased levels of organic acids are suspected of decreasing cerebral oxidative metabolism and interfering with proper neural transmission. The calcium and phosphorous levels in the nervous system also become abnormal and contribute to coma and seizures. Other local electrolyte imbalances and acidoses also are suspected of contributing to the encephalopathy.

Uremia is usually readily diagnosed in the data base chemistry profile. The blood urea nitrogen, serum creatinine, and serum phosphorus determinations are elevated above normal.

Uremic encephalopathy rapidly improves after dialysis in humans. If the underlying cause of renal failure can be corrected, the prognosis for the animal with this encephalopathy is good. Often uremic encephalopathy is seen in the terminal stages of renal failure and the prognosis is grave.

Miscellaneous metabolic disorders

Many metabolic disorders alter normal cerebral metabolism and produce behavior abnormalities in dogs.

Hypoglycemia produces confusion, disorientation, and generalized weakness.[62] Seizures are commonly seen associated with the behavioral changes. Hypoglycemia has many causes and is discussed more fully in Chapter 8.

Hyperglycemia as associated with diabetes mellitus can produce a hyperosmolar syndrome and resultant dehydration of the brain. Behavior changes can range from confusion, disorientation, and depression to coma. Other hyperosmolar syndromes may be produced by electrolyte disturbances, particularly hypernatremia. The brain has many built-in protective mechanisms. The blood–brain barrier and astrocytes protect the neurons from electrolyte shifts (see Fig. 1–5). Hyperosmolar syndromes are discussed further in Chapter 10.

Acidosis and alkalosis may produce behavior abnormalities in animals. Acidosis often produces depression, disorientation, and coma, and is discussed in Chapter 10. Alkalosis rarely occurs, but can produce seizures (Chap. 8).

Hypoxia and anoxia can produce depression, disorientation, syncope, seizures (Chap. 8), or blindness (Chap. 9).

Toxicity

Lead poisoning

Incidence: Frequent

Lead is a common intoxicant of puppies, which have a tendency to chew and consume foreign objects. Lead-base paint is the most frequent source of poisoning, but other sources include storage battery plates, asphalt roofing, linoleum tile, caulking compounds, golf balls, lead fish-ing sinkers, rubber boots, ceramic dog dishes containing lead, and plumbers' materials.[95]

Lead interrupts hemoglobin synthesis and interferes with the normal maturation process of red blood cells (RBC). RBCs also become more fragile and have a shortened life span. Immature and abnormal RBCs are in the peripheral blood and have reduced oxygen-carrying capacity. Encephalopathy may be due to ischemic effects on neurons or to cerebral edema.

Signalment and history. Although lead poisoning occurs most frequently in young animals, any age, breed, or sex of dog or cat could potentially be poisoned if the animal ingested toxic amounts of lead.

The primary complaint is often abnormal behavior and seizures. Hysteria, manifested by excessive crying, barking, running in every direction, and biting at everything, is the most common behavioral abnormality, but dementia, compulsive pacing, and blindness also occur.[35,49,95]

Anorexia, vomiting, diarrhea, and constipation may be seen. Possible sources of lead contamination should be discussed with the owner, although sometimes a lead source cannot be determined.

Physical and neurologic examinations. The body temperature may be elevated in an animal that is hysterical or having seizures. The abdomen may be tender when palpated, and there may be a slight pallor of the mucous membranes.

The findings of the neurologic examination vary, but often support diffuse cerebral disease. Along with the behavior changes described, the animal may be ataxic, have a decreased menace-response and dilated pupils, which may have a decreased response to light during hysteria. There are usually no focal signs in lead-induced encephalopathy. Chronic lead poisoning can produce polyneuropathy. The animal with polyneuropathy may be quadriparetic or quadriplegic, and have depressed spinal reflexes (Chap. 16).

Ancillary diagnostic investigations. Lead poisoning may be difficult to differentiate from distemper and rabies virus infections in dogs, and other infections and metabolic disorders in dogs and cats, after the initial physical and neurologic examination. However, the initial clinico-pathologic tests may support a diagnosis of lead poisoning. The CBC often shows nucleated and sometimes stippled RBCs in the peripheral blood, often with no associated anemia; or the CBC may be normal. There may be an increased reticulocyte count. Urinalysis may be normal or show hyaline and granular casts, and small amounts of protein. Occasionally, glucose may be found in the urine, from lead-induced renal damage.

The EEG abnormalities associated with lead poisoning often consist of high-voltage slow-wave activity, which often cannot be differentiated from encephalitis.

CSF analysis is often normal. If cerebral edema is present, the CSF pressure may be elevated. In severe cases, there may be an increase in RBCs and white blood cells (WBCs), which consist mainly of lymphocytes, and the CSF protein content may be elevated.

Radiographs of the abdomen may show lead-containing radiopaque material in the gastrointestinal tract, which must be removed prior to therapy. In young dogs with chronic lead intoxication, a "leadline" may be seen at the metaphysis of long bones on radiographs.

Blood lead analysis is the single best antemortem test.[96] Blood lead greater than 35 µg/100 ml supports a diagnosis of lead poisoning. Urine lead content greater than 75 µg/100 ml is also suggestive of lead poisoning. A challenge may be performed with a chelating agent at 110 mg/kg/day (not to exceed 2 g) calcium disodium–ethylenediaminetetraacetic acid (Ca EDTA) diluted to a concentration of 10 mg/ml in 5% dextrose solution. A pretreatment urine lead sample is taken. The Ca EDTA diluted solution is divided into 4 doses and given every 6 hours. A 24-hour urine lead sample is collected. A urine lead sample greater than 821 μg/100 ml, 24 hours after chelation therapy is begun, is diagnostic of lead poisoning. An analysis of lead in the liver is the most reliable test, but antemortem biopsy is rarely performed in animals.

Therapy and prognosis. The therapy of lead poisoning is a chelating agent such as Ca EDTA at the dosage recommended for the urine challenge test (110 mg/kg/Ca EDTA diluted in 5% dextrose to 10 mg/ml) divided into 4 subcutaneous injections daily. Ca EDTA may be continued 4 to 7 days, depending on the response. A normal blood lead level 1 week after therapy is discontinued indicates that therapy was successful. If the blood lead level is still elevated, consider persistent or reintoxication and repeat therapy.

Penicillamine, an oral chelating agent, may be used in place of Ca EDTA in animals that cannot be hospitalized. A daily dose of 33 mg/kg may be divided and given every 6 hours, for 1 week. Then the drug is withdrawn for 1 week and the dose repeated for 1 more week. Penicillamine should be given when the stomach is empty. If vomiting occurs, antiemetic drugs may be used. A normal blood lead level 1 week after therapy indicates that therapy was successful.

Anticonvulsive therapy may be useful to control seizures (Chaps. 6 and 8). If the animal has signs of acute cerebral edema and cerebral inflammation on CSF analysis, 20% mannitol and corticosteroid therapy should be administered.

If lead poisoning is diagnosed and corrected early, the prognosis for recovery is good. If the signs are severe and chronic, or CSF is abnormal, there may be severe brain damage. Serial neurologic examina-

tions and evaluations of the EEG can aid in determining the longterm prognosis in these animals. In time, they may be able to compensate for their deficits and be functional pets.

If the lead source can be removed, an animal with polyneuropathy associated with chronic lead poisoning can potentially recover.

Owners should consult their physicians concerning lead poisoning in family members, especially children.

Pathology. On histologic examination of the cerebrum in dogs with chronic lead poisoning, laminar necrosis, gliosis, proliferation of capillaries, and hemorrhages may be seen.

Miscellaneous toxicities

Many drugs can produce behavior alterations in animals. The owner should be thoroughly questioned as to the presence in the environment and possible exposure of the animal to prescribed, nonprescribed, and illegal psychotropic drugs. Marijuana is a commonly abused drug that produces alterations in the behavior of dogs when consumed orally or inhaled with the aid of the owner. Amphetamine and cocaine can produce hyperactive behavior and seizures in dogs.[81] Table 7–9 is a list of some drugs that can produce depression with accompanying fatigue and somnolence. Other drugs may produce stupor and coma (Chap. 10). The local poison control center should be contacted in cases of unknown drug effects.

Nutritional disorders

Thiamine deficiency

Incidence: Occasional

Thiamine (B₁) deficiency often occurs in cats fed all-fish diets, which contain thia-

Table 7–9
Drugs that can produce behavior changes of depression with fatigue and somnolence

acetanilid
acetone
acetylene
amylacetate
amyl alcohol
amyl nitrite
ameline
antipyrine
Arnica
arsine
barbiturates
benzene
bromides
carbon dioxide
carbon disulfide
carbon monoxide
carbon tetrachloride
chlordiazepoxide
chloral hydrate
chlorobenzene
chloroethane
chloroform
cortisone
Daphne
Delphinium
diazepam
dichloroethane
dichlorohydrin
dichloromethane
diethylstilbestrol
diisopropyl fluorophosphate
diphenylhydantoin
diphenhydramine hydrochloride
ethanol
ether
ethorphine
ethylacetate
ethylene chlorohydrin
ethylene oxide
Euonymus
gasoline
Helvella
hydrogen sulfide
hyoscyamine
iodides
isoniazid
kerosene
ketamine
ketene
lithium chloride
Lolium temulentum
marijuana
meprobamate

mercaptan
methyl bromide
methyl chloride
methyl iodine
methyl salicylate
morphine
naphazoline
naphthalene
nerve gas
nickel carbonyl
nitrite
nitroaniline
nitrobenzene
nitrogen oxide
nitrous oxide
opium
oxygen (100%, 3 centimeters)
perchlorethylene
phencyclidine
phenylenediamine
phenothiazine tranquilizer
phenylhydrazine
phenylhydroxylamine
Phytolacca
pokeweed
primidone
Pyrethrum
pyridine
pyrogallol
quinine
reserpine
richweed
saffron
salicylamide
salicylate
Solanum
scopolamine
strychnine
styrene
sulfaphridine
tetrachloroethane
tetrahydronaphthalene
thiocyanates
Thuja
toluene
tribromoethanol
trichloroethylene
trimethadione
Veratrum
hypervitaminosis D
water-hemlock
xylene

Courtesy of Dr. Roger Yeary, the Ohio State University, Dept. of Veterinary Physiology and Pharmacology.

minase. It may also occur occasionally in young cats, following a chronic disease such as a severe respiratory infection, in which the cat is anorexic and receives no vitamin supplementation. Occasionally, dogs fed only cooked-meat diets will develop signs of thiamine deficiency.[69] Thiamine deficiency produces abnormal glucose metabolism in the brain and resultant encephalopathy.

Thiamine deficiency-induced polyneuropathy occurs commonly in humans and may be seen in cats, presented with ventral neck flexion and weakness (Chap. 16).

Signalment and history. Any age, breed, or sex of dog or cat can be affected by thiamine deficiency. The most common signalment is a young or young adult cat.

The presenting complaint may be depression and ataxia. The cat may be disoriented and continually crying. Convulsions, with a marked ventroflexion of the neck, have been reported. The animal may be presented only with ataxia (Chap. 13).

The type of diet, all fish or all cooked meat, may be ascertained from the history. The loss of equilibrium and ataxia may also follow a period of anorexia associated with a chronic disease such as an upper respiratory infection.

Physical and neurologic examinations. As discussed with the history, the neurologic abnormalities vary depending on the part of the nervous system involved. Abnormal behavior and seizures are due to disease rostral to the midbrain. Coma or semicoma and extensor rigidity is due to midbrain involvement (Chap. 10). Ataxia and loss of equilibrium are due to pontine–medullary brain stem involvement of the vestibular nuclei. A flaccid quadriparesis may be due to diffuse peripheral nerve involvement.

Ancillary diagnostic investigations. The diagnosis is suspected from the history and signalment, and further sup-ported by complete remission of the signs following intramuscular injections of 50 to 100 mg of thiamine every 12 hours.

Blood thiamine levels can be measured and will be lower in thiamine-deficient animals than in control animals.

Therapy and prognosis. Daily injections or oral dosage of 50 to 100 mg of thiamine every 12 hours may be administered for several days, but the clinical signs should improve in 24 hours in acute cases presenting with dementia and seizures. Seizures may be controlled with anticonvulsant therapy (Chaps. 6 and 8). If the diet is corrected, the prognosis may be good.

If the animal is in a coma and demonstrating extensor rigidity, thiamine injections may be given, but brain stem damage can be permanent and may result in death.

The ataxia that is manifested following chronic anorexia in kittens may never improve with therapy or age, but the animal may be an acceptable pet.

Animals with polyneuropathy can potentially recover if thiamine supplementation is provided.

Pathology. Thiamine deficiency can produce cerebrocortical necrosis. In cats, however, the common lesions seen terminally are symmetric, bilateral hemorrhage of brain stem nuclei.

Trauma and vascular disorders

Trauma

Incidence: Common

Trauma is a common cause of behavior abnormalities in animals. Immediately following a head injury, the animal may be confused, demented, disoriented, and hysterical. Seizures also may be seen. Semicoma and coma are common signs. A further description of the diagnosis and management of cranial trauma is found in Chapter 10.

Cerebrovascular disease

Incidence: Rare

Many acute neurologic syndromes are erroneously referred to as "stroke" in dogs and cats. Compared with man, cerebrovascular disease is very rare in animals. On occasion, atherosclerotic thrombosis or an arteriovenous malformation may produce acute behavior changes. A CT or MRI scan may be useful to differentiate these from other lesions. Most cerebrovascular disease in dogs and cats producing focal signs are associated with neoplasia or coagulopathy.[41]

Feline cerebral infarct

Incidence: Occasional

A cerebral infarct syndrome of unknown etiology has been reported to occur occasionally in cats.[94]

Signalment and History. Adult cats of any breed and sex can be affected. The onset of neurologic deficit is peracute. The primary complaint is often a behavior change of severe dementia with compulsive circling. The animal may also display aggressive behavior or seizures. There is no history of previous illness or trauma that is related to the onset of the signs. The signs do not progress, but either remain the same or improve slightly.

Physical and neurologic examinations. The main abnormalities are discovered on the neurologic examination. Brain tissue in the middle cerebral artery distribution is often primarily involved and the neurologic examination findings are comparable with a lesion in that region.

The cats are demented and compulsively circle toward the side of the infarct. Partial seizures of the contralateral face and limbs also can be observed because of frontal lobe involvement. Transient contralateral hemiparesis may be seen in the first 24 hours after the onset of signs. Placing, hopping, and conscious proprioception are often abnormal in the contralateral limbs. Tendon reflexes in the contralateral limbs also can be exaggerated. A contralateral facial hypalgesia is suspected of being associated with parietal lobe cerebral cortex disease. Aggressive behavior and hysteria are associated with temporal lobe cerebral cortex, amygdala, and hippocampus disease.

The cat may have contralateral blindness with normal pupillary light reflexes, which are associated with occipital lobe cerebral cortex disease. Occasionally, infarction in the region of the optic chiasm produces bilateral blindness with dilated unresponsive pupils (Chap. 9).

Ancillary diagnostic investigations. The clinicopathologic tests included in the data base are usually normal. The EEG is abnormal and may show an asymmetry between right and left sides. CSF may have no increase in cells, but a mild increase in protein content. Skull radiographs are normal. Cerebral angiography, nuclear brain scans, magnetic resonance imaging, and computerized axial tomography may demonstrate the lesion.

The diagnosis is often suspected from the acute onset of nonprogressive unilateral cerebral disease with no associated illness or trauma.

Therapy and prognosis. Seizures may be controlled acutely with anticonvulsant therapy (Chap. 6). Longterm anticonvulsant maintenance therapy may also be needed (Chap. 8). Cats have been reported to die within the first 24 hours, but this is rarely a fatal disease.

There is no specific therapy for the infarct. Because this is not a progressive disorder, the cats may be acceptable pets unless aggressive behavior is persistent or seizures are uncontrollable. In these cases, many cats are euthanized.

Pathology. Lesions consist of variable degrees of unilateral or bilateral ischemic necrosis of the cerebral cortex and subcortical limbic system structures. In some cases, venous thrombosis and vasculitis are present. The major infarction is frequently in the middle cerebral artery distribution. The cause of the disease is presently unknown.

Degeneration

Multisystem neuronal degeneration

Cocker spaniels 10 to 14 months of age may be presented for lethargy, loss of recognition of the owner, hypersexuality, aggressiveness, and anorexia.[36] Along with the behavior abnormalities, ataxia, hypermetria, and tremors of the head may occur. The signs progress and the dogs are often euthanized. Diffuse neuronal loss is present in subcortical, brain stem, and cerebellar nuclei. Cerebellar and subcortical white matter gliosis are also present. An inherited degeneration is thought to be the cause.

Neoplasia

Cerebral

Incidence: Frequent

Primary or metastatic neoplasia involving the telencephalon and diencephalon commonly produces behavior changes in animals.[10,47]

Signalment and history. Neoplastic processes can occur in any age, breed, or sex, but is most common after 5 years of age.[11,74] Glial cell tumors are common in Boxers and Boston terriers over 5 years of age. Meningiomas are common in aged cats.[60]

Behavior abnormalities will vary with the area affected by the tumor (see Table 7–1). The signs may have an insidious onset, and progress as the tumor and secondary nervous tissue edema surrounding the tumor involve more structures. The rate of progression of the signs varies with the rate of growth and location of the tumor.

Partial seizures or partial seizures that secondarily generalize often are associated with tumors of the cerebral cortex (Chap. 8).

Physical and neurologic examinations. Evidence of neoplasia in other systems may appear on the physical examination in cases of metastatic neoplasia to the brain.

Neurologic examination findings support the presence of focal telencephalic or diencephalic disease. Compulsive circling toward the lesion, dementia and hopping, placing and proprioceptive deficits in the contralateral limbs may be seen, and suggest unilateral or asymmetric brain disease (Fig. 7–5A, B, C). The neurologic examination may be normal except for some behavior changes with diencephalic tumors (Fig. 7–6A, B).

A pituitary tumor may result in one or more endocrinopathies and rarely bilateral blindness with dilated unresponsive pupils from invasion of the optic chiasm (Chap. 9).

Ancillary diagnostic investigations. The EEG is often slow and increased in amplitude and asymmetric in tumors of the cerebral cortex. Pituitary and small hypothalamic tumors may produce a normal alert EEG, which becomes abnormal as relaxation occurs. The EEG may become very slow, with reduced voltages in severe

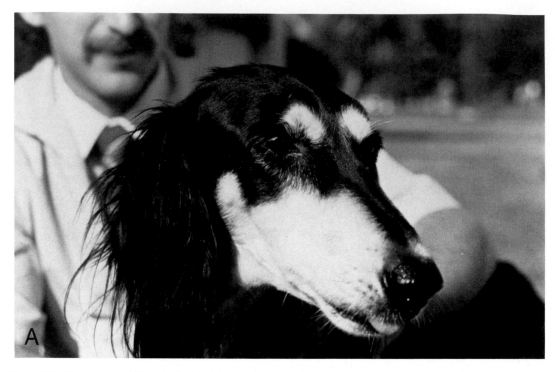

Figure 7–5. *(A)* A 10-year-old female Saluki with progressive dementia and loss of recognition of the owner. Note the blank facial expression and slight tongue protrusion.

cerebral edema secondary to a neoplastic process (see Fig. 5–9).

CSF analysis can further support the suspicion of cerebral neoplasia. In most cerebral tumors except meningiomas, the CSF pressure is elevated because of the secondary edema of the surrounding nervous tissue. The CSF cell number may be normal or can be elevated as high as 500 cells per microliter in other cases. Usually there is a mixed cell population. Meningiomas most often produce the greatest CSF pleocytosis and must be differentiated from meningoencephalitis.[2,15] The cell number is rarely increased, but the CSF protein content is elevated.

Thoracic radiographs should be evaluated if metastatic neoplasia is thought to be present. Skull radiographs are often normal unless the neoplastic process involves the bone or is calcified itself. Menin-

giomas are occasionally calcified and visualized on scout radiographs.

Cerebral angiography and brain scans can aid in the visualization of the tumor. Computerized axial tomography (CT) scans and magnetic resonance imaging (MRI) scans can localize the tumor and determine its size and extent[85] (see Fig. 5–24A–D), (Fig. 7–6A, B).

Therapy and prognosis. Surgical removal combined with radiation therapy is the current therapy used for brain tumors.[48] Some experimental investigations of chemotherapy regimens, boron neutron capture therapy and radioactive implants, are being performed. The prognosis for an animal with a meningioma that can be completely removed is good. The prognosis for animals with any of the other neoplastic processes is often grave.

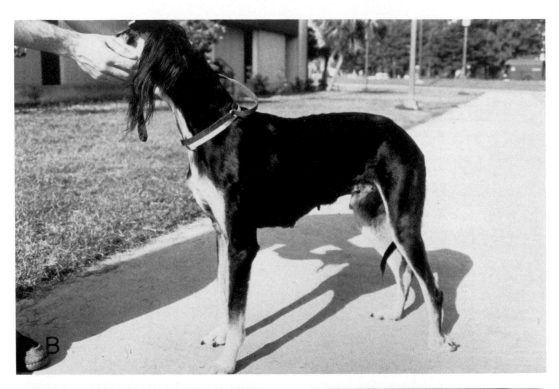

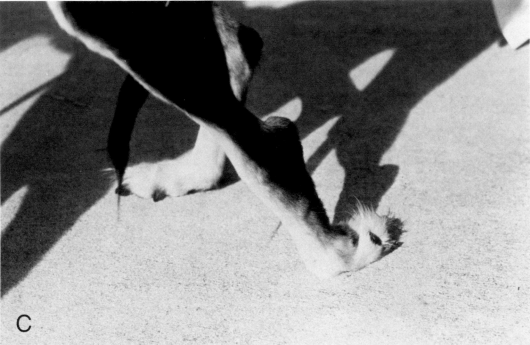

Figure 7–5. *(B)* and *(C)* This Saluki also had conscious proprioceptive deficit of the left pelvic limb only. Because of the progressive course of the disease process and the asymmetry of neurologic signs, a focal lesion of the right cerebrum or diencephalon was suspected. A right frontal lobe meningioma was found.

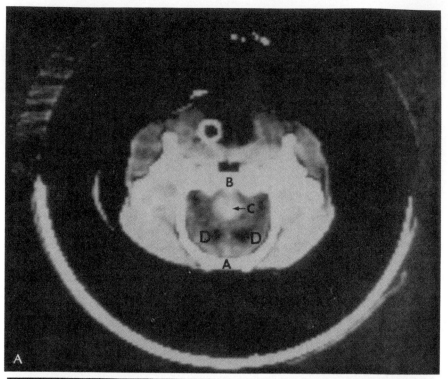

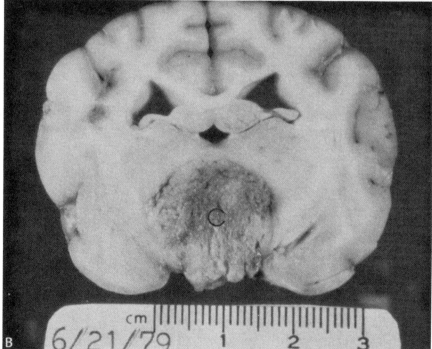

Figure 7–6. *(A)*, CT scan of a 9-year-old Boston terrier. The dog had an abnormal personality but no other deficits on the neurologic examination. (A) dorsal cranial vault, (B) floor of cranial vault, (C) enhanced tumor, (D) enlarged ventricles. *(B)* Gross necropsy of the brain of the dog in Figure *A*. The location of the tumor (C) on necropsy coincides with the location on the CT scan. Histologic diagnosis was ependymoma.

The current medical therapy for cerebral neoplasia is mainly aimed at the control of secondary cerebral edema. Mannitol 20% (1–2 mg/kg) and 10–15 mg/kg intravenous methylprednisolone sodium succinate (Solu-Medrol) therapy may be given immediately if the signs are severe (Chap. 6). Longterm management of cerebral edema may be maintained by oral prednisone administered daily or every other day as the needs of the individual patient dictate. (Chap. 6) The management of secondary cerebral edema may improve the neurologic deficit and prolong the life of the animal, but the longterm prognosis is grave. The neoplastic process may eventually be fatal, or debilitate the animal so severely that euthanasia is performed.

Pathology. The common primary tumors of the nervous system include astrocytomas, oligodendrogliomas, ependymomas, choroid plexus papillomas, glioblastomas, spongioblastomas, meningiomas, and chromophobe adenomas. The histologic characteristics of these tumors are described elsewhere.

Metastatic or invasive neoplasms originating in tissue outside the nervous system include lymphosarcomas, mammary gland adenocarcinomas, prostatic adenocarcinomas, hemangiosarcomas, osteosarcomas, fibrosarcomas, chondrosarcomas, and malignant melanomas.

Types of cerebral neoplasia

Astrocytoma. Astrocytomas are commonly located in the pyriform area of the temporal lobe, in other regions of the cerebral hemispheres, the thalamus, hypothalamus, and midbrain. On rare occasions, astrocytomas occur in the cerebellum or spinal cord.

Astrocytomas are solid gray-white tumors that are poorly demarcated from the surrounding parenchyma. Astrocytomas

do not penetrate the ventricular system or metastasize.

Oligodendroglioma. Oligodendrogliomas are most often located in the cerebral hemispheres and seem to originate from white matter. The tumors have a soft gelatinous consistency, and are often red, red-pink, or gray in color. Oligodendrogliomas often erode through to ventricular or meningeal surfaces.

Ependymoma. Ependymomas are most commonly found in ependymal surfaces of the lateral ventricles. Occasionally, they are located in the third or fourth ventricle. They are large, soft, gray-white to red neoplasms that infiltrate and produce extensive damage. They are invasive into the ventricular system and metastasize in cerebrospinal fluid pathways.

Choroid plexus papilloma. Choroid plexus papillomas develop in the third, fourth, and lateral ventricles. They are well circumscribed with a gray-white to red, granular to papillomatous appearance. On rare occasions, they are invasive and metastasize along cerebrospinal fluid pathways.

Glioblastoma. Glioblastomas are most commonly located in the cerebral hemispheres, in the pyriform area of the temporal lobe, the thalamus, and hypothalamus. These tumors are often vascular and contain hemorrhages. They may appear large and somewhat circumscribed.

Spongioblastoma. Spongioblastomas are rare neoplasms located near ependymal surfaces or the midline in the brain stem or cerebellum.

Meningioma. Meningiomas are slow-growing tumors, which often grow under the dura and expand toward the brain. Solitary tumors occur in dogs. Cats may have multiple tumors. Calcification may occur. The tumors are often solid to very firm, gray-white, yellow, or red in color. They may contain cholesterol crystals or deposits of lipid pigment.

Chromophobe adenoma. A chromophobe adenoma or pituitary adenoma is a neoplasm that arises in the pituitary gland.

References

1. Bailey, C.S. and Higgins, R.I.: Characteristics of cerebrospinal fluid associated with canine granulomatous meningoencephalitis: A retrospective study. J. Am. Vet. Med. Assoc., *188*:418, 1986.
2. Bailey, C.S. and Higgens, R.J.: Characteristics of cisternal cerebrospinal fluid associated with primary brain tumors in the dog: A retrospective study. J. Am. Vet. Med. Assoc., *188*:414, 1986.
3. Barker, C.G., et al.: Fucosidosis in English Springer Spaniels: Results of a trial screening program. J. Small Anim. Pract., *29*:623, 1988.
4. Baumgartner, W.K., et al.: Acute encephalitis and hydrocephalus in dogs caused by canine parainfluenza virus. Vet. Pathol., *19*:79, 1982.
5. Bedford, P.G.C.: Diagnosis of rabies in animals. Vet. Rec., *99*:160, 1976.
6. Berger, B., et al.: Congenital feline portosystemic shunts. L. Am. Vet. Med. Assoc., *188*:517, 1986.
7. Bestetti, G., Fatzer, R., and Frankhauser, R.: Encephalitis following vaccination against distemper and infectious hepatitis in the dog. Acta Neuropathol., *43*:69, 1978.
8. Blaxter, A.C., et al.: Congenital portosystemic shunts in the cat: A report of nine cases. J. Small Anim. Pract., *29*:631, 1988.
9. Braund, K.G., et al.: Granulomatous meningoencephalomyelitis in six dogs. J. Am. Vet. Med. Assoc., *172(10)*:1195, 1978.
10. Braund, K.G.: Neoplasia of the nervous system. Compendium on Continuing Education, *6*:717, 1984.
11. Braund, K.G.: Central nervous system meningiomas. Compendium on Continuing Education, *8*:241, 1986.
12. Braund, K.G., Brewer, R.D., and Mayhew, I.G.: Inflammatory, infectious, immune, parasitic and vascular diseases. *In* Veterinary Neurology. Edited by J.E. Oliver, B.F. Hoerlein, and I.G. Mayhew. Philadelphia, W.B. Saunders, 1987.
13. Breider, M.A., et al.: Blastomycosis in cats: Five cases (1979–1986). J. Am. Vet. Med. Assoc., *193*:570, 1988.
14. Breznock, E.M.: Surgical manipulation of portosystemic shunts in dogs. J. Am. Vet. Med. Assoc., *174(8)*:819, 1978.
15. Carillo, J.M., et al.: Intracranial neoplasm and associated inflammatory response from the central nervous system. J. Am. Anim. Hosp. Assoc., *22*:367, 1986.
16. Cook, J.R., et al.: Intracranial cuterebral myiasis causing acute lateralizing meningoencephalitis in two cats. J. Am. Anim. Hosp. Assoc., *21*:279, 1985.
17. Cordy, D.R.: Canine granulomatous meningoencephalomyelitis. Vet. Pathol., *16*:325, 1979.
18. Cordy, D.R. and Holliday, T.A.: A necrotizing meningoencephalitis of pug dogs. Vet. Pathol., *26*:191, 1989.
19. Cornwell, H.I.C., et al.: Encephalitis in dogs associated with a batch of canine distemper (Rockborn) vaccine. Vet. Rec., *112*:54, 1988.
20. Cuddon, P.A. and Smith-Maxie, L.: Reticulosis of the central nervous system in the dog. Compendium on Continuing Education, *6*:23, 1984.
21. Cummings, J.F., et al.: The clinical and pathologic heterogeneity of feline alpha mannosidosis. J. Vet. Intern. Med., *2*:163, 1988.
22. Cusick, P.K., Cameron, A.M. and Parker, A.L.: Canine neuronal glycoproteinosis—Lafora's disease in the dog. Am. Anim. Hosp. Assoc. J., *12*:518, 1976.
23. Dow, S.W., et al.: Central nervous system infection associated with anaerobic bacteria in two dogs and two cats. J. Vet. Intern. Med., *2*:171, 1988.
24. Dubey, J.P.: Toxoplasmosis. J. Am. Vet. Med. Assoc., *189*:166, 1986.
25. Dubey, J.P., et al.: Newly recognized fatal protozoan disease of dogs. J. Am. Vet. Med. Assoc., *192*:1269, 1988.
26. Evermann, J.E., et al.: Isolation of a paramyxovirus from the cerebrospinal fluid of

a dog with posterior paresis. J. Am. Vet. Med. Assoc., *177*:1132, 1980.

27. Fenner, W.R.: Meningitis. *In* Current Veterinary Therapy IX. Edited by R.W. Kirk. Philadelphia, W.B. Saunders, 1986.

28. Fiske, R.A., et al.: Phaeohyphomycotic encephalitis in two dogs. J. Am. Anim. Hosp. Assoc., *22*:327, 1986.

29. Fletcher, T.F., Suzuki, K., and Martin, F.B.: Galactocerebrosidase activity in canine globoid leukodystrophy. Neurology (NY), *27*:758, 1977.

30. Greene, C.E.: Infectious disease affecting the central nervous system. *In* Neurologic Disorders. Edited by J.N. Kornegay. New York, Churchill Livingstone, 1986.

31. Greene, C.E., Vandevelde, M., and Braund, K.: Lissencephaly in two Lhasa Apso dogs. J. Am. Vet. Med. Assoc., *169(4)*:405, 1976.

32. Gustafson, D.P.: Pseudorabies in dogs and cats. *In* Current Veterinary Therapy VI. Edited by R.W. Kirk. Philadelphia, W.B. Saunders, 1977.

33. Higgins, R.J., Vandevelde, M., and Braund, K.B.: Internal hydrocephalus and associated periventricular encephalitis in young dogs. Vet. Pathol., *14*:236, 1977.

34. Hoff, E.J. and Vandevelde, M.: Non-suppurative encephalomyelitis in cats suggestive of a viral origin. Vet. Pathol., *18*:170, 1981.

35. Hoffheimer, M.S.: Lead poisoning in a cat. Compendium on Continuing Education, *10*:724, 1988.

36. Jaggy, A. and Vandevelde, M.: Multisystem neuronal degeneration in cocker spaniels. J. Vet. Intern. Med., *2*:117, 1988.

37. Jauregui, P.H. and Marquez-Monter, H.: Cysticercosis of the brain in dogs in Mexico City. Am. J. Vet. Res., *38(10)*:1641, 1977.

38. Johnson, B.J. and Castro, A.E.: Isolation of canine parvovirus from a dog brain with severe necrotizing vasculitis and encephalomalacia. J. Am. Vet. Med. Assoc., *184*:1398, 1984.

39. Johnson, C.A., et al.: Congenital portosystemic shunts in dogs: 46 cases (1979–1986). J. Am. Vet. Med. Assoc., *191*:1478, 1987.

40. Johnson, S.E.: Hepatic encephalopathy in two aged dogs secondary to a presumed congenital portal azygous shunt. J. Am. Hosp. Assoc., *25*:129, 1989.

41. Joseph, R.J., et al.: Canine cerebrovascular disease: Clinical and pathological findings in 17 cases. J. Am. Vet. Med. Assoc., *27*:569, 1988.

42. Kabay, M.J.: The pathology of disseminated Aspergillus terreus infection in dogs. Vet. Pathol., *22*:540, 1985.

43. Kay, N.D., et al.: Diagnosis and management of an atypical case of canine hydrocephalus, using computed tomography, ventriculoperitoneal shunting and nuclear scintigraphy. J. Am. Vet. Med. Assoc., *188*:423, 1986.

44. Keenan, K.P., et al.: Studies on the pathogenesis of Rickettsia rickettsii in the dog: Clinical and clincopathologic changes in experimental infection. Am. J. Vet. Res., *38*:851, 1977.

45. Kornegay, J.N.: Feline infectious peritonitis: The central nervous system form. Am. Anim. Hosp. Assoc. J., *14*:580, 1978.

46. Kornegay, J.N., Lorenz, M.D., and Zenoble, R.D.: Bacterial meningoencephalitis in two dogs. J. Am. Vet. Med. Assoc., *173(10)*: 1334, 1978.

47. Kornegay, J.N.: Central nervous system neoplasia. *In* Neurologic Disorders. Edited by J.N. Kornegay. New York, Churchill Livingstone, 1986.

48. Kostolich, M. and Dulish, M.L.: A surgical approach to the canine olfactory bulb for meningioma removal. Vet. Surg., *16*:273, 1987.

49. Kowalczyk, D.F.: Lead poisoning in dogs at the University of Pennsylvania Veterinary Hospital. J. Am. Vet. Med. Assoc., *168(5)*: 428, 1976.

50. Laflamme, D.P.: Dietary management of canine hepatic encephalopathy. Compendium on Continuing Education, *10*:1258, 1988.

51. Luttgen, P.J.: Inflammatory disease of the central nervous system. Vet. Clin. North Am., *18*:623, 1988.

52. MacDonald, J.M., et al.: Cuterebra encephalitis in a dog. Cornell Vet., *66*:372, 1976.

53. Maenhout, T., et al.: Mannosidosis in a litter of persian cats. Vet. Rec., *122*:351, 1988.

54. Mathews, K. and Gofton, N.: Congenital extrahepatic portosystemic shunt occlusion in the dog: Gross observations during surgical correction. J. Am. Anim. Hosp. Assoc., *24*:387, 1988.

55. McKenzie, B.E., Lyles, D.I., and Clink-scales, J.A.: Intracerebral migration of Cuterebra larva in a kitten. J. Am. Vet. Med. Assoc., *172*:173, 1978.
56. Meric, S.M.: Corticosteroid responsive meningitis in ten dogs. J. Am. Anim. Hosp. Assoc., *21*:677, 1985.
57. Meric, S.M.: Canine meningitis, a changing emphasis. J. Vet. Intern. Med., *2*:26, 1988.
58. Meyer, D.J., et al.: Ammonia tolerance test in clinically normal dogs and in dogs with portosystemic shunts. J. Am. Vet. Med. Assoc., *173*:377, 1978.
59. Minor, R.: Rabies in the dog. Vet. Rec., *101*:516, 1977.
60. Nafe, L.A.: Meningiomas in cats. J. Am. Vet. Med. Assoc., *174*:1224, 1979.
61. Nafe, L.A., et al.: Central nervous system involvement of blastomycosis in the dog. J. Am. Anim. Hosp. Assoc., *19*:933, 1983.
62. Nafe, L.A.: Metabolic neurologic diseases. *In* Neurologic Disorders. Edited by J.N. Kornegay. New York, Churchill Livingstone, 1986.
63. Neer, T.M.: Disseminated aspergillosis. Compendium on Continuing Education, *10*:465, 1988.
64. Pearce, J.R., et al.: Amoebic meningoencephalitis caused by Acanthamoeba castellani in a dog. J. Am. Vet. Med. Assoc., *187*:951, 1985.
65. Pederson, N.C., et al.: Rabies vaccine virus infection in three dogs. J. Am. Vet. Med. Assoc., *172*:1092, 1978.
66. Pryor, W.H., et al.: Coccidioides immitis encephalitis in two dogs. J. Am. Vet. Med. Assoc., *161*:1108, 1972.
67. Rand, J.S., et al.: Portosystemic vascular shunts in a family of American Cocker Spaniels. J. Am. Anim. Hosp. Assoc., *24*:265, 1988.
68. Raskin, N.H. and Fishman, R.A.: Neurologic disorders in renal failure (first of two parts). N. Engl. J. Med., *294(3)*:143, 1976.
69. Read, D.H., et al.: Polioencephalomalacia of dogs with thiamine deficiency. Vet. Pathol., *14*:103, 1977.
70. Rhoades, H.E., et al.: Nocardiosis in a dog with multiple lesions of the central nervous system. J. Am. Vet. Med. Assoc., *142*:278, 1963.
71. Rogers, W.A., et al.: Intrahepatic arterio-venous fistulae in a dog resulting in portal hypertension, portacaval shunts, and reversal of portal blood flow. Am. Anim. Hosp. Assoc. J., *13*:470, 1977.
72. Russo, M.E.: Primary reticulosis of the central nervous system in dogs. J. Am. Vet. med. Assoc., *174*:492, 1979.
73. Sarfaty, D. et al.: Differential diagnosis of granulomatous meningoencephalomyelitis, distemper, and suppurative meningoencephalitis in the dog. J. Am. Vet. Med. Assoc., *188*:387, 1986.
74. Safarty, D., et al.: Cerebral astrocytoma in four cats: Clinical and pathologic findings. J. Am. Vet. Med. Assoc., *191*:976, 1987.
75. Scavelli, T.D., et al.: Portosystemic shunts in cats: Seven cases (1976–1984). J. Am. Vet. Med. Assoc., *189*:317, 1986.
76. Schultze, A.E., et al.: Eosinophilic meningoencephalitis in a cat. J. Am. Anim. Hosp. Assoc., *22*:623, 1986.
77. Segedy, A.K. and Hayden, D.W.: Cerebral vascular accident caused by Dirofilaria immitis in a dog. Am. Anim. Hosp. Assoc. J., *14*:752, 1978.
78. Sherding, R.G.: Hepatic encephalopathy in the dog. Compendium on Continuing Education, *1*:55, 1979.
79. Stevens, D.R. and Osburn, B.I.: Immune deficiency in a dog with distemper. J. Am. Vet. Med. Assoc., *168*:493, 1976.
80. Stone, A.B.: Variant lesions in the central nervous system of dogs and cats. J. Small Anim. Pract., *10*:287, 1969.
81. Stowe, C.M., et al.: Amphetamine poisoning in dogs. J. Am. Vet. Med. Assoc., *168*:504, 1976.
82. Strombeck, D.R., et al.: Hyperammonemia and hepatic encephalopathy in the dog. J. Am. Vet. Med. Assoc., *166*:1105, 1975.
83. Sutton, R.H.: Cryptococcosus in dogs: A report on 6 cases. Aust. Vet. J., *57*:558, 1981.
84. Thomas J.B. and Eger C. Granulomatous meningoencephalomyelitis in 21 dogs. J. Sm. Anim. Pract. *30*:287, 1989.
85. Turrel, J.M.: Computed tomographic characteristics of primary brain tumors in 50 dogs. J. Am. Vet. Med. Assoc., *188*:851, 1986.
86. Tyler, D.E., et al.: Disseminated protothecosis with central nervous system involve-

ment in a dog. J. Am. Vet. Med. Assoc., *176*:987, 1980.

87. USDHEW CDC: Suspected vaccine induced rabies in cats. Morbid. Mortal. Weekly Report, *29*:86, 1980.

88. Vandevelde, M. and Kristensen, B.: Observations on the distribution of canine distemper virus in the central nervous system of dogs with demyelinating encephalitis. Acta Neuropathol., *40*:233, 1977.

89. Vandevelde M., et al.: Immunohistological studies on primary reticulosis of the canine brain. Vet. Pathol., *18*:577, 1981.

90. Wilkinson, G.T.: Feline crytpococcosis: A review and seven case reports. J. Small Anim. Pract., *20*:749, 1979.

91. Wilson, R.B., et al.: A neurologic syndrome associated with use of a canine coronavirus-parvovirus vaccine in dogs. Compendium on Continuing Education, *8*:117, 1986.

92. Wood, G.L., et al.: Disseminated aspergillosis in a dog. J. Am. Vet. Med. Assoc., *172*:704, 1978.

93. Wrigley, R.H., et al.: Ultrasonographic diagnosis of portacaval shunts in young dogs. J. Am. Vet. Med. Assoc., *191*:421, 1987.

94. Zaki, F.A. and Nafe, L.E.: Ischaemic encephalopathy and focal granulomatous meningoencephalitis in the cat. J. Small Anim. Pract., *21*:429, 1980.

95. Zook, B.C., Carpenter, J.L., and Roberts, R.M.: Lead poisoning in dogs: Occurrence, source, clinical pathology and electroencephalography. Am. J. Vet. Res., *33*:891, 1972.

96. Zook, B.C., et al.: Lead poisoning in dogs: Analysis of blood, urine, hair, and liver for lead. Am. J. Vet. Res., *33*:903, 1972.

Epilepsy can be defined as a disorder characterized by recurrent seizures with no active underlying disease process occurring in the brain. Epilepsy may be caused by an inherited biochemical defect or may be acquired because of some cerebral insult resulting in a focus of neurons with altered thresholds.

Types of seizures

Seizures may be classified into three basic types: generalized, partial, and partial with secondary generalization. These seizures are classified by the electric changes in the cerebral cortex, detected on the electroencephalogram (EEG) examination, and the clinical signs the animal demonstrates.[17,22] If the cerebral cortical discharge is diffuse and there is symmetric involvement of the entire brain bilaterally, the seizure is termed a generalized seizure (Fig. 8–2). During the seizure, there is a diffuse synchronous spike and spike-wave activity occurring in all leads on the EEG. Generalized seizures are most often associated with metabolic disturbances, toxicities, nutritional deficiencies, and true or inherited epilepsy. Generalized seizures may be mild, without loss of consciousness, or severe, with a total loss of consciousness. The latter have been called grand mal seizures in humans.

Mild generalized

A mild generalized seizure is often associated with true or inherited epilepsy of Poodles, but is also seen in metabolic and toxic disturbances. In epilepsy of Poodles, the animal may have an aura, or a feeling the seizure is going to happen, and try to hide or to seek out the owner for comfort. Shortly following the behavior change, uncontrollable clonic jerking of the limbs, neck, and head spontaneously begins. The animal usually maintains sternal recum-

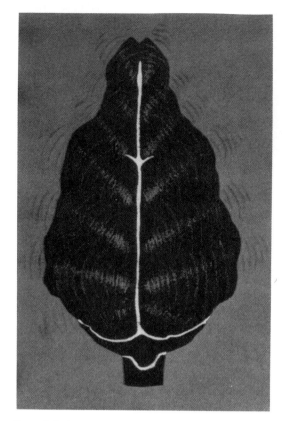

Figure 8–2. A generalized seizure with symmetric cerebral cortex discharges.

bency. Mild or excessive salivation, and occasionally vomiting, may occur during this period. The animal may be anxious and confused, but not unconscious, and it often attempts to crawl to the owner. Owners have reported that during this type of seizure, the seizure time can be shortened by comforting and reassuring the animal. The ictal period usually lasts from 1 to 10 minutes, but can continue up to 1 hour in some animals. The animal is often exhausted in the postictal period, and may vomit then if it did not do so during the ictus.

A mild generalized seizure in humans, characterized by a specific three-per-second spike and dome EEG pattern, is called petit mal. During a petit mal seizure, there is a loss of consciousness for 1 to 2 seconds, with no motor signs other than a few eye blinks, and little observable clinical change. This type of seizure may occur in dogs and cats, but the EEG change is not a 3-per-second spike and dome pattern, so should not be called petit mal.

Severe generalized

A severe generalized seizure may or may not have an aura. The animal may suddenly fall on its side unconscious, and cry out as it falls. This has been called the epileptic cry in humans, and is caused by air rushing past the contracting larynx. The eyes are generally open and the pupils dilated. The limbs, neck, face, and jaw muscles may become symmetrically rigid during the tonic phase. A clonic phase with jerking of the limbs, neck, face, and jaw muscles may occur. During these two periods, the animal is usually unable to respire properly and becomes cyanotic. Dogs' and cats' respiratory passages rarely become obstructed by their tongues, and owners should be warned to keep their fingers out of the animal's mouth during the seizure or they may get bitten or further obstruct respirations. If severe tongue lacerations occur during the clonic phase of the seizure, the owner may prevent this by carefully wedging a small object between the teeth on one side. During the tonic and clonic phases of the severe generalized seizure, the animal usually salivates excessively. As the animal relaxes it may also urinate and defecate. The animal may paddle or lie quietly before recovery begins. The interval from the onset of the seizure to the onset of recovery is about 30 to 90 seconds for most severe generalized seizures. Longer severe generalized seizures may be associated with toxicities and metabolic disorders. During the recovery period, the animal may be exhausted, and want to sleep, or be hyperactive, continually pace, and appear disoriented. Some

animals may injure themselves during a hyperactive recovery period and require sedation. Other animals may want to urinate or defecate if they did not do so during the seizure, or may be hungry or thirsty. The recovery period most commonly lasts a few minutes to an hour, but may continue all day in some animals. If an active disease process is present, such as encephalitis, toxicity, nutritional deficiency, metabolic disturbance, or neoplasia, the animal may never recover to a completely normal state.

Partial

If the seizure discharge is focal and involves only one portion of the brain, the result is a partial seizure (Fig. 8–3). Paroxysmal spike and spike-wave complexes on the EEG occur primarily in the leads closest to the focus. Partial seizures are most

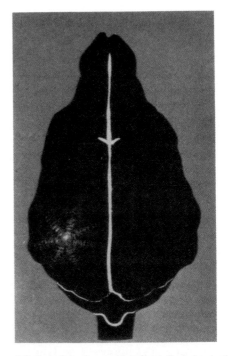

Figure 8-3. A partial seizure with a focal discharge in the cerebral cortex.

commonly associated with a focus of brain damage caused by an infection, metabolic insult, traumatic insult, or neoplasia. Partial seizures may have no prodrome or aura. The actual seizure or ictal period may have a variety of appearances, depending on the location of seizure discharges.[10,12] Partial seizures may vary in length, and the recovery period may be short. Table 8–1 is a list of some partial seizures described in dogs and cats and a possible location of the focus. There have been a few studies in animals comparing the appearance of the seizure with a proven location of a focus on histologic examination, and much of the information has been extrapolated from studies on epileptic foci in humans.

Unilateral neuronal discharges in the frontal lobe of the cerebral cortex produce twitching of the muscles on the opposite side of the body (contralateral). The head may turn away from the side of the focal discharge, and only the face muscles or forelimb muscles on the contralateral side may be affected. The seizure may remain in the region of the focus or may spread throughout the cortex and down through the brain stem and spinal cord, and produce secondary generalization.

Periodic abnormal behavior, associated with disorientation and confusion, or hysterical running may be associated with temporal lobe and limbic system neuronal discharges. During the seizure, the animals may also lick their lips, chew, and swallow excessively. Periodic abnormal behavior may also be a psychologic disorder that must be differentiated from a seizure.

"Fly biting," "star gazing," and other behavior suggesting that an animal is hallucinating have been seen in Schnauzers and King Charles spaniels as well as in mixed breed dogs. Although the exact location has not been determined in these animals, a temporal or occipital lobe dysfunction is suspected, as these regions can produce hallucinations in humans.

Episodic tail-chasing and self-mutilation may have many causes (Chap. 20). A

Table 8–1
Types of partial seizures and possible locations of lesions

Seizure description	Location of lesion
Unilateral muscle twitching of the face, limb, or limbs; focal motor seizure	Contralateral frontal lobe of cerebral cortex (motor region)
Bizarre, aggressive behavior, chewing, lip smacking, excessive swallowing, running, confusion; psychomotor seizure	Temporal lobe of cerebral cortex and limbic system structures
"Fly biting," "star gazing;" hallucinations	Temporal or occipital lobes of cerebral cortex
Episodic tail chasing and self-mutilation	Parietal lobe of cerebral cortex (if true seizure activity)
Chronic episodic vomiting and diarrhea	Limbic system and hypothalamus (if true seizure activity)

few of the animals that exhibit this behavior have an abnormal EEG and may respond to anticonvulsant therapy. A focus in the sensory region of the parietal lobe cerebral cortex is suspected.

A few cases of episodic chronic vomiting and diarrhea have been suspected of being caused by abnormal neuronal discharges in the limbic system, which includes the hypothalamus.[2] Spike discharges have been reported in the EEG tracings of these animals, and there is clinical improvement with anticonvulsant therapy. This is probably a rare cause of gastrointestinal upset in the dog.

Partial with secondary generalization

A partial seizure can secondarily generalize to involve other parts of the brain (Fig. 8–4). The secondary generalization may occur so rapidly that the partial phase of the seizure lasts only seconds and may not be observed. Partial seizures that secondarily generalize, like partial seizures that do not, are associated with focal lesions in the brain. If the focus is in a motor area of the frontal lobe cerebral cortex, the animal may show a contralateral motor sign, such as turning the head and lifting a forelimb, before collapsing into lateral recumbency in a severe generalized seizure. This brief motor sign of the partial seizure is referred to as a localizing sign.

If the seizure discharge begins in a nonmotor area of the brain, the partial part of the seizure may be overlooked. By careful observation of the animal during the severe generalized part of the seizure, one may detect some asymmetric motor activity. One side of the face may be contracted more severely than the other, or there may be a difference of tone or movement in the limbs. The owner should be instructed to observe the animal for any asymmetric involvement of the body during the seizure, as this information will aid

in determining the type of seizure and underlying disease process. The generalized portion of the seizure usually lasts from 30 to 90 seconds, and the recovery may be similar to the severe generalized seizure. The animal should be observed during the recovery for any signs that might indicate residual activity in a focus of the brain. Continual compulsive circling to one side during the recovery period may indicate a focal lesion.

Patient evaluation

Signalment and history

The importance of the signalment and history of an animal was discussed in Chapter 2. The type and duration of the seizure itself and the onset, course, frequency, and duration of the seizure disorder should be described to help determine whether an active disease process is affecting the brain or if the animal has epilepsy. An acute onset of severe, frequent seizures could indicate an infectious, toxic, nutritional, metabolic, or neoplastic process. An intermittent seizure disorder, with no other neurologic abnormalities in between the seizures, which has been going on for a year or more, is most likely epilepsy. One seizure with no previous history of seizures may be the beginning of an active disease process in an older animal, but may be a one-time idiopathic event in a young animal. Table 8–2 outlines common causes of seizures in various age groups.

Physical and neurologic examinations

The physical examination can be useful to detect disease in other body systems, which might secondarily or concurrently be affecting the brain and producing seizures (Chap. 3). A new, concurrent neurologic deficit reported in the history and con-

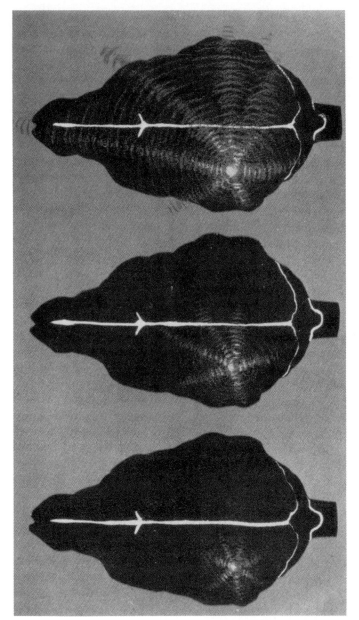

Figure 8–4. A partial seizure that secondarily generalizes as the discharge spreads over the cerebral cortex.

Table 8–2
Differential diagnosis of seizures in dogs and cats

Young (under 9 months of age)
1. Congenital hydrocephalus
2. Lissencephaly
3. Lysosomal storage disorders
4. Distemper and FIP virus and other causes of encephalitis
5. Trauma
6. Toxicity—lead, organophosphates, etc.
7. Hypoglycemia
8. Hepatic encephalopathy—portacaval shunt
9. Other congenital defects with associated metabolic disorders
10. Thiamine deficiency

Adult (9 months to 5 years)
1. Distemper and FIP virus and other causes of encephalitis
2. Trauma
3. Toxicity—organophosphates, etc.
4. Hypoglycemia
5. Hepatic encephalopathy—portacaval shunt, acquired cirrhosis
6. Other acquired metabolic disorders
7. True epilepsy
8. Acquired epilepsy
9. Cerebral neoplasia—rare

Old (5 years and older)
1. Distemper and FIP virus and other causes of encephalitis
2. Trauma
3. Toxicity—organophosphates, etc.
4. Hypoglycemia—insulinoma
5. Hepatic encephalopathy—acquired cirrhosis
6. Other acquired metabolic disorders
7. Acquired epilepsy
8. Cerebral neoplasia

firmed on the neurologic examination may be a sign of an active nervous system disease, such as infection or tumor.

A neurologic deficit found on the examination, which was not reported in the history, could be a new development associated with an active disease process or an old lesion due to residual damage from some previous insult, which also produced the seizure focus. Transient neurologic deficits may be found during the postictal period. The physical and neurologic examinations in animals with epilepsy are often normal.

Ancillary diagnostic investigations

The ancillary diagnostic investigations used to evaluate animals with seizures are basically the same as those used to evaluate animals with lesions above the foramen magnum (Chap. 4) and with behavior disorders (Chap. 7). A complete blood count (CBC), chemistry profile, EEG, cerebrospinal fluid (CSF), and neuroradiology of the skull all can be used to determine the underlying cause of the seizures[24] (Chap. 5).

Table 8–3 outlines the diagnostic approach to the evaluation of seizures in dogs and cats.

Congenital and familial disorders

Hydrocephalus, lissencephaly, and the lysosomal storage diseases, such as GM_2 gangliosidosis, ceroid lipofuscinosis, neuronal glycoproteinosis, and fucosidosis have seizures as one of the signs of neurologic dysfunction. Animals with these disorders also have behavior changes of dementia and irritability. These are discussed in Chapter 7. True epilepsy is a familial disorder in dogs and is discussed later in this chapter.

Infections and other inflammations

Viral cerebral infections with distemper virus in dogs and feline infectious peritonitis (FIP) virus in cats may have seizures as one of the clinical signs of neurologic dysfunction (Chap. 7). Possible abnormal findings on the physical and neurologic examinations may support the diagnosis, or the animals can appear normal. EEG, CSF analysis, and serum and CSF distemper and FIP virus titer determinations may aid in the diagnosis (Chap. 7). Because there

are so many different organisms that produce encephalitis, serum and CSF titers and cultures may help in the differential diagnosis (see Table 7–8). If no organism is found, but there is pleocytosis of the cerebrospinal fluid, a steroid-responsive meningoencephalitis is possible and glucocorticoid therapy should be given. A complete discussion of differential diagnosis and therapy of encephalitis is found in Chapter 7. Causes of meningoencephalitis in dogs and cats that might produce seizures are listed in Tables 7–6 and 7–7.

Granulomatous meningoencephalitis may also occasionally produce seizures in dogs and cats, but often, brain stem signs predominate (Chaps. 7 and 12).

Seizures may continue periodically even after the infection or inflammation has passed, because of the residual damage from the encephalitis process, producing an epileptic focus. This postinfection epilepsy is another form of acquired epilepsy discussed later in this chapter.

Metabolic disorders

Seizures may be associated with several metabolic disorders such as hypoglycemia, hypocalcemia, hypomagnesemia, hypoxia, hepatic disorders, end-stage renal failure, acid-base imbalances, particularly alkalosis, and osmolality disturbances.

Hypoglycemia

Incidence: Frequent

The most common metabolic cause of seizures in small animals is hypoglycemia. There are several different underlying causes of hypoglycemia in animals, and hypoglycemia can be included in the differential diagnosis of seizures in any age dog or cat (see Table 8–2).

In puppies. Severe infestation with parasites and an inadequate diet is a com-

Table 8–3
Diagnostic approach for the evaluation of seizures

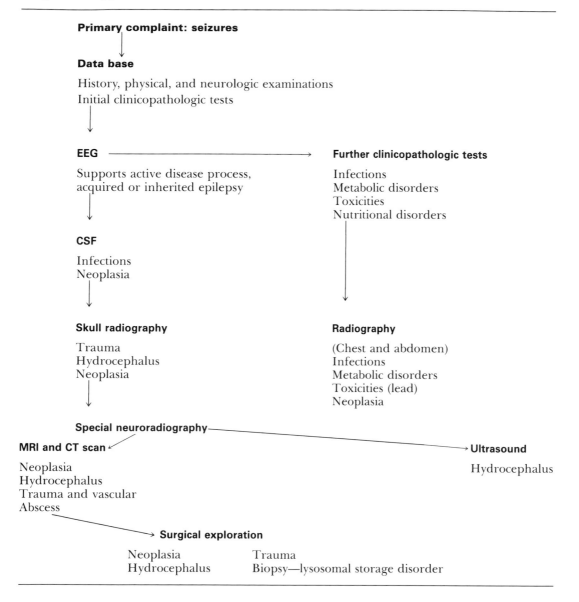

Primary complaint: seizures

Data base

History, physical, and neurologic examinations
Initial clinicopathologic tests

EEG ⟶ **Further clinicopathologic tests**

Supports active disease process,
acquired or inherited epilepsy

Infections
Metabolic disorders
Toxicities
Nutritional disorders

CSF

Infections
Neoplasia

Skull radiography

Trauma
Hydrocephalus
Neoplasia

Radiography

(Chest and abdomen)
Infections
Metabolic disorders
Toxicities (lead)
Neoplasia

Special neuroradiography

MRI and CT scan

Neoplasia
Hydrocephalus
Trauma and vascular
Abscess

Ultrasound

Hydrocephalus

Surgical exploration

Neoplasia   Trauma
Hydrocephalus   Biopsy—lysosomal storage disorder

mon cause of hypoglycemia in young puppies. The puppies may be depressed and weak in between the seizures. Anemia and hypocalcemia may further compound the problems. Serum glucose determinations are usually below 50 mg/dl. Fifty percent dextrose therapy may be administered in-travenously or orally at a dose of 1–4 mg/kg of body weight or to effect. If the animal is severely anemic, a transfusion may also be necessary. If serum calcium determinations are also low (below 7.0 mg/dl), 2.2 ml/kg of body weight of a 10% calcium gluconate solution should be

Table 8–5
Chemicals that cause convulsions

- absinthe
- acetanilide
- acetone cyanohydrin
- acetonitrile
- acetylsalicylic acid
- aconite
- acridium Cl
- acrylonitrile
- aldrin
- *Amanita pantherona*
- 2-aminopyrine
- amphetamine
- apomorphine
- arecoline
- arsenic trioxide
- arsine
- *Aspidium*
- atropine
- barium
- bromates
- butacaine
- caffeine
- camphor
- carbon dioxide
- castor beans
- cedar oil
- *chenopodium oil*
- chloramine T
- chlordane
- chlorinated camphene
- chloronaphthalene
- chlorpromazine
- choke cherry
- cocaine
- coniine
- corticotrophin
- cortisone
- cresol
- creosote
- cyanide
- cyclotrimethylene
- DDT
- DFP

- digitalis
- dimenhydrinate
- dimercaprol
- dinitrobenzene
- dinitrocresol
- dinitrophenol
- diphenhydramine
- disulfiram
- dulcamara
- endrin
- ephedrine
- ergot
- ethylene glycol
- *Eucalyptus oil*
- fluorides
- *Galerina venerata*
- gasoline
- *Gloriosa superba*
- *Gymnothorax flavimarginatus*
  Helvella
- heroin
- hexachlorophene
- hydrogen sulfide
- insulin
- isoniazid
- kerosene
- ketamine
- lead
- lobeline
- meperidine
- mercaptan
- metaldehyde
- methapyrilene HCl
- methyl bromide
- methyl chloride
- methyl formate
- methyl salicylate
- monochloroacetic acid
- morphine
- naphthol
- *Narcissus bulb*
- neostigmine
- nicotine

- nitrogen oxide
- *Oenanthe crocata*
- oxygen (100%, 3 atm)
- pantopon
- parathion
- phencyclidene
- phenol
- phosphorus
- physostigmine
- picrotoxin
- pilocarpine
- procaine
- pyridamine maleate
- pyrimidine
- quinine
- resorcinol
- *Rhodotypos* (berries)
- Rosemary oil
- saffron
- sage, oil of
- salicylates
- santonin
- *Senecio canicida*
- sodium fluoroacetate
- squill
- streptomycin
- strychnine
- *Tanacetum vulgare*
- *Taxus baccata*
- tetracaine
- tetrachloroethane
- tetraethyl pyrophosphate
- *Tetraodontia*
- thallium
- thiocyanates
- *Thuja*
- trinitrotoluene
- tripelennamine HCl
- veratrum
- Vitamin D
- water hemlock
- zinc cyanide

Courtesy of Dr. Roger Yeary. The Ohio State University, Dept. of Veterinary Physiology and Pharmacology.

known, the vital functions of the animal should be stabilized and a poison control center contacted for further information.

Nutritional disorders

Seizures may be seen in the late stages of thiamine deficiency in cats. Thiamine deficiency is rare in dogs. The seizures are preceded by ataxia, ventral neck flexion, and abnormal behavior (Chap. 7).

Pyridoxine (vitamin B_6) deficiency is a cause of seizures in humans, but this is not a confirmed cause in dogs and cats.

Trauma and vascular disorders

Animals may have a seizure immediately or within a few days after a severe head injury. Seizures may be only one of the signs of nervous system dysfunction. A traumatic incident is often known from the history, and signs of trauma may be apparent on the physical examination. The management of head trauma and accompanying seizures is discussed in Chapter 10. Animals may also begin seizures up to 6 months to 2 years following a head injury. Post-traumatic epilepsy is a type of acquired epilepsy that will be discussed later in the chapter.

Neoplasia

Primary and metastatic neoplastic processes affecting the cerebral cortex and rostral brain stem can result in seizures, along with behavior abnormalities. Neoplasia can occur at any age, but is more common in older animals (see Table 8–2). The diagnosis and management of cerebral neoplasia is discussed in Chapter 7.

Epilepsy

The terms epilepsy and seizures are used interchangeably by some authors. Epilepsy is categorized as symptomatic, having an underlying disease process, or as true and idiopathic, and not having an underlying disease process. For simplification, epilepsy is defined in this book as a disorder of recurrent seizures with no underlying disease process, and other causes of seizures are discussed in terms of the underlying disease process. Seizures are then a sign of epilepsy as well as of the other differential diagnoses discussed. Seizures from any causes may be similar in appearance. It is important to differentiate epilepsy from the other causes of seizures, because the prognosis for the animal may be better if it has epilepsy.

Epilepsy can be classified as true, idiopathic, and inherited or as acquired and noninherited.[39,40] The treatment of true and acquired epilepsy may be the same. The differentiation of true and acquired epilepsy becomes important when determining the desirability of breeding a purebred animal that has seizures, or when a prognosis is needed of seizure control for certain purebred dogs with inherited epilepsy, such as German Shepherds, Saint Bernards, and Irish Setters. Table 8–6 outlines some differences in true and acquired epilepsy.

True Epilepsy

Incidence: Frequent in certain breeds

True or inherited epilepsy is often suspected in purebred dogs, but rarely in dogs of mixed breeds.[14] Inherited epilepsy has been studied in Beagles, German Shepherds (Alsatians), Keeshonds, Tervueren Shepherds, and Irish Setters.[14,17,48,49] Other breeds that are sus-

Table 8–7
Guide to anticonvulsant therapy

1. Select a single drug such as phenobarbital or primidone.
2. Begin at the recommended dose and adjust the dosage until the seizures are controlled with no toxic side effects.
3. If persistent side effects are seen or seizures are not controlled after 2 weeks, measure serum anticonvulsant levels and adjust dosage until levels are within the therapeutic range.
4. If seizures are not satisfactorally controlled when the serum level of drug is in the therapeutic range, switch to either primidone or phenobarbital and repeat steps 2 and 3.
5. Once seizures are controlled, monitor serum liver enzymes and liver function (bile acids) every 1–3 months if on primidone or 6–9 months if on phenobarbital.
6. If there are no toxic side effects seen, do not begin decreasing the dose or altering the frequency of medication until the animal has been free of seizures for 6 months.
7. Monitor the levels of anticonvulsants in the serum on those animals that are difficult to control, as increasing doses of anticonvulsant may be required to maintain a given serum level.
8. If the routine anticonvulsants fail, less commonly used anticonvulsants may be tried with caution, as dosages are not standardized and longterm side effects are unknown (see Table 8–12). Rule out a progressive underlying disease process producing the seizures by repeating the neurologic examination, clinicopathologic tests, CSF analysis, and CT or MRI scans.

When to begin anticonvulsant therapy

Unlike humans, a few seizures a year in a dog or cat may have no disastrous effect on its daily life. Infrequent, mild generalized and partial seizures may have little longterm effect on the animal.

If the seizures are severe, generalized, and occur in multiples several times a year or the owner is very upset about them, control with anticonvulsant therapy should be attempted.

Maintenance anticonvulsant therapy is often not initiated if the frequency of seizures is less than once a month, if the seizures are single, brief (30 to 90 seconds), with a rapid uneventful recovery, and if the animal has an understanding owner.

Owners must understand from the beginning that the goal of anticonvulsant therapy is to reduce the frequency and severity of seizures and the response will vary with each animal. The seizures are only controlled, not cured, and the success of drug therapy will depend primarily on the owners. They must make a commitment to follow directions explicitly and administer the drug at the proper dose and frequency. The owner also must understand that each animal is an individual, and several attempts with various doses and drugs may be made until the proper program is found for the animal. The owner should be warned about possible side effects and informed that many are transient and will disappear as the animal either adjusts to the drug dose or as the dose is decreased. For best results, the owner should be instructed to obtain a calendar and each day write down the time and dose of medication, any side effects, and the time and severity of any seizures. The veterinarian can then periodically review the calendar with the owner and decide a rational change of therapy if needed. The owner should understand that occasional seizures may still occur. If educated properly, most owners are willing to work closely with their veterinarian, and are not upset if a few seizures continue during the adjustment period.

What anticonvulsant to select

Phenobarbital 2 mg/kg every 12 hours orally is often the first anticonvulsant of choice in dogs and cats[5,17,19] (Table 8–8). Many seizures will be controlled within 24 to 48 hours. Phenobarbital has a wide margin of safety and few side effects. If seizures continue after 48 hours, the dosage should be increased and the serum phenobarbital level monitored. The serum phenobarbital level may have to be maintained between 30 and 40 μg/ml in dogs and cats whose seizures are difficult to control.[16,18,46] If the seizures continue when the serum level is over 40 μg/ml or the animal is sedated, another anticonvulsant such as primidone should be tried. Serum phenobarbital steady state is reached in 10–18 days and the sample is drawn 2–4 hours following administration.

A few dogs become hyperactive instead of sedated with phenobarbital. If hyperactivity occurs, mephobarbital, a longer acting barbiturate, may be substituted at the same dosage to reduce the hyperactivity. On rare occasions, phenobarbital produces polyuria, polydipsia, and polyphagia, but this is usually less than with primidone. Some animals become tolerant to phenobarbital and the dose must be increased and administered every 6 to 8 hours to maintain a therapeutic serum level. All longterm anticonvulsant therapy has some negative effect on liver function, but phenobarbital may have the least effect.[6] Phenobarbital is a controlled substance, widely abused by humans, so careful monitoring of the amount of drug dispensed is necessary.

Primidone (Table 8–9) metabolizes to phenobarbital and phenylethylmalonic acid (PEMA). Primidone and its metabolites all have anticonvulsant properties and may control seizures better in certain dogs than phenobarbital alone.[15,44] Primidone is toxic to cats and not recommended. A dose of 14.3 mg/kg of primidone may be given to dogs orally every 12 hours initially. The dosage may be increased to control the seizures, and serum levels of both phenobarbital and primidone can be monitored.[13] The effective serum primidone level is between 5 and 15 μg/ml.[16,50] Primidone takes 6–8 days to reach a steady state in the serum. Serum primidone levels are obtained 2–4 hours after administration.

Sedation, hyperexcitability, bizzare behavior, polyuria, polydipsia, and polyphagia may be side effects of primidone. Hepatic necrosis leading to cirrhosis can be a fatal complication in individual dogs.[4,7,31] All dogs on primidone should have serum liver enzymes monitored, and if they continue to elevate, the drug should be discontinued. A mild elevation of liver enzymes is expected with any anticonvulsant drug.[47] Anemia and dermatitis are rare side effects of primidone.[21]

In some dogs a combination of phenobarbital and primidone may control seizures better than either single drug. A combination of drugs should be used only after each drug alone has been unsuccessful.

Diphenylhydantoin (Table 8–10) produces little sedation and may be the drug of choice in working or show dogs. Because the drug is so rapidly metabolized by dogs, a dose of 20 to 35 mg/kg or more every 6 to 8 hours or more may be necessary to maintain a therapeutic blood level and control seizures.[36,41] The high and frequent dosage makes the drug expensive and inconvenient to give to dogs. Diphenylhydantoin is toxic to cats because it is very slowly metabolized.

Diphenylhydantoin may produce toxic hepatopathy and intrahepatic cholestasis in dogs, especially in combination with other anticonvulsant drugs.[8,33] The therapeutic success is rarely improved when diphenylhydantoin and phenobarbital are combined in dogs. Diphenylhydantoin in-

(Continued on page 199)

Table 8–8
Phenobarbital

Action:

Depresses repetitive electrical activity of multineuronal networks

Metabolism:

Serum levels stable in 7–10 days
Half-life in dogs 36–46 hours
Detoxified by the liver and excreted by the kidneys
A powerful enzyme-inducer for itself and other drugs
Dependence and tolerance developed in the animal

Type of Patient:

Cats
Dogs experiencing seizures several times weekly
Dogs that have seizures when excited
Animals in which cost of therapy is a factor

Supplied (oral):

Elixir—4 mg/ml (good for cats and puppies)
¼ gr or 16 mg tablets
½ gr or 32 mg tablets
1 gr or 64 mg tablets

Dosage:

Dogs and cats—2 mg/kg every 12 hours

Effective serum level:

15–40 μg/ml

Sample cost (1990—Approximate, varies with pharmacy)

¼ gr $6.00/100 tablets
½ gr $7.00/100 tablets
Elixer 4 mg/ml $8.50/pint
14 kg dog—$0.14/day starting dose

Toxic side effects:

Sedation
Paradoxic hyperactivity (less than primidone)
Polyuria, polydipsia, polyphagia (less than primidone)
Anemia (rare)

Other related oral compounds:

Mephobarbital (Mebaral)—similar to phenobarbital but may be longer acting; use when animal
hyperactive on phenobarbital

Table 8–9
Primidone (Mylepsin or Mysoline)

Action:

Similar to phenobarbital; primidone and its metabolites phenobarbital and phenylethyl malonic acid (PEMA) all have anticonvulsant action.

Metabolism:

Serum levels of phenobarbital stable in 7 days
Metabolized by the liver and excreted by the kidneys

Type of patient:

Dogs experiencing seizures several times weekly
Dogs that have seizures when excited
Dogs in which phenobarbital does not control seizures
Toxic to cats—not recommended

Supplied (oral): Primidone (Mylepsin, Mysoline)

50 mg/ml solution
50 mg tablets
250 mg tablets

Dosage:

Dogs—14.3 mg/kg every 12 hours: half of recommended dose; increase as needed to control seizures (may be less for larger dogs)

Effective serum level

Phenobarbital 15–40 μg/ml; primidone 5–15 μg/ml

Sample cost (1990—Approximate, varies with pharmacy)

250 mg tablets—$12.00/100 tablets
14 kg dog—$0.24 at starting dose

Toxic side effects:

Often greater side effects than phenobarbital
Sedation
Paradoxic hyperactivity
Polyuria, polydipsia, polyphagia
Hepatic necrosis (few individuals)
Anemia (rare)

Comments:

Monitor liver enzymes and liver function monthly for 6 months
Differences in seizure control noticed in individuals when switched from Mysoline to Mylepsin, may be related to product absorption

Table 8–10
Diphenylhydantoin (Dilantin)

Action:

Stabilizes excitable membranes
Reduces post-tetanic potentiation
Limits spread of seizure activity; if seizures still occur, they may be less severe.

Metabolism:

Half-life in the dog is 4 hours
Half-life in cats, 24–108 hours
Metabolized by the liver and excreted by the kidneys

Type of patient:

Rarely used
Dogs having seizures twice a month or less
Show dogs and working dogs
Small dogs or dogs where cost of therapy is not a factor
Dogs that have toxic side effects to or are not controlled by other anticonvulsants
Not recommended in cats

Supplied (oral): Phenytoin, Dilantin, DPH

6 mg/ml solution (mix well with each use)
25 mg/ml solution (mix well with each use)
30 mg capsules
50 mg tablets
100 mg capsules

Dosage:

Dogs—20–35 mg/kg every 6–8 hours

Effective serum level

10–20 µg/ml

Sample cost (1990—Approximate, varies with pharmacy)

100 mg capsules—$11.00/100 capsules
14 kg dog—$1.65/day starting dose

Toxic side effects:

Few side effects
Anemia—rare
Gingival hyperplasia—rare
Liver disease

Other related oral compounds:

Mesantoin—Mephenytoin

teracts with several drugs and can increase to toxic levels if combined with choloramphenicol.

Diazepam (Table 8–11) is not a very effective oral anticonvulsant in dogs, but may be useful in cats. A dose of 1 to 2 mg diazepam every 8 hours may be administered to adult cats with few side effects.

When anticonvulsant therapy should be changed

If adequate seizure control is obtained, the therapy should not be altered for at least 6 months, unless seizures recur at an unacceptable frequency and severity or tox-

icities such as hepatopathy, dermatitis, or anemia develop.

The serum alkaline phosphatase levels mildly increase in many dogs on anticonvulsant therapy, particularly primidone.[47] If all the liver enzymes elevate grossly, the drug should be tapered and replaced by another anticonvulsant. Anemia rarely occurs secondarily to anticonvulsant therapy in animals.

If the animal has been seizure-free for 6 months, a decrease in dosage of the medication can be tried. Some veterinarians try a decreased frequency of medication once daily. This is not recommended. The animal develops a physical dependence on

Table 8–11
Diazepam (Valium)

Action:

Limits the spread of seizure activity
Elevates seizure threshold

Metabolism:

Metabolized by liver and excreted by kidney

Type of patient:

Used intravenously to arrest status epilepticus in dogs and cats
May be used as an oral anticonvulsant in cats if phenobarbital not effective; may be combined with phenobarbital
Not effective as a single anticonvulsant in dogs

Supplied (oral):

2 mg tablets
5 mg tablets

Dosage:

Cats—1–2 mg every 8 hours

Sample cost (1990—Approximate, varies with pharmacy)

2 mg—$25.00/100 tablets; 5 mg—$40.00/100 tablets
5 kg cat—$0.38–$0.75/day

Toxic side effects:

Sedation
Polyphagia

phenobarbital and primidone. An abrupt withdrawal of either drug may result in status epilepticus.

Individual animals may also develop a tolerance to a particular drug, especially to phenobarbital or primidone, and the dose and frequency of medication may have to be increased over time or another anticonvulsant added.

If the routine anticonvulsant therapy is not effective, there are some other drugs available that have had limited use in veterinary medicine.[5,19,27,32,43] The longterm side effects of these drugs are not known in animals. These drugs should, therefore, be used as a last resort, with the owner's permission. Table 8–12 lists less frequently used anticonvulsant drugs and their dosages and side effects.

When serum phenobarbital concentrations are between 25 and 30 μg/ml and dogs are still seizuring frequently or in clusters, then clonazepam (Klonopin) or potassium bromide may be combined with the phenobarbital (see Table 8–12). If sedation occurs, the phenobarbital dosage can be slightly decreased. Clonazepam may improve the seizure frequency, but is expensive to use in large dogs and must be given every 8 hours.[1,27] Potassium bromide (KBr) reduces seizure frequency and often stops clusters of seizures from occurring when added to phenobarbital.[27,37] There currently is no pharmaceutical grade of KBr available and excessive handling of the raw chemical* may produce toxicities in man. Both clonazepam and KBr, however, have helped many dogs whose seizures were intractable when treated by standard protocols.

Valproic acid (Depakene) and carbamazepine (Tegretol) may be combined with phenobarbital to attempt control of intractable seizures; however, these appear to be less effective than clonazepam and

KBr in the limited studies available. Paramethadione (Paradione) may control seizures in some dogs better than standard anticonvulsants, but the longterm side effects are not known. Chlorazepate dipotassium (Tranxene) has also had limited use in the dog.

Reasons for anticonvulsant failures

The most common reason for anticonvulsant failure is improper administration of the medication. Often, owners are lax in giving the correct dosage on schedule. Some veterinarians try to use the drugs once daily, when the recommended dosage is 2 or 3 times daily. Other veterinarians may try one drug at one dose, get no response, then try another drug at one dose and get no response, and not give either drug a fair trial. In these instances, the owner and veterinarian have failed, not the anticonvulsant.

A true anticonvulsant failure exists if control of the seizures is not achieved when the drugs are prescribed correctly by the veterinarian, the dose increased slowly until the serum level reaches the maximum therapeutic range, and the owner administers medication faithfully.

The seizures associated with true epilepsy of German Shepherds, Saint Bernards, and Irish Setters are often only partially controlled regardless of the anticonvulsant tried. True epilepsy may be considered in these breeds when routine anticonvulsants fail.

The original diagnosis may be incorrect for seizures that do not respond to anticonvulsant therapy. A metabolic disorder, encephalitis, or cerebral neoplasia may have progressive, uncontrollable seizures.

If the animal has been controlled on a drug and then seems to go out of control, several factors may be considered. If the animal has been on phenobarbital or primidone, perhaps a tolerance to the medica-

---

* Fischer Chemical Company, Springfield, NJ

Table 8–12
Alternative maintenance anticonvulsant therapy for uncontrolled seizures in dogs

1. Clonazepam (Klonopin)

   a. Dosage: 0.06–0.2 mg/kg (divided every 6–8 hours) with phenobarbital or 1.5 mg/kg (divided every 8 hours) if given alone

   b. Side effects: sedation

   c. Effective serum level: 0.02–0.08 μg/ml

   d. Miscellaneous: usually combined with phenobarbital; may be more effective than phenobarbital alone

   e. Cost (1990): 2 mg tablets, $40.59/100 tablets; 14 kg dog—$0.20—$0.60/day

2. Potassium bromide

   a. Dosage: 25 mg/kg orally once daily with food with phenobarbital or twice daily if given alone

   b. Side effects: sedation

   c. Effective serum level: 500–1,000 μg/ml

   d. Miscellaneous: usually combined with phenobarbital; toxic to humans; no pharmaceutical grade currently available; especially affective to decrease cluster seizures in dogs

   e. Cost (1990): Chemical grade crystals 250 mg dissolved in 1 ml water—Cost to client $1.50/30 ml; 14 kg dog $.07/day

3. Valproic acid (Depakene)

   a. Dosage: 15–200 mg/kg/day orally (divided every 6–8 hours.)

   b. Side effects: sedation, hepatopathy

   c. Effective serum level: 500–1,000 μg/ml (man)

   d. Miscellaneous: usually combined with phenobarbital

   e. Cost (1990): 250 mg capsules, $60.00/100 capsules; 14 kg dog—$0.60–$6.00/day

4. Carbamazepine (Tegretol)

   a. Dosage: 4–10 mg/kg/day orally (divided every 8–12 hrs)

   b. Side effects: sedation, nystagmus, vomiting, hepatopathy

   c. Effective serum level: 5–10 μg/ml (man)

   d. Miscellaneous: may be combined with phenobarbital

   e. Cost (1990): 100 mg capsules, $20.00/100; 14 kg dog—$0.20/day

5. Paramethadione (Paradione)

   a. Dosage: 30–50 mg/kg/day orally (divided every 8 hrs)

   b. Side effects: sedation

   c. Effective serum level: unknown

   d. Miscellaneous: longterm side effects are unknown

6. Chlorazepate dipotassium (Tranxene)

   a. Dosage: 2-6 mg/kg/day (divided every 8–12 hours)

   b. Side effects: sedation

   c. Effective serum level: unknown

   d. Miscellaneous: longterm effects and efficacy unknown

   e. Cost (1990): 15 mg tablets, $71.00/100; 14 kg dog—$1.40/day

tion has developed, and the dosage or frequency of drug administration needs to be increased or another anticonvulsant tried or added to the therapy regimen.

Estrus may bring on an increased frequency of seizures in some bitches. If this seems to be the case in an individual animal, perhaps an ovariohysterectomy will solve the problem.

A systemic disease process with vomiting, diarrhea, and fever or a liver disease might result in an alteration of the absorption, metabolism, and efficacy of an anticonvulsant drug, and seizures may recur or go out of control. Once the new disease process is controlled, the seizures may also come back into control.

Several drugs may be given to a dog for treatment of problems unrelated to the seizure disorder, which might alter the absorption or metabolism of the anticonvulsant.[9,38,42] This could result in a sudden recurrence of seizures or toxicity. Phenobarbital enhances the metabolism of digitoxin, dipyrone, griseofulvin, and phenylbutazone. Chloramphenicol may raise serum levels of diphenylhydantoin and phenobarbital and produce toxicity.

Amphetamines, phenothiazine tranquilizers, and organophosphate dips and medications may stimulate seizures in epileptic dogs and cats and should not be administered. Ivermectin monthly for heartworm control may exacerbate seizures in some dogs.

It is possible for a dog or cat that has been a controlled epileptic for many years to develop a second neurologic disorder characterized by seizures, such as hypoglycemia, encephalitis, or brain tumor, and appear to go out of control. Reevaluation will usually indicate a new disease process.

Adjuncts to anticonvulsant therapy

Some dogs have seizures when stressed by bathing, clipping, or guests in the house.

Increasing the anticonvulsant dose 12 hours prior to the stress may abort the seizure.

Some dogs develop a specific pattern to the frequency of their seizures, such as every 8 to 10 weeks or every full moon. Often these seizures can be aborted by increasing the anticonvulsant dose a few days prior to the scheduled time, and then again decreasing the dose a few days past the time. Each dog must be evaluated individually.

Seizure control may be enhanced in an individual dog or cat by the administration of glucocorticoids or adrenocorticotropic hormone (ACTH) along with the anticonvulsants. This should only be used when routine anticonvulsant therapy has been thoroughly tried and found not to be adequate.

In some individual dogs and cats, a low-protein, high-fat diet, or a "ketogenic" diet, along with routine anticonvulsant therapy, may improve seizure control. Some dogs have fewer seizures when placed on a prescription diet for kidney patients such as K/D.*

Special considerations and prognosis for epileptic animals

The veterinarian must take some special considerations into account during the general health care of an epileptic dog or cat. If a tranquilizer is needed for travel or as preanesthesia treatment, diazepam or phenobarbital should be used and not acepromazine. If a dog controlled on diphenylhydantoin or phenobarbital develops an infection, and chloramphenicol is the antibiotic of choice, the dose should be decreased, as chloramphenicol alters its metabolism and the animal may become toxic.

---

*Hill's Division, Riviana Foods, Topeka, Kansas 66601.

If the animal develops liver disease later in life, the anticonvulsant may not be effective or toxic side effects may occur. Concomitant hepatic encephalopathy disrupts the seizure control of an epileptic animal.

The prognosis for epilepsy in most dogs and cats is good except for the examples cited in German Shepherds, Saint Bernards, and Irish Setters. If epilepsy is acquired at a young age, the seizure frequency may decrease with age. In a few individuals, a primary epileptic focus may produce a secondary epileptic focus in the same site on the other side of the brain. The secondary focus can produce seizures that may differ slightly with age. Epileptic foci are rarely localized sufficiently during the clinical evaluation so that surgical removal could be performed.

The majority of epileptic dogs and cats can be controlled adequately on routine anticonvulsant therapy and lead normal lives. The greatest aid to successful treatment of epilepsy in animals is the education and commitment of the animal's owner.

References

1. Blackmore, J; ACVIM—Neurology, Stewart, Florida, personal communications.
2. Breitschwerdt, E.B. Breazile, J.E., and Broadhurst, J.J.: Clinical and electroencephalographic findings associated with ten cases of suspected limbic epilepsy in the dog. J. Am. Anim. Hosp. Assoc., *15*:37, 1979.
3. Breitschwerdt, E.B., et al.: Hypoglycemia in four dogs with sepsis. J. Am. Vet. Assoc., *178*:1072, 1981.
4. Bunch, S.E., et al.: Hepatic cirrhosis associated with long term anticonvulsant drug therapy in dogs. J. Am. Vet. Med. Assoc., *181*:357, 1982.
5. Bunch, S.E.: Anticonvulsant drug therapy in companion animals. *In* Current Veterinary Therapy VIII. Edited by R.W. Kirk. Philadelphia, W.B. Saunders, 1983.
6. Bunch, S.E., et al.: Compromised hepatic function in dogs treated with anticonvulsant drugs. J. Am. Vet. Med. Assoc., *184*:444, 1984.
7. Bunch, S.E., et al.: Effects of long term primidone and phenytoin administration on canine hepatic function and morphology. Am. J. Vet. Res., *46*:105, 1985.
8. Bunch, S.E., et al.: Toxic hepatopathy and intrahepatic cholestasis associated with phenytoin administration in combination with other anticonvulsant drugs in three dogs. J. Am. Anim. Hosp. Assoc., *190*:194, 1987.
9. Campbell, C.L.: Primidone intoxication associated with concurrent use of chloramphenicol. J. Am. Vet. Med. Assoc., *182*:992, 1983.
10. Casey, W.C. and Blaunch, B.S.: Jaw snapping syndrome in eight dogs. J. Am. Vet. Med. Assoc., *175*:709, 1979.
11. Caywood, D.D., et al.: Pancreatic insulin secreting neoplasms: Clinical, diagnostic, and prognostic features in 73 dogs. J. Am. Anim. Hosp. Assoc., *24*:577, 1988.
12. Crowell-Davis, S.L., Lappin, M., and Oliver, J.E.: Stimulus-responsive psychomotor epilepsy in a doberman pinscher. J. Am. Anim. Hosp. Assoc., *25*:57, 1989.
13. Cunningham, J.G., Haidukewych, D., and Jenson, H.A.: Therapeutic serum concentrations of primidone and its metabolites phenobarbital and phenylethylmalonamide in epileptic dogs. J. Am. Vet. Med. Assoc., *182*:1091, 1983.
14. Cunningham, J.G. and Farnbach, G.C.: Inheritance and idiopathic canine epilepsy. J. Am. Anim. Hosp. Assoc., *24*:421, 1988.
15. Farnbach, G.C.: Efficacy of primidone in dogs with seizures unresponsive to phenobarbital. J. Am. Vet. Med. Assoc., *1985*:867, 1984.
16. Farnbach, G.C.: Serum concentrations and efficacy of phenytoin, phenobarbital and primidone in canine epilepsy. J. Am. Anim. Hosp. Assoc., *184*:1117, 1984.
17. Farnbach, G.C.: Seizures in the dog. Part I. Basis, classification and predilection. Compendium or Continuing Education 6:569, 1984.
18. Farnbach, G.C.: Seizures in the dog. Part II. Control. Compendium on Continuing Education, 7:505, 1985.

19. Forrester, S.D., et al.: Current concepts in the management of canine epilepsy. Compendium on Continuing Education, *11*:811, 1989.
20. Frey, H.H. and Loeschen, W.: Pharmacokinetics of antiepileptic drugs in dogs: A review. J. Vet. Pharmacol. Ther., *8*:219, 1985.
21. Henricks, PM.: Dermatitis associated with the use of primidone in a dog. J. Am. Vet. Med. Assoc., *191*:237, 1987.
22. Holliday, T.A.: Seizure Disorders. Vet. Clin. North Am., *10*:3, 1980.
23. Ihle, S.L., Nelson, R.W., and Cook, J.R.: Seizures as a manifestation of primary hyperparathyroidism in a dog. J. Am. Vet. Med. Assoc., *192*:71, 1988.
24. Knecht, C.D., Sorjonen, D.C., and Simpson, S.T.: Ancillary tests in the diagnosis of seizures. J. Am. Anim. Hosp. Assoc., *20*:455, 1984.
25. Knowlen, G.G. and Schall, W.D.: The amended insulin-glucose ratio. Is it really better? J. Am. Vet. Med. Assoc., *185*:397, 1984.
26. Kruth, S.A., et al.: Insulin-secreting islet cell tumors: Establishing a diagnosis and the clinical source for 25 dogs. J. Am. Vet. Med. Assoc., *181*:54, 1982.
27. Lane, S.B. and Bunch S.E.: Medical Management of recurrent seizures in dogs and cats. J. Am. Coll. Vet. Int. Med., *4*:26, 1990.
28. Leifer, C.E., et al.: Hypoglycemia associated with non islet cell tumor in 13 dogs. J. Am. Vet. Med. Assoc., *186*:53, 1985.
29. Leifer, et al.: Insulin secreting tumor: Diagnosis and medical and surgical management in 55 dogs. J. Am. Vet. Med. Assoc., *188*:60, 1986.
30. Mehlhaff, C.E., et al.: Insulin producing islet cell neoplasms: Surgical considerations and general management in 35 dogs. J. Am. Anim. Hosp. Assoc., *21*:607, 1985.
31. Meyer, D.J. and Noonan, N.E.: Liver tests in dogs receiving anticonvulsant drugs (diphenylhydantoin and primidone). J. Am. Anim. Hosp. Assoc., *17*:26, 1981.
32. Nafe, L.A., Parker, A., and Kay, W.J.: Sodium valproate. A preliminary clinical trial in epileptic dogs. J. Am. Anim. Hosp. Assoc., *17*:131, 1981.
33. Nash, A.S., Thompson, H., and Bogan, J.A.: Phenytoin toxicity: A fatal case in a dog with hepatitis and jaundice. Vet. Rec., *100*:280, 1977.
34. Parent, J.M.: Clinical management of seizures Vet. Clin. North Am. 18:605, 1988.
35. Parker, A.J., O'Brien, D., and Musselman, E.E.: Diazoxide treatment of metastatic insulinoma in a dog. J. Am. Anim. Hosp. Assoc., *18*:315, 1982.
36. Pasten, L.: Diphenylhydantoin in the canine: Clinical aspects and determinations of therapeutic blood levels. J. Am. Anim. Hosp. Assoc., *13*:247, 1977.
37. Pearce, L.A.: Potassium bromide as an adjunct to phenobarbital for management of uncontrolled seizures in dogs. Prog. Vet. Neurol., 1:95, 1990.
38. Pedersoli, W.M., Ganjam, V.K., and Nachreiner, R.E: Serum digoxin concentrations in dogs before, during and after concomitant treatment with phenobarbital. Am. J. Vet. Res., *41*:1639, 1980.
39. Raw, M.E. and Gaskell, C.J.: A review of one hundred cases of presumed canine epilepsy. J. Small Anim. Pract., *26*:645, 1985.
40. Russo, M.E.: The pathophysiology of epilepsy. Cornell Vet., *71*:221, 1981.
41. Sanders, J.E. and Yeary, R.A.: Serum concentrations of orally administered diphenylhydantoin in dogs. J. Am. Vet. Med. Assoc., *172*:153, 1978.
42. Sanders, J.E., Yeary, R.A., and Fenner, W.R.: Interaction of phenytoin with chloramphenicol or pentobarbital in the dog. J. Am. Vet. Med. Assoc., *175*:177, 1979.
43. Schulman, J.: Epileptic seizures controlled with paramethadione/primidone. (Vet. Med. Sm. Anim. Clin.) VMSAC, *76*:827, 1981.
44. Schwartz-Porsche, D., Loscher, W., and Frey, H.H.: Treatment of canine epilepsy with primidone. J. Am. Vet. Med. Assoc., *181*:592, 1982.
45. Shell, L.: Antiepileptic drugs. Compendium on Continuing Education, 6:432, 1984.
46. Skinner, S.F., et al.: Longitudinal study of phenobarbital in serum, cerebrospinal fluid, and saliva in the dog. Am. J. Vet. Res., *41*:600, 1980.

47. Sturtevant, F.S., Hoffman, W.E., and Dorner, J.L.: The effect of three anticonvulsant drugs and ACTH on canine serum alkaline phosphatase. J. Am. Anim. Hosp. Assoc., 13:754, 1977.
48. Van Der Velden, N.A.: Fits in Tervueren Shepherd dogs: A presumed hereditary trait. J. Small Anim. Pract., 9:63, 1968.
49. Wallace, M.E.: Keeshonds: A genetic study of epilepsy and EEG readings. J. Small Anim. Pract., 16:1, 1975.
50. Yeary, R.A.: Serum concentrations of primidone and its metabolities, phenyl-ethylamalonamide and phenobarbital, in the dog. Am. J. Vet. Res., 41:1643, 1980.

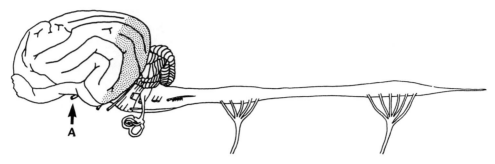

Figure 9–1. Location of a lesion producing a visual deficit. Optic nerve (A), optic tract, lateral geniculate nucleus, and optic radiations are beneath the cerebral cortex. Occipital lobe cerebral cortex is indicated by dotted region.

Location of the lesion (Figure 9–1): **optic nerve, optic tract, lateral geniculate nucleus, optic radiations, occipital lobe, cerebral cortex**

Mechanisms of disease and differential diagnosis

Congenital and familial disorders

Optic nerve hypoplasia
Hydrocephalus
  (Chap. 7)

Lissencephaly
  (Chap. 7)
Lysosomal storage
  diseases (Chap. 7)

Infections, immune-mediated disorders, and other inflammations

Optic neuritis

Meningoencephalitis
  (Chap. 7)

Metabolic disorders

Ischemia—anoxia
Severe hypoglycemia
Hepatoencephalopathy
Osmolality disturbances
Heat stroke

Toxicity

Severe lead poisoning

Nutritional disorders

Severe thiamine deficiency

Trauma and vascular disorders

Hemorrhage and edema   Infarcts

Neoplasia

Primary nervous system
Optic nerve
CNS
  (Chap. 7)

Metastatic nervous
system
  (Chap. 7)

Chapter 9

Visual dysfunction

Visual deficits in animals may be due to lesions within the eyeball itself or be associated with lesions of the innervation to the eye.[3,8] Diseases of the innervation necessary for vision are discussed in this chapter (Fig. 9–1).

The pathway for vision includes the retina, optic nerve, optic chiasm, optic tract, lateral geniculate nucleus, optic radiations, and occipital lobe cortex[4] (Fig. 9–2). Seventy-five percent of optic nerve fibers cross in the optic chiasm in dogs and 65% in cats. The major part of vision, therefore, has a contralateral representation in the cerebral cortex. However, as 25% and 35% of fibers in dogs and cats, respectively, stay on the same side, there can be visual dysfunction from visual field deficits, and this is referred to as hemianopsia or hemianopia. Visual fields can be crudely evaluated using the menace response and response to moving fingers or other objects in the temporal (lateral) or nasal (medial) visual fields. The visual fields and their corresponding retinal region are illustrated in Figure 9–2. The types of hemianopia are illustrated in Figure 9–3, and may occur with some lesions in dogs and cats. In other cases, sparing of the temporal or nasal visual field cannot be appreciated without electroretinography (ERG).

Some optic tract fibers exit and syn-

VISUAL FIELDS

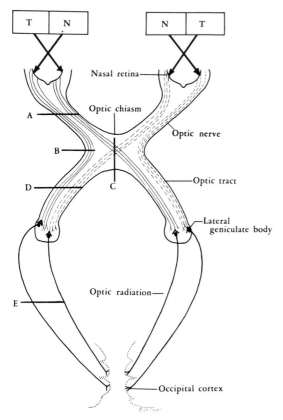

Figure 9–2. The neuroanatomic pathway for vision. (From Jenkins, T.W.: Functional Mamalian Neuroanatomy. Philadelphia, Lea & Febiger, 1978.)

mal is blind and has a loss of pupil response to light, a lesion must be present in the retina, optic nerve, optic chiasm, or optic tract prior to the exit of fibers to the pretectal nucleus (Fig. 9–4). This type of blindness may be referred to as peripheral blindness.

If the animal has a visual deficit and pupils that respond normally to light, the lesion most likely affects the visual pathway after the fibers to the pretectal region have left the optic tracts. These findings indicate a lesion of the caudal optic tracts, lateral geniculate body, optic radiations, and occipital lobe cortex and this type of blindness is called amaurosis or central blindness. As discussed above, total blind-

apse on pretectal nuclei, whereas others continue on and synapse with the lateral geniculate nucleus (Fig. 9–4). Fibers from the pretectal nuclei synapse on the Edinger-Westphal nucleus in the midbrain (Fig. 9–4). Fibers from the Edinger-Westphal nucleus pass through the oculomotor nerve (cranial nerve III) to provide parasympathetic innervation to the circular, smooth muscle of the iris.

When the optic and oculomotor nerve system is stimulated by light shining into the retina, the pupil constricts. If the ani-

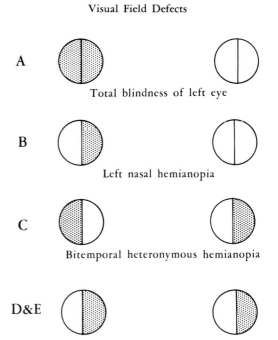

Visual Field Defects

A — Total blindness of left eye

B — Left nasal hemianopia

C — Bitemporal heteronymous hemianopia

D&E — Right homonymous hemianopia

Figure 9–3. A diagram of visual field defects produced by lesions of the visual pathway at levels corresponding to the letter in Figure 9–2. (From Jenkins, T.W.: Functional Mammalian Neuroanatomy. Philadelphia, Lea & Febiger, 1978.)

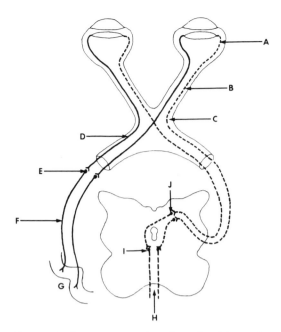

Figure 9–4. The neuroanatomic pathway for vision and pupillary light reflexes. (A) retina, (B) optic nerve, (C) optic chiasm, (D) optic tract, (E) lateral geniculate nucleus, (F) optic radiations, (G) occipital lobe cortex, (H) oculomotor nerve, (I) Edinger-Westphal nucleus, (J) pretectal nucleus. Broken lines outline the pupillary light reflex pathway. Unbroken lines outline the visual pathway. (After Palmer, 1976).

ness may not be present and a hemianopia may be seen (see Fig. 9–3) Animals with partial retinal disease may have reduced vision but the pupils may still be responsive to light, so thorough funduscopic and ERG examinations may be necessary to rule out primary retinal disease.

Patient evaluation

Signalment and history

Blindness from birth in young animals is suggestive of a developmental anomaly of the eye or visual pathway through the nervous system.

Blindness associated with systemic illness may be due to optic neuritis or meningoencephalitis, but sometimes no signs of systemic illness are present with these disorders.

Blindness following an episode of anoxia or other severe metabolic crisis may result from occipital lobe laminar necrosis.

Blindness following trauma may be associated with injury anywhere along the visual pathway.

On rare occasions, an animal may have endocrinopathy and associated blindness suggestive of a pituitary lesion, such as an infection or tumor, also involving the nearby optic chiasm. Most pituitary lesions grow into the hypothalamus and produce behavior changes and not visual deficits.

A history of other neurologic problems may aid in localizing the lesion to a specific region of the visual pathway or may support the presence of a multifocal disease process.

Physical and neurologic examinations

A thorough ophthalmologic examination should always be performed to rule out blindness associated with structural disease within the eye itself. Other information obtained on the physical examination may support infection, trauma, or neoplasia as a mechanism for the blindness (Chap. 3).

The neurologic examination is used to determine whether the animal is blind, whether one side is involved more than the other or whether there is a visual field deficit, and whether the blindness is caused by involvement of structures necessary for the pupillary light reflex or involvement of structures after the optic chiasm.

Vision may be grossly tested by observing the animal's ability to avoid obstacles while walking around an unfamiliar room. The eyes may be separately patched to see whether there is a difference in vision. The mental status of the animal should be carefully evaluated, because a demented, compulsively pacing animal will crash into obstacles because of unresponsiveness to the environment (Chap. 8).

Cotton balls may be tossed into the air: the animal will usually watch them fall silently to the ground if its vision and mental state are normal (Chap. 3).

The hand may be advanced toward the eye in a menacing gesture in nasal and temporal visual fields and blinking or avoidance observed (Chap. 3). A loss of menace-response may be seen in a young animal, a severely demented or blind animal, or an animal with facial paralysis or severe cerebellar disease.

Once the degree of visual deficit, any asymmetry, and the side of primary involvement are determined, the pupillary light reflexes are tested. Light shown in the right eye causes the right and left pupils to constrict because of the crossing of fibers at the optic chiasm and pretectal region.

If the right eye is blind and has no direct pupillary constriction and does not produce simultaneous constriction in the left pupil (consensual response), then the lesion is in the retina or right optic nerve (Table 9–1).

If both eyes are blind and the pupils are dilated and unresponsive to light either directly or consensually, then either bilateral retinal, optic nerve, or optic chiasm disease is present; however, bilateral optic nerve disease is most common (Table 9–1).

If the right eye has decreased vision with normal constriction of the right pupil and normal simultaneous constriction of the left pupil, the lesion is most likely located in the left optic tract (after the exit of fibers to the pretectal nucleus), lateral geniculate body, left optic radiations, or occipital lobe cortex (Table 9–1).

Lesions such as neoplasia of the left internal capsule may produce dementia, compulsive circling to the left, and placing, hopping, and proprioceptive deficits of the right side (Chap. 7). The optic radiations are located near the internal capsule and may also be involved, resulting in a menace-response deficit and decreased vision in the right eye, with a normal pupillary response to light.

If an animal is blind in both eyes and the pupils respond normally to light (amaurosis), a bilateral lesion in the optic tracts (after the exit of fibers to the pretectal nucleus), lateral geniculate bodies, optic radiations, or occipital cortex is present.

The degree of vision may be difficult to judge accurately in animals. Occasionally an animal with a retinal or optic nerve lesion may not respond well to visual tests but may have enough innervation for the pupil constriction to light. Occasionally the opposite is true. However, the combination of signs listed in Table 9–1 can serve as a helpful guide to localize the lesion.

Ancillary diagnostic investigations

The complete blood count (CBC) and chemistry profile findings may be abnormal in central nervous system (CNS) infections or with metabolic causes of blindness. Often the clinicopathologic tests are normal.

The electroencephalogram (EEG) is useful in evaluating diffuse and focal disease of the cerebral cortex. Blindness produced by occipital cerebral cortex disease may have an associated abnormal EEG (Chap. 5).

The cerebrospinal fluid (CSF) analysis may show increased white blood cells and protein in infections producing blindness or may show elevated pressure and protein content in neoplastic processes producing blindness (Chap. 5).

Table 9–1
Visual deficit and pupillary light reflex changes with lesions along the visual pathway

Lesion location	Neurologic exam findings
Unilateral retina or optic nerve	Ipsilateral visual deficit or blindness with no direct or consensual pupil response to light from the ipsilateral eye
Bilateral retina, optic nerves, or optic chiasm	Bilateral visual deficit or blindness with no direct or consensual pupil response to light in either eye.
Unilateral optic tract	Contralateral visual deficit with variable pupil responses, depending on the part of the tract involved, usually normal pupil responses if after fibers have exited to pretectal area (hemianopia)
Unilateral lateral geniculate nucleus, optic radiations, and occipital lobe cortex	Contralateral visual deficit with normal pupil responses (hemianopia)
Bilateral lateral geniculate nucleus, optic radiations, and occipital lobe cortex	Bilateral visual deficit or blindness with normal pupil responses (amaurosis)

Plain skull radiographs may aid in the diagnosis of optic nerve hypoplasia, hydrocephalus, lissencephaly, cranial vault fractures, and tumors producing blindness.

Special neuroradiographic techniques such as optic thecography, MRI, and CT scans can demonstrate changes associated with hydrocephalus, hemorrhage and infarcts, and neoplasia, which may produce blindness.[9,10]

Special electrodiagnostic testing of the visual system may also be performed. An electroretinography (ERG) is a recording of retinal electric alterations in response to a flashing light stimulus.[15] The ERG is an objective method of evaluating retinal function. If blindness is produced by structures behind the retina, the ERG will be normal. If the ERG is abnormal, the retina is diseased, but this does not rule out concomitant disease of the optic nerve or other parts of the visual pathway.

Visual evoked potentials (VEP) are electric alterations recorded from the scalp over the occipital lobe region of the cerebral cortex in response to flashes of light in the eye.[2,15,16] If the visual pathway is intact, a visual evoked potential will be seen. Studies are being performed on the normal and abnormal responses in animals. The VEP may be useful in testing visual acuity. Table 9–2 summarizes the diagnostic approach for evaluation of visual dysfunction.

Congenital and familial disorders

Optic nerve aplasia or hypoplasia

Incidence: Occasional

Bilateral optic nerve aplasia or hypoplasia is a lack of or an incomplete development of the optic nerve, optic chiasm, and optic tracts, respectively.[1,5,7] Optic nerve hypoplasia has a sporadic incidence in dogs and cats.

Affected animals are usually blind from birth with no history of other neurologic problems. The optic discs are smaller than normal on ophthalmoscopic examination, but the retina appears normal. The animals are blind, with bilaterally dilated unresponsive pupils suggestive of bilateral optic nerve disease.

ERG examination is normal, as the outer layers of the retina are normal. Small optic formina have been observed on skull radiographs.

There is no therapy for optic nerve hypoplasia and the animal will never be visual.

Hydrocephalus

Incidence: Frequent

Animals with hydrocephalus may have unilateral and bilateral visual deficits with normal pupillary light reflexes. The visual deficit is caused by reduction in the size of optic radiations and occipital lobe cerebral cortex. Hydrocephalus is described more fully in Chapter 7.

Lissencephaly

Incidence: Rare

Animals with lissencephaly often have bilateral loss of menace-response and may appear to have some visual deficit, although they are not blind. They have a lack of gyral formations in the occipital cortex as well as in other areas of the cerebral cortex. Lissencephaly is more fully described in Chapter 7.

Lysosomal storage disorders

Incidence: Rare

Blindness may be one of the signs associated with lysosomal storage disorders, particularly GM_2 gangliosidosis and ceroid lipofuscinosis. The blindness is most commonly associated with normal pupillary light reflexes. The neuronal changes occur in the lateral geniculate nucleus and occipital lobe cerebral cortex. Lysosomal storage diseases are described more fully in Chapter 7.

Infections, immune-mediated disorders, and other inflammations

Optic neuritis

Incidence: Frequent

Optic neuritis is an inflammation of the optic nerves producing impaired vision or blindness.[3,6,8,11] Optic neuritis has been associated with infections caused by canine distemper virus, toxoplasmosis, feline infectious peritonitis virus, cryptococcosis, blastomycosis, aspergillosis, and bacteremias, and also with granulomatous meningoencephalitis (GME—reticulosis) of the nervous system. Vitamin A deficiency, neoplasia, and reactions to toxic substances also have been incriminated. Cases of optic neuritis in man may be associated with immune-mediated disorders following viral infection. An immunopathologic origin is suspected in some cases of optic neuritis in dogs and cats.

Signalment and history. Several breeds of dogs and cats, ranging in ages from 7 months to 9 years, have been af-

Table 9–2
Diagnostic approach for the evaluation of visual dysfunction

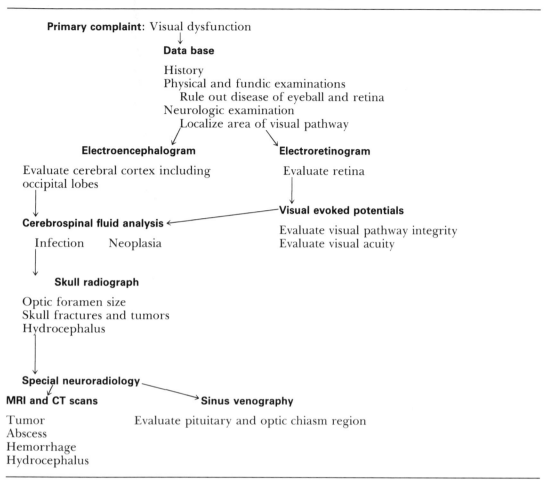

Primary complaint: Visual dysfunction

Data base

History
Physical and fundic examinations
    Rule out disease of eyeball and retina
Neurologic examination
    Localize area of visual pathway

Electroencephalogram

Evaluate cerebral cortex including
occipital lobes

Electroretinogram

Evaluate retina

Visual evoked potentials

Evaluate visual pathway integrity
Evaluate visual acuity

Cerebrospinal fluid analysis

Infection   Neoplasia

Skull radiograph

Optic foramen size
Skull fractures and tumors
Hydrocephalus

Special neuroradiology
MRI and CT scans   **Sinus venography**

Tumor   Evaluate pituitary and optic chiasm region
Abscess
Hemorrhage
Hydrocephalus

---

fected. The visual deficit is acute in onset and often unassociated with other neurologic signs or obvious disease in other systems.

Physical and neurologic examinations. Chorioretinitis lesions and enlarged optic discs from papillitis may be observed on ophthalmologic examination. The optic discs may also appear atrophic or may be normal. The animals may have varying degrees of visual deficit that is asymmetric or symmetric, or the animal may be completely blind. The pupils are often dilated and may have a decreased or absent response to light stimulation, depending on the severity of the optic nerve involvement (see Fig. 9–5). Other signs of neurologic deficit unassociated with the visual system may be seen and suggest a multifocal nervous system disease. In many cases of optic neuritis, the neurologic examination is normal except for the blindness and pupillary light reflex changes.

Ancillary diagnostic investigations. Clinicopathologic tests, including analysis of CSF, are often normal. EEG findings

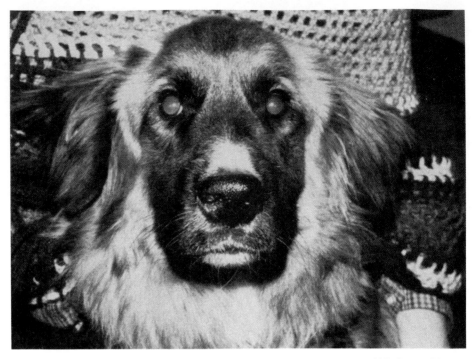

Figure 9–5. A 9-month-old male St. Bernard mix breed dog with an acute onset of blindness with dilated, unresponsive pupils. No abnormalities were found on ophthalmologic examination. Optic neuritis was suspected.

may support the presence of concomitant encephalitis or may be normal. If the outer layers of the retina are diseased, the ERG may be abnormal. The ERG is important to differentiate optic neuritis from sudden acquired retinal degeneration (SARD), another common cause of acute blindness. There may be no funduscopic changes with SARD, but the ERG will be abnormal.[12] There is no treatment for SARD, and the visual deficit is usually permanent. However, the ERG is normal when only the optic nerves are involved.

Therapy and prognosis. Glucocorticoid therapy has been suggested for the treatment of optic neuritis. Therapy may begin with high doses that are decreased over 3 to 5 weeks (Chap. 6). Some cases dramatically improve with glucocorticoids, while others respond little. Recurrence of blindness is common. The prognosis for the disease is often poor because the underlying neurologic disease may be encephalitis or GME. Optic neuritis may progress to optic nerve atrophy, with a permanent loss of vision.

Meningoencephalitis

Viral, protozoal, fungal, bacterial, rickettsial, and parasitic infections and granulomatous meningoencephalitis (reticulosis) and steroid-responsive inflammations of the CNS can produce a visual deficit along with other neurologic signs. These infections and inflammations are described in Chapter 7 and are listed in Tables 7–6 and 7–7. If the optic nerves are affected, the animal will have decreased vision and decreased or absent pupil responses to light. An inflammatory process located at the base of the brain may affect the pituitary gland and nearby optic chiasm, producing endocrine disorders and blindness. The signs produced by involvement of other nervous system structures may help to localize the lesion to a particular region of the visual pathway, or may support the presence of multifocal nervous system disease.

Infections and inflammations most commonly involve the optic tracts, lateral geniculate nucleus, optic radiations, or occipital cortex, and produce unilateral and bilateral visual deficits and normal pupils. EEG and CSF analysis are often the greatest aids in the diagnosis of multifocal CNS infections (Chap. 7).

Metabolic disorders

Ischemia—anoxia

Incidence: Frequent

Cerebral ischemia is a reduction in cerebral blood flow to levels that are insufficient to maintain normal function. Ischemia produces not only a lack of oxygen to tissues and local anoxia, but also a lack of substrates, such as glucose, necessary for energy metabolism (Chap. 1).

Cardiac arrest from anesthetic overdoses and other causes produces cerebral ischemia.[8,13] The areas of the cerebral cortex that suffer the most are those regions supplied by the terminations of the anterior and middle cerebral arteries where there is little collateral circulation. The vessels in the terminal regions referred to as "watershed areas" collapse first in cardiac insufficiency, and cerebrocortical necrosis occurs. Ischemic cerebrocortical necrosis has a laminar distribution in the layers of cerebral cortex and is bilaterally symmetric. The occipital lobe visual cortex is often affected. If the animals are resuscitated and survive, they are often blind with normal pupillary light responses.

Signalment and history. Any age, breed, or sex of dog or cat may suffer an ischemic insult. Total cerebral ischemia of 9 minutes or more usually produces severe brain damage or death in dogs. The animals are usually blind with normal pupils and may be severely demented on recovery.

Therapy and prognosis. Immediate therapy with 1 to 2 g/kg 20% mannitol and 30 mg/kg methylprednisolone sodium succinate (Solu-Medrol), both intravenously, should be given to treat cerebral edema (Chap. 6). The animal should then be maintained on prednisone 2 mg/kg divided every 12 hours for 5 to 7 days orally, then in decreasing doses every 3 to 5 days for 2 to 3 weeks, depending on the clinical response (Chap. 6).

In severe damage, the animals, may be demented, blind, and initially unable to ambulate. They must be hand-fed and given general supportive care. Coma, dilated pupils, and extensor rigidity indicate extensive midbrain damage (Chap. 10). This may be a direct result of ischemia, or may be due to tentorial herniation of the occipital lobes caused by cerebral edema (Chap. 10). If the latter case is true, the midbrain dysfunction may improve following therapy for cerebral edema. After a few days the animals usually begin to ambulate; however, they are often ataxic because of Purkinje cell damage in the cerebellum. Once the animals are ambulatory, they usually can maintain their nutrition and hydration themselves. The animals may be unresponsive to their environment or owners, and may not remember house training or any other training they have had. Over many months, affected animals may develop new personalities, reattach themselves to the owners, be retrained, and be acceptable pets. The blindness may be permanent, but the animals may also recover after many months. The animals may continue to improve clinically for as long as 1 year after the insult. The major limiting factor in the fate of these animals is the owner's unwillingness to commit the time and energy to care for a pet in this condition. Many people elect euthanasia. However, for those owners who absolutely refuse to give up, the animal may become an acceptable pet in time, although it may never be normal.

The animal may have seizures periodically following the ischemic insult, from acquired epilepsy (Chap. 8). The seizures can generally be controlled with routine anticonvulsant therapy and are usually not a severe complicating factor in the recovery of the animal (Chap. 8).

Pathology. On histologic examination of the nervous system, lesions are not confined to the cerebral cortex; they affect the brain stem and cerebellum as well. The amount of recovery an animal will have depends mainly on the severity of involvement of brain stem nuclei and the cerebellum.

Metabolic, toxic, and nutritional disorders

Other severe metabolic, toxic, and nutritional disorders affecting energy metabolism may produce laminar or pseudolaminar cerebrocortical necrosis and cause visual impairment in animals. Some of these are hypoxia, severe hypoglycemia, thiamine deficiency, chronic hepatic encephalopathy, heat stroke (hyperthermia), osmolality disturbances, and lead intoxication. Severe hypoglycemia and thiamine deficiency in small animals usually produce seizures, dementia, and coma (Chaps. 7, 8, and 10). Severe hypoglycemia can produce laminar necrosis with relative sparing of brain stem structures. Thiamine deficiency in large animals may produce a characteristic cerebrocortical laminar ne-

crosis, but brain stem nuclei hemorrhage is common in small animals (Chap. 7). Chronic liver failure and hepatic encephalopathy may produce laminar or pseudolaminar necrosis, but animals are usually presented with dementia and seizures, not blindness.

Trauma and vascular disorders

Hemorrhage and edema

Incidence: Frequent

Cerebral hemorrhage and edema from trauma may produce lesions anywhere along the visual pathway and produce visual deficits. Other neurologic deficits may be useful in localizing the lesion. The management of cerebral trauma is discussed in Chapter 10.

Infarcts

Incidence: Rare in dogs, occasional in cats

Cerebral infarction is rare in dogs and occurs only occasionally in cats. In the feline infarction syndrome, optic radiations or part of the occipital lobe cortex may be involved and result in a contralateral visual impairment with normal pupils. Infarction in the region of the optic chiasm may produce bilateral blindness with dilated, unresponsive pupils. Feline cerebral infarct syndrome usually has associated behavior disturbances, and is discussed in Chapter 7.

Neoplasia

Neoplasia at any site along the visual pathway produces visual deficits. A meningioma of the optic nerve may produce unilateral blindness.[14] Generally, other anatomic structures are affected and the associated signs help to localize the tumor. Visual deficits are often asymmetric.

Pituitary tumors rarely compress the optic chiasm in dogs as they do in man. On rare occasions however, the animal may have endocrinopathies and blindness in both eyes with dilated, unresponsive pupils. Meningiomas or gliomas at the base of the brain may compress the optic chiasm and produce similar signs.[17]

A primary CNS neoplasm, such as an astrocytoma, or neoplastic GME (reticulosis) can involve optic tracts and optic radiations and produce visual deficits. The visual deficit is most commonly asymmetric, as the tumor is often to one side of the midline. The pupils may be responsive to light if the optic tract is affected after the exit of the pretectal fibers, or if secondary cerebral swelling has not resulted in some tentorial herniation and slight midbrain compression. Behavior changes, circling, and contralateral hopping, placing, and proprioceptive deficits localize the lesion to the diencephalon near the internal capsule on one side.

Primary neoplasia of the occipital lobe cerebral cortex, such as an oligodendroglioma, may produce a unilateral visual deficit in the contralateral eye, with normal pupils. These signs may be overlooked, however, until internal capsule or midbrain involvement produces more obvious neurologic deficits.

Cerebral neoplasia and reticulosis are discussed further in Chapter 7.

References

1. Barnett, K.C. and Grimes, T.D.: Bilateral aplasia of the optic nerves in a cat. Br. J. Ophthalmol., 58:663, 1974.
2. Bichsel, P., et al.: Recording of visual evoked potentials in dogs with scalp electrodes. J. Vet. Intern. Med., 2:145, 1988.
3. Braund, K.G., et al.: Central (post retinal) visual impairment in the dog—a clinical–pathologic study. J. Small Anim. Pract., 18:395, 1977

4. DeLahunta, A.: The visual system. In Veterinary Neuroanatomy and Clinical Neurology. Philadelphia, W.B. Saunders, 1983.
5. Gelatt, K.N.: Textbook of Veterinary Ophthalmology. Philadelphia, Lea & Febiger, 1981.
6. Irby, N.L.: Diseases of the retina and optic nerve. In Current Veterinary Therapy IX. Edited by R.W. Kirk. Philadelphia, W.B. Saunders, 1986.
7. Kern, T.J. and Riis, R.C.: Optic nerve hypoplasia in three miniature poodles. J. Am. Vet. Med. Assoc., 178:49, 1981.
8. Kornegay, J.N.: Small Animal Neuro-Ophthalmology. Compendium on Continuing Education, 2:923, 1980.
9. LeCouteur, R.A., et al.: Indirect imaging of the canine optic nerve, using metrizamide (optic thecography). Am. J. Vet. Res., 43:1424, 1982.
10. LeCouteur, R.A., et al.: Computed tomography of orbital tumors in the dog. J. Am. Vet. Med. Assoc., 180:910, 1982.
11. Nafe, L.A.: Canine optic neuritis. Compendium on Continuing Education, 3:987, 1981.
12. Neaderland, M.H.: Sudden blindness. In Current Veterinary Therapy X. Edited by R.W. Kirk. Philadelphia, W.B. Saunders, 1989.
13. Palmer, A.C. and Walker, R.G.: The neuropathological effects of cardiac arrest in animals. J. Small Anim. Pract., 11:779, 1970.
14. Paulsen, M.E., et al.: Primary optic nerve meningioma in a dog. J. Am. Anim. Hosp. Assoc., 25:147, 1989.
15. Redding, R.W. and Myers, L.J.: Electrophysiologic diagnosis: Evoked response in veterinary neurology. Edited by J.R. Oliver, B.F. Hoerlein, and I.G. Mayhew. Philadelphia, W.B. Saunders, 1987.
16. Sims, M.H. and Laratta, L.J.: Visual evoked potentials in cats using a light emitting diode simulator. Am. J. Vet. Res., 49:1876, 1988.
17. Skerritt, G.C., et al.: Bilateral blindness in a dog due to invasion of the optic chiasma by a glioma. J. Small Anim. Pract., 27:97, 1986.

cial and somatic sensory pathways, such as those associated with touch, pain, temperature, hearing, and vision.

Stimulation of the ARAS results in stimulation or arousal of the cerebral cortex and an alert mental state. Decreased stimulation of the ARAS results in drowsiness. Lack of stimulation of the ARAS often results in sleep in the normal animal. Lesions of the ARAS result in decreased cerebral cortex stimulation, and can produce depression, delirium, semicoma, or coma. Diffuse frontal lobe cerebral cortex lesions can also produce these altered states of consciousness.

Sleep is an active physiologic process with several stages and varying electroencephalogram (EEG) patterns. Structures responsible for normal sleep cycles and patterns are located in the reticular formation of the caudal diencephalon, midbrain, pons, and rostral medulla.[8] Although the reticular formation structures of the lower pons and medulla have an important influence on sleep cycles, they are not necessary for the maintenance of consciousness in animals. Sleep is a highly complex mechanism and cannot simply be equated with coma as a loss of ARAS stimulation. Only the sleep disorders narcolepsy and cataplexy will be discussed in this chapter.

Patient evaluation

Acute alterations in consciousness or coma may be considered a neurologic emergency.[15] If diffuse cerebral edema occurs, coma may be due to caudal shifting of the brain and herniation of the occipital lobes of the cerebral cortex under the tentorium cerebelli, with resultant midbrain compression. Concurrently or shortly thereafter, the vermis of the cerebellum herniates through the foramen magnum to compress the caudal medulla oblongata. Alterations of function in vital centers in the medulla oblongata can result in death. A rapid diagnosis and correction of cerebral edema and tentorial and vermal herniation may save the life of the animal.

Diffuse cerebral edema may commonly be associated with head trauma, hypoxia, or anoxia, other metabolic disorders, toxicities, and cerebral neoplasia.

Signalment and history

Mechanisms of disease associated with certain ages, breeds, and sexes of animals are discussed in Chapter 2. The onset, progression, and duration of the altered state of consciousness should be immediately determined. It is important to establish the possibility or known incident of recent head trauma in an animal demonstrating a rapidly deteriorating level of consciousness or coma. Possible exposure to CNS depressant drugs such as barbiturates and other tranquilizers should also be questioned. The environment in which the animal was found in a comatose state might give insight into a possible mechanism of disease.

A history of previous behavior alterations, seizures, or other neurologic signs and of disease in other systems may support a diagnosis of infection, metabolic disturbance, nutritional deficiency, or neoplastic process producing the coma.

Physical and neurologic examinations

The animal should be examined and treated for life-threatening problems associated with trauma, such as an obstructed airway or external hemorrhage or hemorrhage into one of the body cavities. Mucous membranes should be examined for pallor or cyanosis, and therapy for shock or hypoxia administered.[7] Respirations and cardiac rate and rhythm should be carefully examined to rule out cardiopulmonary disease secondarily producing the neurologic signs caused by hypoxia or ischemia. Pulse and respirations should be monitored continually to evaluate vital center functions of the brain stem. Diencephalic and midbrain lesions may produce a rhythmic pattern of shallow, deep, then shallow respirations, followed by a period of apnea (Cheyne-Stokes respirations); midbrain lesions can also produce hyperventilation; and lesions of the pons and medulla oblongata can produce irregular or ataxic shallow respirations.[15] Severe lesions of the medulla oblongata also produce a loss of sinus arrhythmia of the heart. Midbrain lesions may produce bradycardia. Body temperature should be examined and monitored to rule out hyperthermia as a cause of the altered state of consciousness.

The neurologic examination is performed to help localize the lesion to the midbrain or the diencephalic and cerebral cortical portion of the ARAS. The level of consciousnss is determined by the response of the animal to noxious external stimuli. If the animal is violently delirious, 1 to 5 mg intravenous diazepam (Valium) may be administered as suggested for status epilepticus (Chap. 6). No drugs causing heavy sedation, such as barbiturates, or pupil changes, such as atropine, should be administered. The size, symmetry, and responsiveness to light of the pupils are evaluated. The pupils may be equally miotic, and only slightly reactive in diffuse cerebral and diencephalic lesions. Midbrain lesions produce altered states of consciousness, commonly semicoma or coma, with large or midposition fixed pupils that are unresponsive to light. Unilateral mydriasis with an unresponsive dilated pupil and an altered state of consciousness is most often caused by ipsilateral, unilateral midbrain disease, and is most comonly seen with cerebral edema and unilateral herniation of the occipital lobe under the tentorium cerebelli.

Vestibular nystagmus and ocular mobility can be tested to evaluate the integrity of the medial longitudinal fasciculus (MLF) through the medulla oblongata, pons, and midbrain from vestibular nuclei to oculomotor nuclei (Chap. 12). If the semicomatose or comatose animal has had or is suspected of having a head injury, the head and neck should not be moved to test vestibular nystagmus. Head and neck injuries commonly occur together. The signs of a cervical lesion may be masked by the altered state of consciousness and may be worsened by manipulation of the neck. The caloric test may be performed to determine the integrity of the brainstem and oculomotor nucleus and nerves. The external ear canal may be irrigated with hot tap water and the eyeballs observed for horizontal nystagmus with the fast phase toward the side tested (Chap. 12). A loss of vestibular nystagmus or caloric-test-response in a comatose or semicomatose animal supports the diagnosis of a midbrain lesion producing the altered consciousness.

The eyeballs should be observed for strabismus. Oculomotor nerve damage associated with midbrain disease produces a ventrolateral deviation of the eyeball.

The midbrain also contains the red and reticular formation nuclei, the origin of important flexor or voluntary motor tracts in animals (Chap. 1). If this region is damaged flexor muscle tone is decreased and the activity in the vestibulospinal and pontine reticulospinal tracts to extensor muscles of the limbs is unopposed. Rigidity of limb extensor muscles is referred to as decerebrate rigidity. In a comatose animal, decerebrate rigidity usually indicates a severe midbrain lesion.

A summary of physical and neurologic examination findings localizing the lesion in a comatose animal are outlined in Table 10–1. The animal may not have all the signs of dysfunction of a certain region. Consciousness and pupil response to light are lost initially. The other cranial nerves

Table 10–1
Location of the lesion and neurologic examination findings in the comatose animal

Location of lesion	Neurologic signs
Cerebrum, diencephalon	Coma, semicoma Normal or miotic responsive pupils Normal vestibular nystagmus Cheyne-Stokes respiration
Midbrain	Coma, semicoma Dilated unresponsive pupils (unilateral or bilateral) Midpoint fixed unresponsive pupils Loss of vestibular nystagmus Ventrolateral strabismus Hyperventilation Cheyne-Stokes respiration Bradycardia
Pons and medulla	Depressed Miotic or normal pupils Loss of vestibular nystagmus Deficits of cranial nerves V–XII Depressed or ataxic respirations Bradycardia, loss of sinus arrhythmia

may be examined to evaluate the integrity of the pons and medulla oblongata (Chap. 11).

Any voluntary movement is noted and spinal reflexes are examined. A traumatized animal should be manipulated as little as possible to prevent further damage to the spinal cord from possibly fractured vertebrae. Absent spinal reflexes most often indicate concurrent spinal cord or peripheral nerve disease.

Serial neurologic examinations should be performed as frequently as needed to evaluate the animal for further deterioration or improvement. The animal is deteriorating and midbrain disease is present if the level of consciousness decreases from semicomatose to comatose, if the pupils go

from normal or miotic to mydriatic or midpoint-fixed, if the caloric test becomes negative, and if ventrolateral strabismus and extensor rigidity of the limbs develops.

The prognosis for recovery from coma due to midbrain disease is generally poorer than recovery from diffuse cerebral or diencephalic disease.

Ancillary diagnostic investigations

In acute coma of unknown cause, initial clinicopathologic tests can be very important to rule out metabolic disease. A complete blood count (CBC) may support a diagnosis of severe anemia, polycythemia, or infection. Immediate serum glucose, blood urea nitrogen (BUN), and electrolyte determinations should be performed. Hyperglycemia, hypoglycemia, uremia, and hypoadrenocorticism may produce collapse and altered states of consciousness.

Serum osmolality may be estimated using the following formula:

$$\text{Serum osmolality} = 2 (Na^+ + K^+)$$
$$+ \frac{\text{Serum glucose}}{18}$$
$$+ \frac{\text{BUN}}{2.8} = \frac{\text{mOsm}}{\text{kg } H_2O}$$

Normal values are approximately 300 mOsm/kg H_2O. Cerebral signs may be seen when serum osmolality is over 350 mOsm/kg H_2O.

Serum bile acids, Bromsulphalein (BSP), and blood ammonia determinations may be useful in evaluating hepatic coma (Chap. 7).

An electrocardiogram (ECG) should be evaluated if arrhythmia and cardiovascular problems are suspected from the findings of the physical examination. Cardiac arrhythmias are commonly associated with head injuries and the heart should be monitored on all dogs and cats who have received a traumatic injury.

An electroencephalogram (EEG) may be helpful in determining the underlying disease process and prognosis (Chap. 5). A slowing and flattening of the EEG with burst suppression is indicative of severe cerebral cortical depression as seen with toxicities, severe metabolic disturbances, and cerebral edema.

Cerebrospinal fluid (CSF) analysis is the greatest aid in the diagnosis of central nervous system (CNS) infections (Chap. 7). Animals with a known head injury should not have CSF collected from the cisterna magna, as this produces a low pressure area at the collection site and causes occipital lobe and cerebellar vermal herniation. If the pressure is elevated on CSF collection in an animal that has not had head trauma, a small amount of fluid is removed for analysis, and 1 to 2 gm/kg 20% mannitol and 30 mg/kg methylprednisolone sodium succinate (Solu-Medrol) are given intravenously for cerebral edema (Chap. 6).

Table 10–2 outlines the diagnostic approach to an animal with an altered state of consciousness or coma.

Congenital and familial disorders

Hydrocephalus

Incidence: Frequent

Animals with hydrocephalus commonly have behavior disorders (Chap. 7) or seizures (Chap. 8). A mild head injury in a hydrocephalic dog can produce severe cerebral hemorrhage with an associated altered state of consciousness or coma. The diagnosis and therapy of hydrocephalus is discussed in Chapter 7.

Lysosomal storage disorders

Incidence: Rare

The lysosomal storage disorders have a variety of clinical signs, depending on the particular enzyme defect (Chap. 7). The end stage of some of these disorders, particularly GM_2 gangliosidosis, ceroid lipofuscinosis, and neuronal glycoproteinosis, may result in more than a demented animal. The animal may become delirious, semicomatose, or comatose.

Narcolepsy

Incidence: Occasional

Narcolepsy is a transient altered state of consciousness and muscle tone that is classified as a disorder of sleep.[2,5,10] An abnormal concentration and turnover of several neurotransmitters in brain stem sleep

Table 10–3
Chemicals affecting the nervous system producing altered states of consciousness

- acetonitrile
- acridium chloride
- acrylonitrile
- *Agrostemma githago*
- *Amanita muscaria*
- *Amanita phalloides*
- alkylmercury
- arsenic trioxide
- arsine
- *Aspidium*
- atropine
- benzalkonium chloride
- benzene
- *Blighia sapida*
- bromate
- camphor
- carbon monoxide
- carbon tetrachloride
- castor beans
- castor oil
- cresol
- cubeb
- dichloroethylene
- dinitrobenzene
- dinitrocresol
- dinitrophenol
- diphenhydramine
- diphenylhydantoin
- endrin
- ethylene glycol
- gasoline
- *Gloriosa suberba*
- *Gymnothorax flavimarginalus*
- homatropine
- insulin
- *Jatrophora ureus*
- Lethane
- lithium chloride
- malathion
- *Melia azedarach*
- metaldehyde
- methanol
- methantheline bromide
- methapyrilene HCl
- methyl formate
- methyl salicylate
- naphthalene
- nerve gas
- nitrobenzene
- organo-phosphate insecticides
- *Parthenocissus quine*
- perchloroethylene
- phenol
- picrotoxin
- *quafolia*
- *Rhoicissus comeifolio* (root)
- *Rhodotypus* (berries)
- saffron
- scopolamine
- *Senecia canicida*
- sodium fluoroacetate
- tetrachloroethane
- toluene
- trichloroethylene
- trinitrotoluene
- urethane
- Vitamin D
- *Zygadenus*

Courtesy of Dr. Roger Yeary. The Ohio State University, Dept. of Veterinary Physiology and Pharmacology

Trauma and vascular disorders

Trauma

Incidence: Frequent

Intracranial injury and resulting cerebral hemorrhage or edema are among the most common causes of an altered state of consciousness dealt with in veterinary practice.[1,4,6]

In many instances, the trauma is witnessed or lacerations and bruising around the head are found on the physical examination.

Intracranial injury often produces a neurologic emergency that must be dealt with immediately. The first steps to take in evaluation and management of the head injury patient are listed in Table 10–4.

Invariably, some degree of cerebral edema develops, which may be fatal unless immediately managed. A patent airway should be established and oxygen therapy given as the first step in control of cerebral edema. The head should be elevated slightly and no pressure should be placed on the jugular veins. The mucous membrane perfusion and color, heart rate and rhythm, signs of external or internal hemorrhage, and body temperature are quickly examined and the animal is treated for life-threatening problems. Cerebral hypoxia and ischemia from lowered cardiac output both contribute to the development of cerebral edema.

Intravenous fluid administration is used to combat shock, but discontinued once shock is controlled, as overhydration may complicate cerebral edema. Methyl-

prednisolone sodium succinate (Solu-Medrol) 30 mg/kg is administered intravenously (Chap. 6). Ampicillin 11 to 22 mg/kg every 8 hours, chloramphenicol 50 mg/kg every 8 hours, or trimethoprim sulfadiazine 15 mg/kg every 12 hours are often given parenterally to prevent endotoxic shock. Antibiotics may be continued if open wounds are present or cranial surgery is performed.

Once acute life-threatening problems and shock are controlled, the initial baseline neurologic examination is performed. If the animal is semicomatose or comatose, it should be manipulated as little as possible until the possibility of concurrent vertebral fractures is ruled out. The level of consciousness is noted. If the animal is delirious or having seizures, diazepam may be administered intravenously, but nothing should be given that will alter the consciousness or affect the pupils.

Pupil size, symmetry, and responsive-

Table 10–4
Management of intracranial injury

1. Establish a patent airway—give oxygen, elevate head
2. Examine for and treat life-threatening problems
3. Treat shock:
   a. Fluids—do not overhydrate (no jugular catheters)
   b. Glucocorticoids (methyl prednisolone sodium succinate 10–30 mg/kg intravenously)—repeat every 8 hours for cerebral edema control
   c. Antibiotics—continue if open wounds or if craniotomy performed
4. Neurologic examination
   a. Monitor level of consciousness.
   b. Monitor pupil size, symmetry, and responsiveness to light.
   c. Evaluate caloric response.
   d. Examine other cranial nerves.
   e. Note posture abnormalities and voluntary movements.
   f. Monitor rate and rhythm of respirations.
   g. Monitor rate and rhythm of heart.
   h. Monitor body temperature.
5. If deterioration is seen on serial neurologic examinations, or midbrain compression suspected on initial exam:
   a. Give 20% mannitol, 1–2.2 g/kg intravenously.
   b. Craniotomy for cerebral edema and hemorrhage control

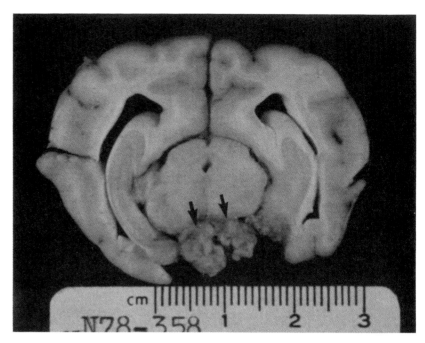

Figure 11–5. A meningioma (arrows) compressing the right oculomotor nerve in a 12-year-old Chihuahua with a dilated nonresponsive right pupil and ventrolateral deviation of the eyeball.

of the eyeball in the periorbital region (Fig. 11–6).

The abducent nerve nucleus is located in the rostral medulla oblongata near the midline just ventral to the floor of the fourth ventricle. The abducent nerve fibers pass ventrally and exit in the rostral portion of the medulla oblongata lateral to the pyramids. The abducent nerve exits through the orbital fissure of the skull to innervate the lateral rectus and retractor oculi muscles of the eyeball (see Fig. 11–6).

Neurologic examination

The direction of eyeball deviation observed when the head is at rest indicates which cranial nerve is affected. If the oculomotor nerve is damaged, the eyeball will deviate ventrolaterally or downward and outward (Fig. 11–7). There may also be a slight ptosis of the eyelid. If the trochlear nerve is damaged, there may be little observable eyeball deviation in dogs, but a lateral deviation of the superior retinal vein may be visualized on a funduscopic examination. When the trochlear nerve is dysfunctional in cats, their vertical pupil rotates such that the dorsal aspect is lateral and the ventral aspect is medial.[4] If the abducent nerve is damaged, a medial or inward deviation of the eyeball occurs and the eyeball may be unable to retract.

When the head is moved and eyeball movement observed, the amount of paresis or paralysis in various planes can be estimated.

Bilateral oculomotor nerve damage produces a divergent strabismus, and each eyeball deviates ventrolaterally. Bilateral abducent nerve disease produces a convergent strabismus, and each eyeball deviates medially.

If strabismus is the only neurologic deficit present in an animal, the lesion prob-

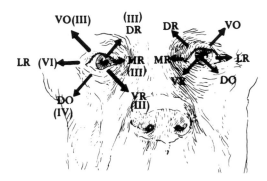

Figure 11–6. Direction the eyeball is pulled by the individual muscles is indicated by the arrows. VO (III), ventral oblique muscles—oculomotor nerve; LR (VI), lateral rectus muscles—abducent nerves; DO (IV), dorsal oblique muscles—trochlear nerve; VR (III) ventral rectus muscles—oculomotor nerve; MR (III) medial rectus muscles—oculomotor nerve; DR (III) dorsal rectus muscles—oculomotor nerve. (From Jenkins, T.: Functional Mammalian Neuroanatomy. Philadelphia, Lea & Febiger, 1978.)

pathways and the medial longitudinal fasciculus, cross to the opposite side, and synapse on the oculomotor, trochlear, and abducent nuclei to produce cooperative conjugate eye movements to the left. The left frontal lobe cortex moves the eyeballs to the right. When the eyeballs are voluntarily moved to the right, the right abducent and left oculomotor nerves are stimulated and the right oculomotor nerves and left abducent are inhibited. In lesions destroying the upper motor neuron influence on conjugate eyeball movement, the eyeballs may deviate toward the side of the lesion and are referred to as adversive eye movements. During a seizure discharge, the eyeballs may deviate away from the side of the focus, as seen with normal stimulation (Chap. 8).

ably involves some site along the peripheral cranial nerve or in the muscle.

If strabismus is caused by involvement of nuclei or fibers within the brain stem, there are often other signs of neurologic deficit from involvement of surrounding neuroanatomic structures.

If a midbrain lesion alters nerve function and produces ventrolateral strabismus, other signs may occur, such as contralateral or ipsilateral hemiparesis with unilateral lesions or alterations in consciousness, and quadriparesis with bilateral lesions (Chap. 10).

If a lesion in the medulla oblongata produces medial strabismus, then limb ataxia, proprioceptive deficits, ipsilateral hemiparesis or quadriparesis, and other cranial nerve signs such as head tilt, nystagmus, and facial paralysis may be seen. Disturbances in vital signs may also occur.

It is important to differentiate peripheral cranial nerve disease from brain stem disease, as the prognosis for the animal with the latter is generally more ominous.

Upper motor neurons originating in the right frontal lobe cerebral cortex descend through corticoreticular ocular

Disease

The mechanisms of disease and differential diagnosis of strabismus include congenital problems, infections, trauma, vascular disorders, and neoplasia, involving either the peripheral cranial nerves and muscles or the brain stem nuclei.[21]

Strabismus is often accompanied by other signs of neurologic dysfunction, but can occasionally be seen alone.

Congenital. Congenital convergent strabismus is commonly seen in Siamese cats. The eyeballs, however, are not paralyzed and there are no abducent nerve lesions. The underlying cause is thought to be an abnormal development of retinal neuronal projections to the lateral geniculate nucleus in the visual pathway. This disorder usually has little clinical significance in the affected Siamese cats (Fig. 11–8).

Occasional cases of congenital convergent strabismus are seen in dogs and are also of little clinical significance.

Divergent strabismus associated with hydrocephalus is usually caused by an ab-

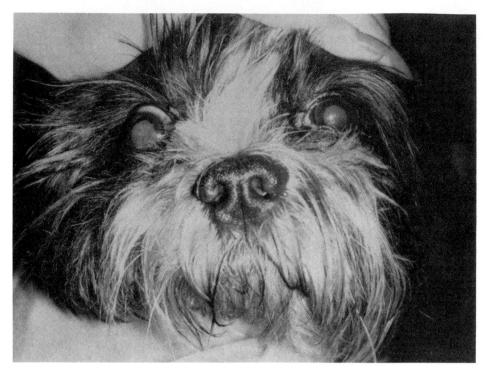

Figure 11–7. Oculomotor nerve paralysis of the right eye. The right eyeball is deviated ventrolaterally and the right pupil is dilated. (Courtesy of Dr. Milton Wyman, Veterinary Medical Teaching Hospital, The Ohio State University.)

normal formation of the skull, and not oculomotor nerve disease (Chap. 7).

Infections. Brain stem infections and inflammations may affect cranial nerves III, IV, and VI and produce strabismus, but will also have conscious proprioceptive deficits, hemiparesis, or quadriparesis or alterations in consciousness from involvement of ascending and descending sensory and motor tracts.

If a brain stem lesion is localized and

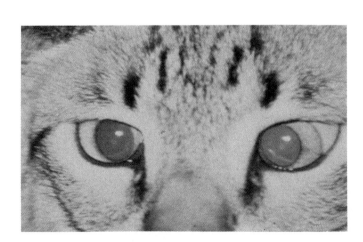

Figure 11–8. Congenital convergent strabismus of Siamese cats. (Courtesy of Dr. Milton Wyman, Veterinary Medical Teaching Hospital, The Ohio State University.)

an infection is suspected, cerebrospinal fluid analysis is the greatest aid to the diagnosis (Chap. 5). Infections of the nervous system are described in Chapters 7 and 12.

Trauma and vascular. Brain stem trauma with hemorrhage and edema can produce strabismus along with other signs of neurologic deficit. Diagnosis and management of cranial trauma are discussed in Chapter 10.

On rare occasions, cerebrovascular disease may produce infarctions of a region of the brain stem, and strabismus and other neurologic signs can result.

Neoplasia. Neurofibrosarcomas, neurofibromas, and neurinomas of individual cranial nerves may produce unilateral strabismus with no other neurologic signs. Neoplasia of peripheral nerves is discussed in Chapter 18. Meningiomas also may occur in a region after the nerve has exited the brain stem. Eventually, these types of tumors slowly enlarge and compress a portion of the brain stem to produce other signs of neurologic deficit (see Fig. 11–5).

Other primary CNS tumors and metastatic tumors may involve cranial nerves III, IV, and VI, as well as the other brain stem structures. Primary CNS and metastatic tumors are described in Chapter 7.

Dropped jaw

Mechanisms of disease and differential diagnosis

Infections and other inflammations. Viral, bacterial, protozoal, or fungal disease and granulomatous meningoencephalitis or other inflammations involving the motor trigeminal nuclei or nerves bilaterally (Chaps. 7 and 12)

Trauma. Bilateral motor trigeminal nerve injury

Idiopathic. Transient trigeminal neuritis

A dropped jaw is usually caused by an inability to close the mouth, and is seen in acute bilateral lesions of the motor portion of the trigeminal nerve. The motor nucleus of the trigeminal nerve is located in the pons at the level of the rostral cerebellar peduncle. The trigeminal motor nerve fibers join the sensory neurons of the trigeminal nerve and pass through the trigeminal canal of the petrosal bone.[4] The fibers then join the mandibular nerve and pass through the oval foramen of the skull to innervate the muscles of mastication, the masseter, temporal, pterygoids, rostral digastricus, and myelohyoid muscles.

Upper motor neurons from the frontal cerebral cortex descend in corticobulbar pathways, cross to the opposite side, and synapse on the motor nucleus of the trigeminal nerve to produce voluntary chewing movements. In severe diffuse cerebral disease with dementia, the jaw may also drop slightly, but the animal can close it occasionally.

Neurologic examinations

A dropped jaw may be the only neurologic deficit in bilateral motor trigeminal nerve disease, or may be associated with proprioceptive deficits and paresis of the limbs in disease of the pons. Persistent bilateral nerve damage can result in atrophy of the temporalis and masseter muscles.

Disease

As listed in the mechanisms of disease and differential diagnosis, a dropped jaw may be associated with infections or trauma. Occasionally, bilateral luxation or subluxation of the temporomandibular joint may be responsible for a bilateral motor trigeminal nerve injury and a dropped jaw.[17]

A transient dropped jaw of unknown origin has been described in dogs.[4,21]

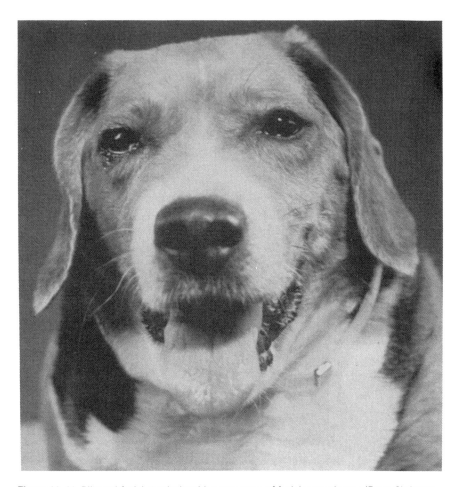

Figure 11–14. Bilateral facial paralysis with contracture of facial musculature. (From Chrisman, C.L.: Disorders of the vestibular system. The Compendium on Continuing Education. *1*(10):747, 1979.)

mone (TSH) test should be performed on all dogs with facial paralysis with no obvious cause (Fig. 11–15).

Trauma. Trauma to the facial nerve superficially on the side of the face, at the base of the ear, or from a skull fracture through the stylomastoid foramen may result in facial nerve paralysis, which can be permanent. EMG examination of facial muscles and nerve stimulation of the facial nerve may be useful in evaluating nerve integrity. The nerve is stimulated at the base of the ear and an evoked response is recorded from muscles of the eyelid, ear, and lips. Peripheral nerve injuries are further discussed in Chapter 18.

Neoplasia. Neurofibrosarcoma, neurofibroma, neurinoma, meningioma, and lymphosarcoma or other metastatic tumors may affect peripheral portions of the facial nerve and initially produce few other signs.[16] Primary and metastatic CNS tumors that may affect the brain stem in this region are discussed in Chapters 7 and 12.

Idiopathic. Acute unilateral or bilateral facial nerve paralysis may be seen in man, and is referred to as Bell's palsy.

Adult dogs, especially Cocker spaniels, may be affected.[10] There are no other signs of neurologic dysfunction. Clinical signs include drooped ear, paralyzed eyelid, and drooped lips. There is no evidence of otitis media on physical or radiographic examination. Positive waves and fibrillation potentials are found in only those muscles innervated by the facial nerve. The facial paralysis is often permanent, and no therapy appears to alter the disease process. Artificial tears may have to be used if sicca is a problem. However, the majority of affected dogs have a normal Schirmer's tear test and tear supplementation is unnecessary. The cornea may be kept moist by retraction of the globe and elevation of the membrane nictitans. The animals can live comfortably with their deficit.

Dysphagia

Mechanisms of disease and differential diagnosis

Infections and other inflammations
Rabies (Chap. 7)
Other viral, bacterial, protozoal, or fungal diseases and granulomatous meningoencephalitis or other inflammations of the medulla oblongata or glossopharyngeal or vagus nerves (Chaps. 7 and 12)

Inflammatory and immune-mediated neuromuscular disorders
Myasthenia gravis (Chap. 16)
Acute polyradiculoneuritis (Chap. 16)
Polymyositis (Chap. 16)

Metabolic and toxic disorders
Other diffuse neuromuscular diseases (Chap. 16)

Trauma and vascular disorders
Hemorrhage, edema, or an infarct involving the medulla oblongata or glossopharyngeal or vagus nerves

Neoplasia
Primary or metastatic CNS or PNS neoplasia involving the medulla oblongata or glossopharyngeal or vagus nerves (Chaps. 7 and 18)

Idiopathic disorders
Cricopharyngeal achalasia
Rule-out non-neurologic disease of the oropharynx

Dysphagia is an inability to swallow properly, which may be caused by disease of the glossopharyngeal nerve, vagus nerve, or associated nuclei of the caudal medulla oblongata.

The glossopharyngeal nerve carries general sensation from the posterior third of the tongue and pharynx. The cell bodies are located in the petrosal ganglion. The axons enter the lateral side of the medulla oblongata caudal to the vestibulocochlear and facial nerves and terminate in the nucleus of the solitary tract.[4] The glossopharyngeal nerve also carries motor fibers, whose cell bodies are located in the rostral two thirds of the nucleus ambiguus in the middle to caudal region of the medulla oblongata. The glossopharyngeal nerve exits the jugular foramen and occipitotympanic fissure of the skull and innervates the stylopharyngeus muscle and some minor pharyngeal musculature. Proper function of sensory and motor components is necessary for swallowing. The glossopharyngeal nerve also innervates the parotid salivary gland.

The vagus nerve innervates the remaining skeletal musculature of the soft palate, larynx, and pharynx. The cell bodies are located in the middle portion of the nucleus ambiguus and axons exit on the lateral aspect of the medulla oblongata caudal to the glossopharyngeal nerve.

Axons of neurons in the caudal portion of the nucleus ambiguus exit the brain stem with the cranial root of the accessory nerve (cranial nerve XI) and join the vagus

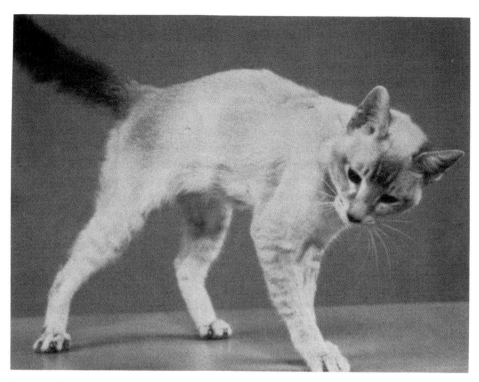

Figure 12–5. A 3-year-old male Lynx point Siamese cat with the idiopathic vestibular syndrome and a left head tilt. (From Chrisman, C.L.: Disorders of the vestibular system. The Compendium on Continuing Education. *1*(10):750, 1979.)

in air by the pelvis, which also causes the head tilt and twisting of the body to become more obvious (Fig. 12–6). A vestibular deficit becomes more obvious if the animal is placed in a water bath, swimming pool, or lake because the forces of gravity are altered. Care must be taken to avoid drowning. If a vestibular deficit is questionable, a small animal can be lifted in the air and dropped onto a heavily padded surface to assess its righting capabilities. With a vestibular deficit, the animal will inappropriately land on its side or back instead of its feet. This test should be used only if vestibular signs are not obvious and with great caution to avoid injury to the animal. The above tests are useful if the vestibular signs on initial examination are subtle, or if a bilateral vestibular deficit is suspected.

Paradoxical vestibular signs have been described with cerebellovestibular lesions. In these cases, the head tilt is directed away from the side of the lesion. Affected animals may have hypermetria of the forelimb on the side of the lesion (opposite the side of the head tilt), which is caused by cerebellar involvement.

With bilateral vestibular deficits, head tilt and nystagmus are frequently absent. The animal may be ataxic from the loss of equilibrium, and the signs may be initially confused with those of cerebellar disease (Chap. 15). However, on close observation, there is no hypermetria, intention tremor, or characteristic head bobbing seen as with cerebellar disease. With bilateral vestibular disease, the animal falls to either side and has a loss of balance with normal strength. Head movements generally consist of wide

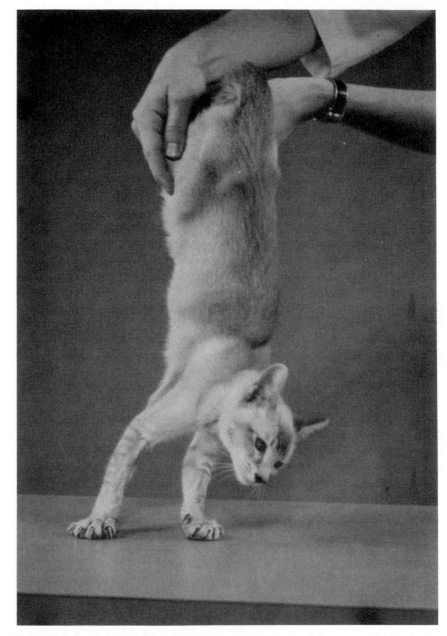

Figure 12–6. Same cat as in Figure 12–5, now suspended by the pelvis, accentuating the head tilt and body twist to the left. (From Chrisman, C.L.: Disorders of the vestibular system. The Compendium on Continuing Education. *1*(10):745, 1979.)

excursions from side to side. If suspended by the pelvis, an animal with bilateral vestibular disease will curl its neck ventrally, and if slowly lowered to the ground, will inappropriately land on the dorsum of the neck instead of the front feet (Chap. 3).

Tight circling to the side of the lesion and a reluctance to turn in the opposite direction may be seen in unilateral vestibular disease. The animal often prefers to lean and walk along a wall on the affected side for support. The animal may bump into objects because of the loss of equilibrium. An animal with a severe acute vestibular disturbance is often so disoriented that continuous rolling and inability to stand can be observed. Serial neurologic evaluations are necessary to determine whether gait deficits are present once the severe rolling stage has passed. Unilateral dysmetria indicates ipsilateral brain stem or cerebellar dysfunction.

In peripheral vestibular dysfunction, there is a decrease in extensor tone on the affected side and an increase in extensor tone on the opposite side. The animal leans toward the side of the lesion. Leaning should not be confused with hemiparesis, where obvious weakness is present. The postural reactions, hopping and placing, and proprioceptive positioning should only reflect a loss of balance, not strength. Brain stem disease is indicated when the animal is too incoordinated or weak to perform the postural reactions or if a conscious proprioceptive deficit is present.

Spinal reflexes can be difficult to assess if the animal is reluctant to lie on one side, struggles, or continually rolls toward the side of the lesion. The spinal reflexes and superficial and deep sensation should be intact, unless concurrent spinal cord or peripheral nerve disease to the limbs is present. Depressed spinal reflexes and obvious muscle atrophy are found if the peripheral nerves to the limbs also are diseased.

After completing the neurologic examination, the examiner should be able to conclude whether the lesion is peripheral (involving only receptors or vestibular nerves) or central (involving vestibular nuclei or the flocculonodular lobe of the cerebellum). The prognosis in peripheral vestibular disorders is generally better than in central vestibular disorders. A summary of the neurologic signs at various anatomic regions differentiating peripheral from central vestibular lesions is found in Table 12–1.

Serial neurologic evaluations over subsequent days are extremely important in determining the prognosis. Idiopathic peripheral vestibular disorders usually appear severe initially, but rapidly improve and have a favorable prognosis.

Ancillary diagnostic investigations

Hematologic and serum biochemical tests frequently do not contribute to the diagnosis of a vestibular problem. Occasionally, neutrophilic leukocytosis is seen with severe inner ear infections, or leukopenia that is suggestive of a viral infection.

In an animal with seizures, behavior changes or signs of a central vestibular disorder, an electroencephalogram (EEG) is used to evaluate cerebral cortex electrical activity. An animal with vestibular signs and an abnormal EEG most likely has a multifocal CNS problem.

CSF analysis may contribute greatly to the diagnosis of a central vestibular problem. Choroid plexus papillomas of the fourth ventricle or astrocytomas of the brain stem may result in elevated CSF pressure and protein with no or a mild increase in cells. Meningiomas affecting the vestibular nerve and compressing the brain stem may produce only an increase in CSF protein but not pressure. Occasionally meningiomas may be associated with CSF pleocytosis (Chap. 5). Viral infections and other nonsuppurative meningoencephalitides typically produce an increase in mononuclear cells and protein within

Table 12–1
Neurologic signs differentiating peripheral from central vestibular disease

Peripheral vestibular disease	Central vestibular disease
Alert	Often depressed
Head tilt	Head tilt
Circling, rolling, leaning	Circling, rolling, leaning
Nystagmus—horizontal or rotary	Nystagmus—horizontal, rotary, or vertical
Positional nystagmus—may change between horizontal and rotary	Positional nystagmus—changing from horizontal or rotary to vertical
Positional strabismus	Positional strabismus
Cranial nerve VII deficit	Cranial nerve V, VI, VII deficits
Horner's syndrome	No Horner's syndrome reported
Gait—mild ataxia and disequillibrium	Gait—severe ataxia
	Ipsilateral hemiparesis or quadriparesis
	Hopping and placing deficits
	Ipsilateral hypermetria
	Conscious proprioceptive deficits
	Head bobbing with cerebellar involvement

the CSF. Bacterial meningitis from extension of inner ear infections up the vestibular nerve or septicemia results in an increase of neutrophils and protein within the CSF. The bacteria can be cultured from the CSF in severe infections. Granulomatous meningoencephalitis may have a predilection for the pontine medullary junction and have an associated pleocytosis of monocytes, lymphocytes, and neutrophils and an elevated protein.

Tympanometry and evaluation of the acoustic reflex is a special technique to evaluate tympanic membrane integrity and middle ear function[11,15] (Chap. 13).

Radiographic examination of the tympanic bullae and bony labyrinth should be performed in peripheral vestibular disease when infection, trauma, or neoplasia are suspected. Ventrodorsal, left and right lateral obliques, and open mouth positions are all used to evaluate any bony changes in the skull.

Cerebral angiography via the vertebral artery is helpful in outlining brain stem mass lesions when neoplasia is thought present. Magnetic resonance imaging (MRI) and computerized axial tomography (CT) scans are more often used to demonstrate brain stem mass lesions in large dogs. In small dogs and cats, the brain stem is so small that visualization may be difficult. Exploratory craniotomy into the dorsal occipitoatlantal space may allow examination, biopsy, and removal of masses from the fourth ventricle. Exploration of the ventral pontine medullary brainstem is very difficult.

Serial evaluations of the clinical data are often necessary to determine the cause of the disease and prognosis for an individual patient. Ancillary diagnostic investigations are normal in most idiopathic peripheral vestibular disorders. Because the prognosis in these disorders is favorable and most animals recover, repeated neurologic examinations are used to monitor the improvement. Table 12–2 outlines the diagnostic approach for disorders of the vestibular system.

Table 12-2
Diagnostic approach for the evaluation of vestibular deficits

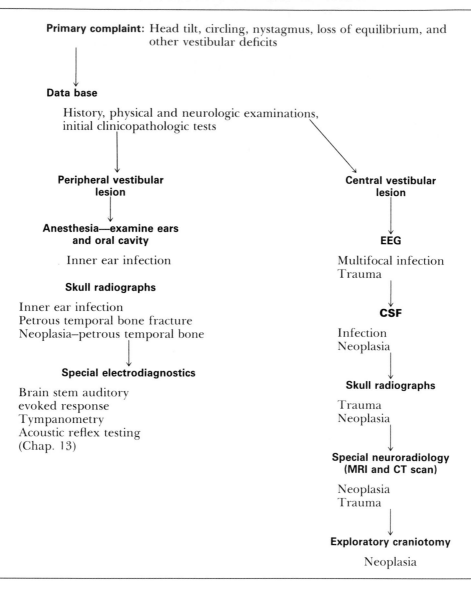

Primary complaint: Head tilt, circling, nystagmus, loss of equilibrium, and other vestibular deficits

Data base

History, physical and neurologic examinations, initial clinicopathologic tests

Peripheral vestibular lesion

Anesthesia—examine ears and oral cavity

Inner ear infection

Skull radiographs

Inner ear infection
Petrous temporal bone fracture
Neoplasia–petrous temporal bone

Special electrodiagnostics

Brain stem auditory
evoked response
Tympanometry
Acoustic reflex testing
(Chap. 13)

Central vestibular lesion

EEG

Multifocal infection
Trauma

CSF

Infection
Neoplasia

Skull radiographs

Trauma
Neoplasia

Special neuroradiology (MRI and CT scan)

Neoplasia
Trauma

Exploratory craniotomy

Neoplasia

Congenital and familial disorders

An acute onset of head tilt, circling, or rolling may occur in German Shepherds, Smooth Haired Fox terriers, Beagles, Doberman Pinschers, and other pure-bred dogs, as well as in Siamese, Burmese, and Tonkanese cats, between 3 and 12 weeks of age.[6,7,19] A transient, spontaneous horizontal nystagmus may also be seen on the neurologic examination as well as positional strabismus on the side of the head tilt. Occasionally, the animals are also deaf. Except for the circling and mild ataxia, the gait is usually normal. The electroencephalogram, skull radiographs, and cerebrospinal fluid have been normal in the few cases examined. Many affected puppies and kittens compensate and become normal within a few weeks or months. In other cases, the head tilt persists, but the circling decreases and only becomes apparent when the animal is excited. If the animal is deaf on presentation, the deafness usually persists. Because the symptoms never progress and are often not debilitating to the animal, many are acceptable pets. The few cases that have been examined histologically have been normal. A congenital possibly inherited developmental abnormality is believed to be the cause.

A congenital bilateral vestibular disturbance has been reported in Beagles, Collies, Akitas, and other breeds of puppies at birth. The animals are ataxic when they begin to walk and demonstrate bobbing or rotary movements of the head. The puppies are also deaf. An abnormal development of both vestibular and auditory receptors is suspected. Affected animals usually do not improve but may be acceptable pets.

A congenital, pendulous nystagmus is common in Siamese and Siamese-mixed cats, and has been seen sporadically in certain breeds of dogs. The movements of the eyes are equal in both directions. Frequently, the head oscillates in rhythm with the eye movements. There are no other symptoms related to vestibular dysfunction. In Siamese cats, the abnormality is localized to the visual pathways and not the vestibular system (Chap. 9).

Infections

Middle and inner ear infections

Incidence: Frequent

The most common cause of peripheral vestibular inflammation is an extension of an infection of the middle ear (otitis media) into the inner ear structures (otitis interna).[9,13,18]

Signalment and history. Any age, breed, or sex of dog or cat can exhibit vestibular signs from an inner ear infection. Cocker spaniels and other long-eared breeds with chronic otitis externa are often affected. Poodles with chronic otitis or pharyngitis are also commonly affected. The signs can appear acutely or insidiously over a period of several weeks. A history of previous otitis externa produced by parasites, bacteria, or fungus is often obtained. Some ear cleaning solutions are irritating to the middle and inner ear and vestibular signs may appear or worsen after application. The tympanic membrane may rupture and produce infection of the middle and inner ears. A history of chronic tonsillitis or pharyngitis is sometimes obtained from the owner. In these cases, extension of the infection through the eustachian or auditory tube into the middle ear and then the inner ear can result. Otitis interna can also result from the hematogenous spread of an infection from elsewhere in the body. The animal may have pain when the mouth is opened and be reluctant to chew.

Physical and neurologic examinations. The external ear canal should be cleaned and thoroughly examined. The tympanic membranes are examined more easily when the animal is anesthetized. The presence of otitis externa and the integrity of the tympanic membrane should be noted. Typanometry may be a more accurate way to evaluate membrane integrity.[11] A gray, dull, opaque and bulging tympanic membrane indicates an exudate in the middle ear. If the tympanic membranes are abnormal, myringotomy may be carefully performed by inserting a 2½ to 3½-inch spinal needle through the otoscope, puncturing the tympanic membrane, and aspirating fluid from the middle ear for cytologic examination and culture. Ipsilateral mandibular lymphadenopathy can occur if the infection is severe. The pharynx should be examined and palpated thoroughly for masses.

On neurologic examination, the vestibular signs may vary in severity, depending on the extent of the lesion. A head tilt is most often present. The animal may circle, lean, or fall toward the affected side. Rolling is rare. Spontaneous nystagmus is occasionally seen, and if present, is horizontal or rotary with the fast component directed away from the side of the lesion. A positional strabismus or eye drop is often present on the affected side, but the eyeballs are not paralyzed. Bilateral inner ear infections also occur, and wide excursions of the head, truncal ataxia, and deafness are the prominent clinical abnormalities. Unilateral facial nerve paralysis is often seen if the middle ear or petrous temporal bone is involved (Chap. 11). The facial paralysis is characterized by an inability to close the eyelid and move the ear or lip on the affected side (Chap. 11). The lip droops and the atonic nose deviates away from the affected side. Occasionally, tear production is reduced, and the mucous membranes may be drier on the affected side, if the salivary glands are denervated. A Schirmer's tear test can be useful to detect mild facial nerve involvement and to monitor progression or regression of the dysfunction. In chronic facial nerve paralysis, contracture and fibrosis of the denervated muscles result in deviation of the nose toward the affected side and elevation of the lip and ear carriage. Bilateral middle ear involvement can result in bilateral facial paralysis (see Figs. 11–13 and 11–14).

Horner's syndrome on the side of the lesion is caused by interruption of sympathetic innervation within the middle ear (Chap. 11). A miotic pupil or an excessive constriction of the pupil to light stimulation is the most consistently observed component of Horner's syndrome.

In a simple inner ear infection, the animal's gait is only mildly ataxic, and it may stumble to the side of the lesion. Occasionally in dogs and more frequently in cats, especially when treated with glucocorticoids, the infection will ascend the vestibular nerve and cause a brain stem abscess or meningitis. If an ascending infection occurs, ipsilateral hypermetria, obvious hemiparesis, and postural deficits can be seen. Secondary edema and cerebellar coning can result in death. Clinicopathologic tests on animals with inner ear infections are often normal. In severe infections, neutrophilic leukocytosis is seen on the complete blood count.

At the time the animal is anesthetized for examination of the tympanic membranes, myringotomy, and tympanometry, radiographs of the skull are taken. If the infection is chronic, thickening of the bony structures may be observed in the middle and inner ears on the radiographs (Fig. 12–7). In severe cases, osteomyelitis and lysis of bone may be seen. If exudate is present in the middle ear, the tympanic bullae will appear cloudy on the skull radiographs. Sometimes in acute cases, radiographic examination is normal.

If signs of brain stem involvement are present, cerebrospinal fluid analysis should be obtained. The cerebrospinal fluid often contains increased neutrophils and protein in ascending infections, and should be cultured to identify the bacteria and determine the sensitivity of the bacteria to antibiotics.

Therapy and prognosis. The treatment of inner ear infections varies with the clinical and radiographic findings. If an early and aggressive medical approach is implemented in animals with mild peripheral vestibular deficits and only mild radiographic changes in the osseous bullae and petrous temporal bone, most infections resolve, do not recur, and rarely need surgical drainage. A combination of trimeth-

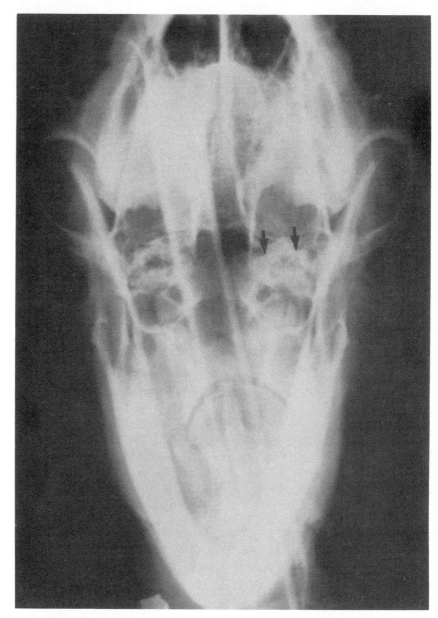

Figure 12–7. Thickening of the left petrous temporal bone (arrows) from an inner ear infection of a dog with a left head tilt (open-mouth radiographic view). (From Chrisman, C.L.: Disorders of the vestibular system. The Compendium on Continuing Education. *1*(10):748, 1979.)

oprim sulfadiazine (Tribrissen) 15 mg/kg every 12 hours and Cephradine (Velosef) 20 mg/kg every 8 hours are given orally for 4 to 6 weeks. Glucocorticoids should be avoided, as they suppress the animal's ability to fight the bacterial or fungal infection that is present and may cause ascending infections into the brain stem.[9] In mild cases, the signs often resolve in 1 to 2 weeks, but will recur if the antibiotic is withdrawn at that time. If a specific bacteria is cultured, a more appropriate antibiotic is administered, depending on the results of the sensitivity tests.

If otitis externa is present, the ears should be cultured and cleaned. Care should be taken in the selection of a topical medication if the tympanic membrane is ruptured. Oil-based or irritating external ear preparations are avoided. Gentamicin otic may produce toxicity to the inner ear structures and should be avoided.[21] Water-based or ophthalmic solutions of antibiotics may be used. Topical medication may be discontinued in a week if the infection is controlled.

Radiographic evidence of exudate in the tympanic bullae frequently indicates that surgical exploration and drainage is required.[9] Nasopharyngeal polyps of the middle ear may result in recurring infections and should be surgically removed.[2,10]

If the inner ear infection is detected early and treated for a sufficient length of time, the prognosis for recovery is good. In cases in which surgical intervention is necessary, the prognosis becomes more guarded. Many cases recover well once surgical drainage is done. The prognosis is guarded or grave in cases of osteomyelitis involving the tympanic bullae and bony labyrinth. In cases in which the otitis interna ascends and produces a brain stem infection, the prognosis is also guarded or grave. Cerebrospinal fluid culture, aggressive therapy with an appropriate systemic antibiotic, and serial neurologic evaluations are of paramount importance.

Facial nerve paralysis and Horner's syndrome are often permanent sequelae of middle ear infections. Keratitis sicca can result from tear gland denervation from the facial nerve paralysis. Corneal ulceration is a frequent complication produced by the lack of tear production and inability to close the eyelid. The administration of artificial tear preparations prevents corneal ulcers. If the animal has proper tear production, it may retract the globe periodically and allow the membrane nictitans to lubricate and protect the cornea. Some animals learn to sleep with a paw covering the affected eye to prevent drying of the cornea.

In cases of resolved simple inner ear infection, the animal should be carefully watched for recurrences of the problem. It is not uncommon for the other ear to become infected, and in many breeds, this is a chronic problem. Ruptured tympanic membranes only occasionally produce detectable hearing deficits. Eventually, they heal, though they may appear scarred. Deafness can result from chronic bilateral inner ear infections.

Miscellaneous infections

Incidence: Occasional

Any cause of meningoencephalitis (Chap. 7 and Tables 7–6 and 7–7) can result in involvement of central vestibular structures.[6,7] Canine distemper virus and feline infectious peritonitis virus infections are the most common. With canine distemper virus infections, the dogs may or may not have a history of systemic illness. Affected animals often have a history of symptoms unrelated to the vestibular system, such as behavior changes, seizures, paresis, or paralysis. Ophthalmic examination sometimes shows evidence of chorioretinitis. A head tilt and circling can be seen on neurologic examination. Ataxia is often pronounced, indicating concurrent brain stem or cerebellar disease. Spontaneous or positional vertical nystagmus may be present in central vestibular lesions. Motor and sensory brain stem tract involvement produce paresis and severe ataxia. High-amplitude slow-wave activity on EEG examination supports a diagnosis of concurrent cerebral involvement. Hematologic evaluation can be normal or show lymphopenia in acute cases. Radiographs of the tympanic bullae and bony labyrinth are normal. Cerebrospinal fluid pleocytosis and elevated protein and titers can help to differentiate viral infections from bacterial and fungal infections as well as other inflammations or tumors (Chap. 5, Chap. 7, and Table 7–8).

Feline infectious peritonitis (FIP) infections may produce signs of central vestibular problems, but neurologic deficits from involvement of other sites within the nervous system are often also present. Slowing and increases in amplitude are seen on the EEG. A serum polyclonal gammopathy and positive serum and CSF FIP titers may be found. Results of radiographic examination of the skull are normal. CSF analysis is either normal or shows an increase in mononuclear cells and protein. The prognosis is often grave.

Other viral, fungal, bacterial, protozoal, rickettsial, and parasitic infections as well as steroid-responsive inflammations found in the CNS of dogs and cats may on rare occasions produce vestibular signs. Central nervous system infections and inflammations are discussed in Chapter 7.

Granulomatous meningoencephalitis

Incidence: Occasional

A granulomatous meningoencephalomyelitis (GME) of unknown cause is seen in dogs, and rarely, cats.[4,16,17] Although GME may occur in focal or multifocal sites throughout the cerebrum, cerebellum, and spinal cord, the pontomedullary brain stem region is a predilection site for this condition, and central vestibular signs are common. Dogs between 8 months and 10 years of age, especially Poodles and terriers, are usually involved. A fever may be found on physical examination early in the course of the disease, but most often affected dogs are afebrile. Affected dogs may or may not have chorioretinitis on ophthalmologic exam. Head tilt, nystagmus, and circling indicate vestibular dysfunction. Other signs indicative of brain stem disease include facial paralysis, facial spasm, loss of facial sensation, auditory deficits, dysmetria, or ipsilateral hemiparesis, hemiplegia, or quadriparesis. Convulsions, depression, and aggressive behavior indicate involvement in cortical or subcortical regions (Chaps. 7 and 8). A diffuse slowing and increased amplitude, compatible with an encephalitis process, are seen on the EEG. A mild to marked increase in leukocytes, particularly lymphocytes and monocytes, is seen in the CSF.[1,17] Granulomatous meningoencephalomyelitis may be difficult to differentiate from canine distemper virus infections or other causes of meningoencephalitis. If CSF titers and cultures are negative and no organism is apparent, aggressive glucocorticoid therapy should be attempted. For the first 24 to 48 hours, 30 mg/kg methylprednisolone sodium succinate (Solu-Medrol) may be administered intravenously every 8 to 12 hours, followed by oral prednisone 2 mg/kg for the next week. If there is some improvement, therapy should be continued, but prednisone doses reduced to avoid gastrointestinal ulcers and pancreatitis (Chap. 6). Most commonly, GME progresses regardless of therapy and the diagnosis is confirmed at necropsy. At necropsy, granulomatous lesions are characteristically found in the brain stem in the region of the vestibular nuclei. An immune-mediated disease is indicated. Some focal GME becomes neoplastic, and it has been referred to as neoplastic reticulosis.

Metabolic disorders

Hypothyroidism

Incidence: Rare

Hypothyroidism may produce signs of peripheral and central vestibular disease with or without involvement of other cranial or

ties. Vertical nystagmus associated with central vestibular disease may be seen. The animals can die from involvement of vital centers in the medulla oblongata and pons. The diagnosis is made only by excluding other causes. In the acute stages, glucocorticoid therapy may be helpful for the first 24 hours. Methylprednisolone sodium succinate (Solu-Medrol) 15 to 30 mg/kg may be given intravenously every 8 to 12 hours, followed by 1 to 2 mg/kg prednisolone daily, divided every 12 hours, given and reduced every 3 to 5 days over the next 2 weeks (Chapter 6). If serial neurologic examinations show improvements, the animal may again be an acceptable pet, but it may require several weeks or months of nursing care.

Neoplasia

Neoplasms arise in peripheral and central vestibular structures in dogs and cats and produce signs of vestibular dysfunction.[6,7]

Peripheral neoplasia

Incidence: Occasional

Neurofibrosarcoma, neurofibromas, and neurinomas can develop on the vestibulocochlear nerve, but occur only occasionally in dogs and cats. The animals are usually adults and often initially have a mild head tilt. The head tilt slowly becomes more marked. No abnormalities may be detected on the physical examination. On initial neurologic examination, only signs of peripheral vestibular involvement (a head tilt, stumbling, circling, and leaning toward the affected side) may be apparent. Nystagmus is usually absent. Skull radiographs are normal initially, but later lysis in the petrous temporal bone may be seen. Tomography may aid in the visualization of bone lysis. MRI and CT scans may enable visualization of masses of the middle and inner ear structures. A neurofibrosarcoma may be difficult to differentiate from a mild inner ear infection initially. The signs continue to progress over several months, despite the use of antibiotics and glucocorticoids. Facial nerve paralysis often develops on the affected side. The tumor can grow along the vestibulocochlear nerve, eventually compress the brain stem, and produce signs of ipsilateral hemiparesis and conscious proprioceptive deficits. A neurofibrosarcoma should be considered in the differential diagnosis of a vestibular disturbance that begins peripherally and slowly progresses over a 6- to 9-month period despite all attempts at medical therapy. There are no reports of surgical removal of these tumors in animals. They are often confirmed only at necropsy.

Osteosarcomas, chondrosarcomas, or fibrosarcomas may affect the osseous bullae and bony labyrinth, and secondarily affect peripheral vestibular structures. These are usually easily demonstrated on routine radiographs (see Figure 11–17A, B). Squamous cell carcinoma of the external and middle ear structures can progress and produce vestibular deficits.[12,14] Tumors arising from tonsillar tissue or metastasis from thyroid adenocarcinomas may involve the peripheral vestibular structures. Nasopharyngeal polyps are benign tumors that occur in the external and middle ears, especially in cats. These are surgically removed and in most cases the prognosis is good.[10]

CNS neoplasia

Incidence: Occasional

Meningioma is another slow-growing tumor, which can compress the brain stem and produce unilateral vestibular signs, particularly in cats. Initially many dogs and cats display only a head tilt and mild ataxia similar to that of animals with neurofibrosarcoma. Facial nerve paralysis is often also present on the affected side. Again, the signs progress slowly over a several-month period regardless of therapy. Trigeminal nerve paralysis resulting in ipsilateral masseter and temporal muscle atrophy can develop as well as diminished sensation to the face (see Figure 11–16). Gait and postural reaction abnormalities are seen as brain stem compression occurs. CSF analysis may be normal or show elevated protein with no increase in cells. Routine radiographs of the skull are usually normal, but MRI and CT scans may demonstrate the lesion. Slow, progressive signs of brain stem dysfunction over many months are suggestive of a meningioma. This region of the brain stem is extremely difficult to explore surgically. No reports of attempted removal of meningiomas from this region are in the veterinary literature. Radiation therapy may improve the prognosis in some cases.

Primary central nervous system tumors (astrocytomas, ependymomas, choroid plexus papillomas, oligodendrogliomas, and other gliomas) of the brain stem can occur in dogs and cats. Boxers and Boston terriers are the breeds most commonly affected. The animals are usually over 5 years of age at the time of presentation. A head tilt, ataxia, hemiparesis, and postural deficits may be seen. Vertical nystagmus may also occur. On occasion a paradoxical head tilt will be produced from flocculonodular cerebellar dysfunction.[20] Facial, abducent, and trigeminal nerve deficits often accompany the vestibular signs. The EEG is often normal. Typical CSF abnormalities include elevated pressure and protein with no increase in cells. Routine skull radiographs are normal; MRI and CT scans usually demonstrate the lesion. The progression of signs occurs over several weeks to a few months, and is usually more rapid than the devel-

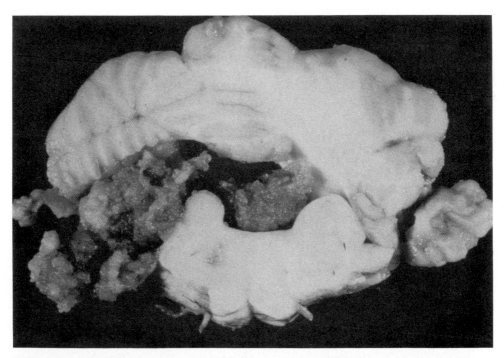

Figure 12–8. A choroid plexus papilloma of the fourth ventricle found at necropsy on a 3-year-old Irish Setter with vestibular deficits. (From Chrisman, C.L.: Vestibular diseases. Vet. Clin. North Am. p. 126, February, 1980.)

Table 12–3
Differential diagnosis of vestibular disease of dogs and cats

	Signalment	Onset	Course	Vestibular and other signs	Ancillary aids	Therapy	Prognosis
Congenital	Doberman, Beagle, German Shepherd, Siamese, Burmese, Tonkanese birth to 12 wks	Acute	Regressive	Peripheral, deafness possible	Negative	None	Compensate
Otitis interna	Cocker Spaniels, Poodles, any dog or cat, any age	Acute or subacute	Progressive	Peripheral, cranial nerve VII, or Horner's syndrome	Myringotomy; skull radiographs tympanometry	Antibiotics; surgical drainage if necessary	Good if treated early and aggressively with antibiotics
Encephalitis							
Viral	Dog or cat any age	Subacute	Progressive	Central, other CNS signs	EEG—Encephalitis; CSF—increased lymphocytes and protein (typical)	Glucocorticoids	Fair to poor
Fungal	Dog or cat any age	Subacute	Progressive	Central, other CNS signs	EEG—meningitis; CSF—increased lymphocytes, monocytes, neutrophils, eosinophils, and protein	Amphotericin B	Poor to grave
Bacterial	Dog or cat any age	Subacute	Progressive	Central, other CNS signs	EEG—may be normal; CSF—increased neutrophils and protein (typical)	Antibiotics	Fair to poor

	Signalment	Onset	Course	Signs	Diagnostic Tests	Treatment	Prognosis
GME	Dog or cat adult	Acute and subacute	Progressive	Central, other CNS signs	EEG—Encephalitis; CSF—increased lymphocytes, monocytes, and neutrophils	None	Grave
Toxicities							
Aminoglycoside antibiotics	Dog or cat any age	Acute, subacute	Progressive	Peripheral, deafness possible	Negative	Withdraw antibiotic	Compensation, deafness permanent
Metronidazole	Dog	Acute	Progressive	Central, seizures, coma	CSF—increased protein	Withdraw drug	Mildly affected; may recover
Nutritional Thiamine	Cats any age	Acute, subacute	Progressive	Central, other CNS signs	EEG; response to thiamine	Thiamine	Good to poor
Trauma and **Vascular**	Dog or cat any age	Acute	Regressive or static	Peripheral or central	EEG—may show concussion; skull radiographs	Steroids	Peripheral good; central
Neoplasia	Boxer, Boston other dogs or cats over 5 yrs	Subacute, chronic	Progressive	Peripheral or central	CSF—increased pressure and protein; CT and MRI scans	Glucocorticoids may improve signs temporarily	Grave
Idiopathic	Adult cats or dogs, aged dogs	Peracute	Regressive	Peripheral	Negative	None	Good

opment of a neurofibrosarcoma or meningioma. Again, the prognosis is grave, and most tumors are confirmed at necropsy.

Neoplastic GME (reticulosis) can also be a neoplastic process affecting the brain stem of dogs. The salient features of the disease are discussed in Chapter 7.

Animals with choroid plexus papillomas of the fourth ventricle may initially have a head tilt and later develop other signs associated with involvement of other brain stem structures (Fig. 12–8). Radiographs of the skull are usually normal. CSF pressure and protein are both greatly elevated.

Metastatic neoplasms occasionally involve the brain stem and produce central vestibular signs. Routine chest radiographs may be examined on animals when neoplasia is suspected and metastatic neoplasia found. As with the other cases of brain stem neoplasia, the prognosis is grave.

Idiopathic disorders

Vestibular syndrome of cats

Incidence: Frequent

An idiopathic vestibular disorder is common in adult cats of any age.[5,19] There is an acute onset of severe head tilt and rolling or falling to one side (see Fig. 12–5). The cat often cries continuously, leans against the wall for support, or remains in a crouched position, not wanting to move. There is no associated illness or history of trauma. In the southern states, it has been suspected that eating blue-tail lizards produces the syndrome in cats. However, the toxicity has never been reproducible experimentally, and a similar syndrome occurs in other parts of the country where blue-tail lizards are not found.

Only signs associated with a peripheral vestibular nerve deficit are found on the neurologic examination. Head tilt, disori-

entation, circling, or rolling are frequently present. A horizontal or rotary nystagmus with the fast phase directed away from the side of the head tilt is often present initially, but subsides after a few days. In the acute stages, evaluation of the gait and postural reactions is difficult, because the animal is struggling from the severe disorientation. The cats are often frightened, and should be observed closely. Excess handling should be avoided. Serial neurologic examinations are extremely important. After 72 hours, the nystagmus usually resolves, although a positional nystagmus may still be elicited. The cat is often ambulatory by 72 hours, but retains its head tilt and continues to circle. No other cranial nerve deficits, hemiparesis, or proprioceptive deficits are found on the neurologic examination. In some cats, bilateral vestibular dysfunction occurs. Affected cats fall to either side with a staggering gait. Wide excursions of the head and loss of normal vestibular nystagmus occur. Affected cats may have diminished or no postrotatory nystagmus on either side and are often deaf.

Clinical laboratory tests, EEG, skull radiographs, and CSF analysis are normal. The diagnosis is made by ruling out other causes of vestibular disease and observing a rapid improvement of signs in cases of unilateral vestibular involvement on serial neurologic examinations. There has been no evidence that glucocorticoid therapy speeds recovery. During the acute phase, if the animal is rolling severely, diazepam 1 to 2 mg every 6 to 8 hours may be administered intramuscularly. Regardless of therapy, the prognosis is good in cats with unilateral disease and the cats often return to normal within 2 to 3 weeks. Some cats will have a residual head tilt. In cats with bilateral disease, recovery occurs slowly over several months and there is often residual equilibrium and hearing deficits. No lesions have been described in the vestibular system on necropsy, and the cause of the syndrome is unknown.

Idiopathic vestibular syndromes of dogs

Incidence: Frequent

Idiopathic vestibular syndromes occur sporadically in dogs of all ages. An acute onset of severe vestibular signs is common, but improvement is noted within 72 hours. The animals will spontaneously return to normal within 1 to 3 weeks.

A specific idiopathic vestibular syndrome is common in geriatric dogs.[6,7,18] An acute onset of head tilt, falling, rolling, or circling is seen. Horizontal or rotary nystagmus is initially present with the fast phase away from the head tilt. The dogs, like the cats, are frequently so disoriented that they are unable to stand. Because of the age and acute onset of the signs, this syndrome has erroneously been called "stroke," or a brain stem hemorrhage or infarct. However, on serial neurologic examinations, no signs of brain stem involvement can be found, and a peripheral vestibular lesion is indicated. Clinicopathologic testing and EEG are normal. Many affected dogs are old, and should not be anesthetized for skull radiographs. The few cases that have been radiographed were normal. The animals improve within a few days, and may be normal in a week. Sometimes the head tilt may be permanent.

Because of the age of the animal and the initial severity of the vestibular deficit, many of these animals are erroneously euthanized because a severe nervous system disease is believed present. However, the rapid improvement on serial neurologic examinations should alert the clinician that a diagnosis of idiopathic vestibular syndrome is likely and the prognosis for recovery is good. No specific therapy seems to alter the speed of recovery. As in the other idiopathic vestibular disturbances, no lesions have been found at necropsy.

A review of the differential diagnosis of vestibular disorders and the salient feature of each are outlined in Table 12–3.

References

1. Bailey, C.S. and Higgins, R.J.: Characteristics of cerebrospinal fluid associated with canine granulomatous meningoencephalitis: A retrospective study. J. Am. Vet. Med. Assoc., *188*:418, 1986.
2. Berzon, J.L. and Bunch, S.E.: Recurrent otitis externa/media secondary to a fibroma in the middle ear. J. Am. Anim. Hosp. Assoc., *16*:73, 1980.
3. Bichsel, P., et al.: Neurologic manifestations associated with hypothyroidism in four dogs. J. Am. Vet. Med. Assoc., *192*:1745, 1988.
4. Braund, K.G.: Granulomatous meningoencephalitis. *In* Current Veterinary Therapy X. Edited by R.W. Kirk. Philadelphia, W. B. Saunders, 1989.
5. Burke, E.E., at al.: Review of idiopathic feline vestibular syndrome in 75 cats. J. Am. Vet. Med. Assoc., *187*:941, 1985.
6. Chrisman, C.L.: Vestibular disease. Vet. Clin. North Am., *10*:103, 1980.
7. deLahunta, A.: Vestibular System—Special Proprioception Veterinary Neuroanatomy and Clinical Neurology. Philadelphia, W.B. Saunders, 1983.
8. Dow, S.W., et al.: Central nervous system toxicosis associated with metronidazole treatment of dogs: Five cases (1984–1987). J. Am. Vet. Med. Assoc., *195*:365, 1989.
9. Howard, P.E., et al.: Otitis media. Part II. Surgical consideration. Compendium on Continuing Education, *5*:18, 1983.
10. Lane, J.G.: Nasopharyngeal polyps arising in the middle ear of the cat. J. Small Anim. Pract., *22*:511, 1981.
11. Little, C.I.L. and Lane, J.G.: An evaluation of tympanometry, otoscopy and palpation for assessment of the canine tympanic membrane. Vet. Rec., *124*:5, 1989.
12. Little, C.J.L., et al.: Neoplasia involving the middle ear cavity of dogs. Vet. Rec., *124*:54, 1989.
13. Neer, T.M. and Howard, P.E.: Otitis media. Compendium on Continuing Education, *4*:410, 1982.
14. Pentlarge, V.M.: Peripheral vestibular diseases in a cat with middle and inner ear squamous cell carcinoma. Compendium on Continuing Education, *6*:731, 1984.
15. Penrod, J.P. and Coulter, D.B.: The diag-

that is not rhythmic or continuous, as is myoclonus.

Opisthotonos and tetanus are discussed together, as are tetany and tremors. Myoclonus and other muscle spasms are discussed separately. Loss of consciousness and opisthotonos are caused by midbrain disease. Mechanisms of diseases, such as severe infections, trauma, and neoplasia, which produce midbrain disease and loss of consciousness, may terminally produce this form of opisthotonos called decerebrate rigidity (Chap. 10).

The most common causes of opisthotonos and tetanus with no altered state of consciousness are infections with Clostridium tetani, mild strychnine and other poisonings, and trauma to the rostral cerebellum. Diseases producing opisthotonos with altered consciousness are discussed in Chapter 10 and will not be dealt with in this chapter.

Opisthotonos and tetanus

Mechanisms of disease and differential diagnosis

Infections and other inflammations
Clostridium tetani
Other severe viral, bacterial, protozoal, or fungal disease and granulomatous meningoencephalitis, and other inflammations (Chaps. 7 and 12)

Toxicity
Strychnine
Metronizadole (Chap. 12)
Other toxicities

Trauma
Midbrain hemorrhage or compression (Chap. 10)
Rostral cerebellar injury

Neoplasia
Midbrain compression (Chap. 10)

Clostridium tetani infections

Incidence: Rare

Deep wounds may provide an anaerobic environment for the multiplication of Clostridium tetani (Cl. tetani) organisms, which are found throughout the environment.[12,15] The organisms produce two exotoxins, tetanospasm, and tetanolysin. The exotoxins are absorbed systemically and are inhibitory to the inhibitory interneurons in the gray matter of the spinal cord and brain stem. The net result is a release of inhibition on motor neurons and a rigidity of muscles all over the head and body.

Signalment and history. Dogs and cats are more resistant to the organism than are horses, so the disease is rare in small animals; however, any age, breed, or sex might be affected. Generalized muscle stiffness may begin 2 to 20 days following the initial wound.

Physical and neurologic examinations. A healed or open wound may be found on physical examination, but occasionally no wound at all is discovered. The clinical appearance of the animal, however, is characteristic. Because of released inhibition of the facial nerve and spasm of facial musculature, the ears are pulled erect on the head and the forehead is wrinkled (Fig. 14–2A,B). The lips are drawn up, giving a sneering expression (called "risus sardonicus"). Release of inhibition of the abducent nerve and spasms of the retractor oculi muscles result in protrusion of the membrane nictitans. Spasms of the masticatory and pharyngeal muscles result in trismus and dysphagia, respectively. The extensor rigidity of the limbs and tail gives the animal a characteristic "saw horse" stance when standing. Clinical signs in dogs and cats may be milder than those seen in horses. If signs are severe, the animal may be presented in opisthotonos

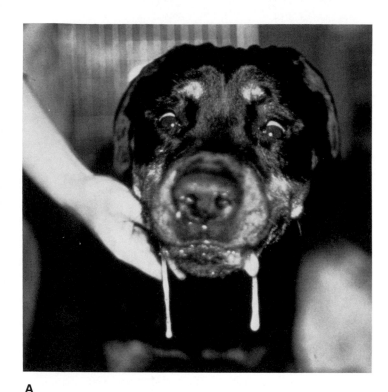

A

Figure 14–2. *(A)* Spasm of facial musculature in a Rottweiler with tetanus. *(B)* A view of the dorsum of the head showing muscle spasms of the same Rottweiler.

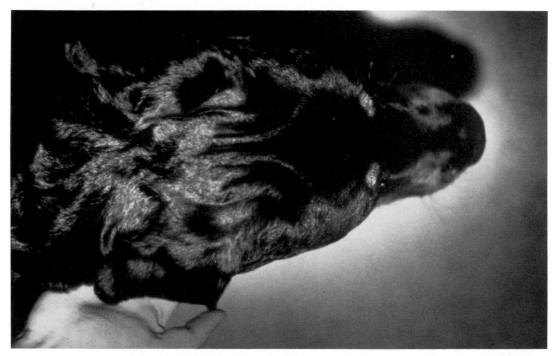

B

with severe respiratory distress from laryngeal, intercostal, and diaphragm muscle spasms. Noise or handling can provoke tetanic spasms. Exotoxins may also affect the sympathetic nervous system and produce arrhythmias, increased blood pressure, pyrexia, and peripheral vasoconstriction.

Ancillary diagnostic investigations. The diagnosis is made primarily by the characteristic appearance on presentation of an animal with no history of strychnine poisoning. Mild cases may be difficult to differentiate from other neuromuscular diseases producing a stiff gait, as there are no specific ancillary investigations that enable a definitive diagnosis to be made (Chap. 16).

Therapy and prognosis. Therapy is aimed at killing the organism, neutralizing the toxin, suppressing the effects of the toxin, and giving supportive care. Penicillin G at 40,000 units/kg is given initially intravenously, followed by daily intramuscular injections of 20,000 units/kg every 12 hours. Tetanus antitoxin (equine origin) should be first given in a test dose of 0.1 or 0.2 ml subcutaneously to see whether anaphylaxis occurs. If no adverse reactions occur within 30 minutes, then 30,000 to 100,000 units daily may be given intravenously or subcutaneously to dogs, and approximately 5,000 units daily to cats for several days, depending on the severity of the signs.

Muscle spasms may be controlled with injections of diazepam or methocarbamol (Chap. 6). Chlorpromazine and phenobarbital are also used.

Wounds should be opened and debrided and flushed thoroughly with an antibacterial agent. If laryngeal spasms are severe, tracheostomy may be performed, but the prognosis is guarded. If pharyngeal spasms and trismus preclude normal eating and drinking, then a pharyngostomy tube may be inserted.

The animal should be placed in a quiet, dark environment and handled as little as possible. Monitoring of cardiac rate and rhythm should be performed in severe cases. The animal should be kept on padding to prevent decubital ulcers and should be turned to the opposite side every 4 hours, if in lateral recumbency, to prevent hypostatic congestion of the lungs. Hydration should be maintained with fluid therapy if needed.

The prognosis is poor if the signs rapidly become severe. Most severely affected animals die within 5 days of respiratory failure or cardiac arrhythmias and hypotension. If the signs are mild or the animal can be maintained for 1 week, then the prognosis for recovery may be better. The therapy of antibiotics and antispasmodic drugs is continued as long as signs are present, which may be several weeks. It may be 30 days or longer before all signs of muscle rigidity disappear. Once the animal has recovered, there are no permanent neurologic deficits; however, tetanus infections produce no lasting immunity.

Prevention. Dogs and cats are rarely routinely vaccinated with tetanus toxoid. If a deep wound is sustained, tetanus may be prevented by thoroughly cleansing the wound and providing immunity either with an antitoxin or toxoid injection.

Strychnine poisoning

Incidence: Rare

Strychnine is a toxic substance that acts on inhibitory interneurons in the spinal cord and brain stem gray matter, and produces opisthotonos and tetanus similar to Cl. tetani infections.[4]

There is no history of a wound. When the animal is presented, the signs of opisthotonos or tetanus are usually severe, although mild cases may mimic Cl. tetani infections. Noise and handling provoke tetanic spasms or convulsions. The animal may be presented in status epilepticus (Chap. 8). Death is usually of respiratory failure from laryngeal, intercostal, and diaphragm muscle spasms.

Treatment is aimed at reducing the muscle spasms and maintaining a patent and functional airway. Diazepam, sodium pentobarbital, or phenobarbital injections may be used to control the muscle spasms and seizures (Chap. 6). An endotracheal tube may be inserted and oxygen therapy administered if the animal is hypoxic. If adequately hydrated, mannitol may be used for diuresis and urinary acidifiers administered to promote excretion of the drug. Gastric lavage may prevent further absorption of the toxic chemical. Stomach contents may be saved and tested for strychnine. The animal should be placed in a quiet, dark environment. The rectal temperature may be severely elevated during the muscle spasms, but usually returns to normal rapidly once the muscle spasms are under control. The animal should be placed on soft padding and turned to the opposite side very 4 hours. Recovery may be complete in 24 to 48 hours. If detected early and clinical signs controlled, the prognosis for recovery may be good. Strychnine is a difficult chemical to obtain.

Rostral cerebellar trauma

Incidence: Occasional

The rostral cerebellum has a descending inhibitory influence on motor neurons, and when this inhibition is acutely interrupted, as with a traumatic insult, opisthotonos results.[4] The management of animals with cranial trauma is described in Chapter 10. If opisthotonos is the main neurologic sign with no other evidence of brain stem or spinal cord dysfunction, the prognosis for eventual relaxation of muscle tone is good. It may take several months of nursing care, and once the an-

imal is ambulatory, severe incoordination may be seen from the cerebellar damage of other areas (Chap. 15).

Tetany and tremors

Mechanisms of disease and differential diagnosis

Congenital and familial disorders
Dysmyelinogenesis

Infections
Nonsuppurative encephalitis
Clostridium tetani

Metabolic disorders
Hypocalcemia
Hypoglycemia (Chap. 7)
Uremic encephalopathy (Chap. 7)

Toxicity
Metaldehyde
Strychnine
Organophosphate
Lead
Ivermectin (Chap. 10)
Many others (Table 14–1)

Idiopathic
Idiopathic tremors of adult dogs

Dysmyelinogenesis

Incidence: Occasional

Dysmyelinogenesis is an abnormal formation of myelin at or near birth that produces whole body and head tremors in puppies. It has been described in the Chow Chow, but has been sporadically seen in other breeds as well,[7,9,13,22] such as Springer Spaniels, Samoyeds, Weimaraners, Bernese Mountain dogs, and Lurchers.

Signs may begin from 2 to 8 weeks of age. Tremors of the head, neck, body, and limbs of varying severity are present when the animal is awake and are absent when

Table 14–1
Chemicals producing tremors or muscle twitching

• acetanilide	• lead
• acetophenetidin	• lethane
• aconite	• leucanthone HCl
• *Amanita pantherona*	• lithium Cl
• *Amanita phalloides*	• manganese (chronic)
• arsanilic acid	• meperidine
• arsine	• mercury
• asterol dihydrochloride	• methyl bromide
• atropine	• metaldehyde
• *Belladonna*	• methanol
• brucine	• methylene blue
• caffeine	• morphine
• calcium cyanamide	• muscarine
• carbon disulfide	• myristicine
• *Chenopodium oil*	• neostigmine
• chlordane	• nerve gas
• chlorobenzene	• nicotine
• chloronaphthalene	• nitrobenzene
• choke cherry	• opium
• cocaine (chronic)	• oxygen (100% 3 atm)
• codeine	• paraldehyde (chronic)
• colchicine	• parathion
• cresol	• pelletierine
• cubeb	• penethamate
• cystine	• pentaborane
• *Daphne*	• phenol
• DDT	• phenylhydroxylamine
• dichloroethane	• physostigmine
• digitalis	• *Phytolacca*
• dinitrobenzene	• picrotoxin
• diphenylhydantoin	• pilocarpine
• diphenhydramine	• pyrilamine maleate
• disulfiram	• pyrilium maleate
• dog parsley	• reserpine
• emetine	• saccharin
• ethyl chloride	• santonin
• ethylene glycol	• scorpion sting
• *Eupatorium urticaefolium*	• Solanum
• fluorides	• strychnine
• gasoline	• tetracaine HCl
• gelsemine	• tetrachloroethane
• hexachlorophene	• tetraethyl pyrophosphate
• hydroquinone	• thallium
• insulin	• thiocyanates
• iproniazid	• vanadium pentoxide
• isoproterenol	• water hemlock

Courtesy of Dr. Roger Yeary, The Ohio State University, Dept. of Veterinary Physiology and Pharmacology.

the animal is asleep or not moving. Excitement or cold temperature makes the tremors worse. There are no other neurologic deficits.

All ancillary diagnostic investigations are normal; the diagnosis is suspected from the signalment and signs. Diazepam (Valium) administered at a dose of 0.5 mg/kg orally every 8 hours may decrease the tremors. The prognosis for recovery is good in most instances, and the puppies may be normal in 1 to 3 months. The cause of the disorder is presently unknown, but an inherited problem is suspected in Chow Chows. Hypomyelinogenesis throughout the nervous system is seen on necropsy examination.

Nonsuppurative encephalitis

Incidence: Occasional

Some adult dogs with whole body tremors and no other neurologic abnormalities are found to have mild, diffuse nonsuppurative encephalitis on necropsy examination.[4] The underlying cause is unknown. This may be the same disorder as the idiopathic tremors of adult dogs discussed later in this chapter, but dogs with the latter are rarely euthanized because they recover from their tremor disorder.

Other dogs with whole body tremors have limb weakness and conscious proprioceptive deficits. A diffuse slowing and increased amplitude may be present on the EEG. CSF mononuclear pleocytosis and increased protein also may be found. Prednisone 2 mg/kg orally may be begun and the dosage reduced over the following month (Chap. 6). Diazepam (Valium) 0.5 mg/kg orally every 8 hours will control the tremors in most cases. Most dogs recover after 6 to 8 weeks and a definitive diagnosis is not made. A nonsuppurative meningoencephalitis is believed to be the cause.

Hypocalcemia

Incidence: Frequent

Calcium acts at the neural membrane to stabilize it. Low calcium in the body often results in excessive membrane depolarization, with tetany or tremors.

Small breed bitches and queens that are near parturition or have whelped and are heavily lactating may be presented with whole body tremors and elevated body temperatures.[1,14] Serum calcium determinations below 7 mg/dl support a diagnosis of hypocalcemia. Animals may also be presented in status epilepticus or complete collapse. This condition is rarely seen in large breed dogs. Hypoparathyroidism is a rare parathyroid malfunction that can produce hypocalcemia and tremors in dogs.[19,20] Hypocalcemia has also been reported with ethylene glycol toxicity, pancreatitis, and canine distemper infections.[23,25] The diagnosis is made based on the clinical examination findings of tremors associated with low serum calcium values.

Calcium gluconate injections and oral calcium supplementation correct the imbalance and control signs.

Hypoglycemia and uremic encephalopathy may also produce tremors and muscle weakness, and are discussed in Chapters 7 and 8.

Toxicity

Table 14–1 lists the many toxic agents that produce tremors in dogs and cats. Many of them also produce seizures (Chap. 8). Organophosphate toxicity should be evaluated with a serum cholinesterase determination.[16] Tremors may appear with serum cholinesterase levels below 500 IU. Ivermectin and ethylene glycol toxicity also should be considered.[18,25] Information on specific antidotes for a given toxic agent may be obtained from a poison control center.

Idiopathic tremors of adult dogs

Incidence: Occasional

An acute onset of head and whole body tremors unassociated with a metabolic or toxic disorder is seen in adult dogs.[4] Small breeds of white dogs are often affected, but these idiopathic tremors may occur in any breed or color. The tremors begin spontaneously, and occur continually while the animal is awake and ambulating and disappear when the animal is asleep or quiet. The tremors become worse with excitement. There is usually little ataxia or weakness of the limbs or other neurologic deficit. All clinicopathologic tests are normal. The EEG may be normal or, on occasion, may be characterized by diffuse slow-wave activity. CSF is normal.

Diazepam (Valium) 0.5 mg/kg orally every 8 hours usually controls the tremors (Chapter 6). Periodically the diazepam is reduced to see if the tremors are still present. The tremors decrease and eventually subside 1 to 3 months after the onset. The cause is presently unknown, as these dogs are rarely euthanized.

Myoclonus

Mechanism of disease and differential diagnosis

Infection
Distemper myoclonus

Distemper myoclonus

Incidence: Frequent

A spontaneous, rhythmic, repetitive myoclonus, also called "canine chorea," has to date been reported only as associated with distemper virus infections of the nervous system.[2] Myoclonus may be associated with other disorders in humans.[10]

It is believed that a neuronal pacemaker is established in the area of the cell bodies of lower motor neurons of the brain stem and spinal cord. Experimental studies of myoclonus involving a limb showed that the myoclonus persisted with spinal cord transection above the segments to the limb and with dorsal root transection at the segments to the limb.[2] The myoclonus was only abolished when the lower motor neurons to the limb were transected.

Distemper-related myoclonus may appear alone or with other neurologic signs. Groups of muscles in the limbs and the temporalis and masseter muscles of the head are most commonly affected. The muscle contraction is rhythmic and repetitive, up to one per second, and persistent even during sleep. The myoclonus may become more severe and involve several muscle groups.

The prognosis for the resolution of myoclonus is grave. No medications that could be given as a daily therapeutic regimen will control the signs. If the myoclonus is severe, the animals are usually euthanized. In mild cases, the dog may be kept as an acceptable pet, but the myoclonus generally persists for years.

Other muscle spasms

Mechanism of disease and differential diagnosis

Congenital and familial disorders
Myotonia

Metabolic disorders
Greyhound cramp

Idiopathic disorders
Scottie cramp

Dancing Doberman disease
Miscellaneous spastic syndrome

Myotonia

Incidence: Rare

Myotonia is a disorder of the muscle characterized by a failure of the muscle to relax once it has contracted. Congenital myotonia has been reported in Chow Chows, Staffordshire terriers, Irish terriers, and Golden Retrievers, as well as other breeds of dogs.[6,8]

The primary complaint is usually a stilted gait and stiff limbs. Stiffness often disappears with exercise in mildly affected dogs. On physical examination, the muscles feel firm. When tapped with a percussion hammer, the muscle sustains a local contraction and produces a visible and palpable dimple. Clinicopathologic testing, including serum CPK determination, is often normal. In other cases serum CPK may be elevated.

The diagnosis is made on needle EMG examination. When the exploring electrode is inserted into the muscle, myotonic discharges are seen and heard and continue after the electrode ceases movement. Myotonic discharges are bizarre high-frequency discharges that wax and wane in amplitude and sound spontaneously, with no electrode movement. The waxing and waning discharge differentiate myotonia from bizarre high-frequency discharges seen associated with denervation.

A marked variation in size between type I and type II fibers and internal nuclei, and angular atrophic fibers are found on muscle biopsy.

Mildly affected animals may make acceptable pets. Congenital myotonia is suspected to arise from an autosomal recessive inheritance. Acquired myotonia may be associated with hyperadrenocorticism and hypothyroidism.[5,6] Myotonic myopathy is further discussed in Chapter 16.

Greyhound cramp

Incidence: Frequent

Muscle cramping in racing greyhounds is thought to be similar to paralytic myoglobinuria or "tying-up" syndrome in horses.[11] It may be caused by an increased deposition of glycogen in the muscle during periods of rest. When the animal exercises, excessive amounts of lactic acid are released, which produce severe muscle cramping and muscle fiber damage with myoglobin release.

The racing greyhound may cramp with varying degrees of severity. If the dog cramps in one limb, the muscles often degenerate and atrophy, and the animal may no longer be useful for racing. In severe episodes, the limb and body muscles cramp during the race and the animal stops and stands rigidly or falls over in a severely distressed and cyanotic state. The animal may die. Proper conditioning and exercising prior to racing seem to prevent this condition. Rhabdomyolysis secondary to status epilepticus has been reported in dogs.[21]

Scottie cramp

Incidence: Occasional

A muscle cramping syndrome has been reported as an inherited problem in Scottish terriers.[3] A similar condition has been reported in Dalmatians.[24] The underlying cause is unknown, but is suspected of being a CNS neurotransmitter disorder and not a primary neuromuscular disorder.[17]

The clinical signs are first noticed from 6 weeks to 18 months of age, but an onset as late as 3 years of age has been reported. The muscle spasms seem to be aggravated by excess activity and excitement. The frequency and severity of signs vary with the individual dog. The muscle rigidity does not appear to be painful. The pelvic limbs alone may be involved in mild attacks. Severe attacks may produce rigidity in all muscles, including the face, and the animal may fall on its side, curl into a ball, and apparently cease respiration. Consciousness is maintained throughout. After approximately 15 seconds, the animal usually relaxes and returns to normal. Mild attacks may appear as periodic pelvic limb stiffness.

Clinicopathologic tests are within normal limits. The needle EMG examination between episodes is normal. During the episode, motor unit activity associated with the muscle spasm is seen. Amphetamine administration aggravates the muscle cramping.

If the clinical signs are frequent and severe, they may be controlled with daily oral dosing of acepromazine maleate (0.1 to 0.75 mg/kg every 12 hours), diazepam (0.5 mg/kg every 8 hours), primidone (12.5 mg/kg every 12 hours), or phenobarbital (0.5 mg/kg every 12 hours). Dogs with mild, infrequent signs are usually not treated.

Breeding studies have supported a recessive inheritance in Scottish terriers.

Dancing Doberman disease

Incidence: Occasional

Doberman Pinchers from 6 months to 7 years of age may be presented for a complaint of flexing one pelvic limb when standing. No orthopedic problem is present and the animal is not lame during ambulation. No response to glucocorticoid or diazepam therapy is seen. Often within 3 to 7 months the opposite pelvic limb becomes affected and while standing the dog will alternately flex and extend each pelvic limb in a dancing motion, then sit down.

Clinicopathologic tests are usually within normal limits. Serum CPK may be slightly elevated or normal. T_3, T_4, and

TSH stimulation tests should be performed to rule out hypothyroidism, but may be normal.

Electromyographic (EMG) studies of the gastrocnemius muscles of one or both pelvic limbs are abnormal. Trains of positive waves, fibrillation potentials, and bizarre high-frequency discharges are present and suggest neuromuscular disease. Nerve conduction studies are normal.

Biopsy of affected gastrocnemius muscles have Type I and II atrophy, internalized nuclei, and fiber necrosis. A primary myopathy is suspected.

The clinical signs slowly progress over the following months to years. Pelvic limb muscle atrophy, mild weakness, hyperactive tendon and muscle reflexes, and conscious proprioceptive deficits may develop. A neurologic component to the disease is thought to exist as well from limited studies of biopsy and necropsy material on affected dogs.

No dogs have been known to spontaneously recover and all dogs insidiously progress but are usually acceptable pets for many years. There is no known treatment.

A neuromuscular disorder of the gastrocnemius muscle is present, but the underlying cause is unknown.

Miscellaneous spastic syndromes

Occasionally, dogs develop an involuntary extension or flexion of one limb of unknown cause. Affected dogs may be presented for extending a rear limb behind them when they stand quietly or when they ambulate. No other neurologic signs are apparent. All clinicopathologic tests and routine needle EMG and motor nerve conduction velocity tests may be normal. The underlying cause is unknown, but these cases appear similar to the spastic paresis and spastic syndrome of cattle. An imbalance in the myotatic reflex has been suggested. Sometimes oral diazepam (Valium)

0.5 mg/kg every 8 hours will improve the signs, but many dogs are not given daily medication because the signs are relatively mild and do not interfere with the animal's ability to ambulate.

References

1. Bjerkas, E.: Eclampsia in the cat. J. Small Anim. Pract., 15:412, 1974.
2. Breazile, J.E., Blough, B.D., and Nail, N.: Experimental study of canine distemper myoclonus. Am. J. Vet. Res., 28:1483, 1967.
3. Clemmons, R.G., et al.: Scotty cramp. A review of cause, characteristics, diagnosis and treatment. Compendium on Continuing Education, 5:395, 1980.
4. DeLahunta, A.: Veterinary Neuroanatomy and Clinical Neurology. Philadelphia, W.B. Saunders, 1983.
5. Duncan, I.D., Griffiths, I.R., and Nash, A.S.: Myotonia in canine Cushing's disease. Vet. Rec., 100:30, 1977.
6. Duncan, I.D. and Griffiths, I.R.: Neuromuscular diseases in neurologic disorders. In Contemporary Issues of Small Animal Practice. Edited by J.N. Kornegay. New York, Churchill-Livingston, 1986.
7. Duncan, I.D.: Abnormalities of myelination of the central nervous system associated with congenital tremor. J. Vet. Intern. Med., 1:10, 1987.
8. Farrow, B.R.H., Malik, R.: Hereditary myotonia in the Chow Chow. J. Small Anim. Pract., 22:451, 1981.
9. Farrow, B.R.H.: Generalized tremor syndrome. In Current Veterinary Therapy IX. Edited by R.W. Kirk. Philadelphia. W.B. Saunders, 1986.
10. Frenken, C.W., et al.: Myoclonic disorders of spinal cord origin. Clin. Neurol. Neurosurg., 79:107, 1975.
11. Gowing, G.M.: An azoturia-like condition in coursing greyhounds. Southwest Vet., 17:183, 1964.
12. Greene, C.G.: Tetanus. In Current Veterinary Therapy VIII. Edited by R.W. Kirk. Philadelphia, W.B. Saunders, 1983.
13. Jackson, K.F. and Duncan, I.D.: Hypomyelination in dogs. In Current Veterinary

Therapy X. Edited by R.W. Kirk. Philadelphia, W. B. Saunders, 1989.
14. Johnston, S.D.: Management of the postpartum bitch and queen. In Current Veterinary Therapy VIII. Edited by R.W. Kirk. Philadelphia, W.B. Saunders, 1983.
15. Killingsworth, C., Chiapella, A., Veralli, P., and DeLahunta, A.: Feline tetanus. Am. Anim. Hosp. Assoc. J., 13:209, 1977.
16. Meerdin, G.L.: Organophosphorus and carbamate insecticide poisoning. In Current Veterinary Therapy X. Edited by R.W. Kirk. Philadelphia, W.B. Saunders, 1989.
17. Meyers, K.M. and Clemmons, R.M.: Scotty cramp. In Current Veterinary Therapy VIII. Edited by R.W. Kirk. Philadelphia, W.B. Saunders, 1983.
18. Paul, A. and Tranquilli, W.: Ivermectin. In Current Veterinary Therapy X. Edited by R.W. Kirk. Philadelphia, W.B. Saunders, 1989.
19. Peterson, M.E.: Hypoparathyroidism. In Current Veterinary Therapy IX. Edited by R.W. Kirk. Philadelphia, W.B. Saunders, 1983.
20. Sherding, R.G., et al.: Primary hypoparathyroidism in the dog. J. Am. Vet. Med. Assoc., 176(5):439, 1980.
21. Sangler, W.L. and Muggli, F.M.: Seizure-induced rhabdomyolysis accompanied by acute renal failure in a dog. J. Am. Vet. Med. Assoc., 172(10):1190, 1978.
22. Vandevelde, M., Braund, K.G., Walker, T.L., and Kornegay, N.J.: Dysmyelination of the central nervous system in the Chow Chow dog. Acta Neuropathol., 42:211, 1978.
23. Weisbrode, S.F. and Krakowka, S.: Canine distemper virus associated hypocalcemia. Am. J. Vet. Res., 40(1):147, 1979.
24. Woods, C.B.: Hyperkinetic episodes in two Dalmatian dogs. Am. Anim. Hosp. Assoc. J., 13:255, 1977.
25. Zenoble, R.D. and Myers, R.K.: Severe hypocalcemia resulting from ethylene glycol poisoning in the dog. Am. Anim. Hosp. Assoc. J., 13:489, 1977.

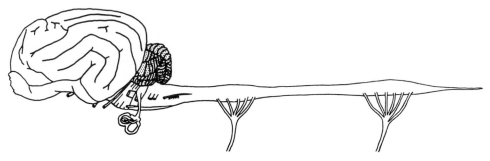

Figure 15–1. Location of the lesion of an animal with ataxia of the head and limbs is the cerebellum (dotted).

Location of the lesion (Figure 15–1): *cerebellum*

Mechanisms of disease and differential diagnosis

Congenital and familial disorders

Panleukopenia virus in kittens
Herpes virus in puppies
Miscellaneous cerebellar hypoplasia and
 degeneration
Cerebellar neuronal abiotrophy
Spongiform degeneration
Lysosomal storage disorders (Chap. 7)
Neuroaxonal dystrophy

Infections and other inflammations (Chaps. 7 and 12)

Distemper virus
Feline infectious peritonitis virus
Toxoplasmosis
Fungal infections
Bacterial infections
Parasites
Granulomatous meningoencephalitis (reticulosis)
Corticosteroid responsive meningoencephalitis

Nutritional

Early thiamine deficiency (Chap. 7)

Trauma and vascular disorders

Cerebellar injury
Spontaneous cerebellar infarct or hemorrhage

Degeneration

Late onset cerebellar degeneration

Neoplasia (Chap. 7)

Meningioma
Astrocytoma
Oligodendroglioma
Medulloblastoma
Reticulosis
Choroid plexus papilloma
Metastatic neoplasia

Chapter 15

Ataxia
of the head
and limbs

Ataxia or incoordination of the head, neck, and all four limbs is most often produced by a lesion in the cerebellum.

The cerebellum, located in the caudal fossa of the skull, is dorsal to the fourth ventricle and attached to the pontine—medullary portion of the brain stem by three pairs of supporting structures referred to as the rostral, middle, and caudal cerebellar peduncles. The cerebellum is composed of two lateral masses, the cerebellar hemispheres, which meet in a center portion called the vermis. Although the cerebellum has many subdivisions, it is organized into three main regions: the rostral, caudal, and flocculonodular lobes. Histologically, the cerebellum consists of a cortical gray matter region of three layers and a subcortical white matter region. The three layers of the cortex consist of an outer molecular layer of stellate and basket cells, a middle layer of Purkinje cells, and an inner layer containing granule cells and other neuron types. The subcortical white matter contains three pairs of deep cerebellar nuclei: the fastigial, interpositus, and lateral nuclei.

One of the main functions of the cerebellum is to coordinate the various muscle groups of the body, so that movements are smooth and accurate. The cerebellum receives continuous, instantaneous information concerning the progress of all muscle activity in order to correct and coordinate this activity. A description of the intricate relationships between the cerebellum and all other parts of the nervous system is beyond the scope of this text, and is discussed in detail elsewhere.[9,11] A simplified version is presented here to explain the role of the cerebellum in the coordination of movement.

Information concerning the position of the limbs and neck is transmitted by way of the spinocerebellar and cuneocerebellar pathways through the caudal and rostral cerebellar peduncles to the cerebellum. Information concerning the initiation of muscle movement is transmitted from the motor areas of the cerebral cortex and subcortical and brain stem motor nuclei through the middle cerebellar peduncle to the cerebellum. The cerebellum processes the information concerning position and movement that is received, and the Purkinje cells transmit signals to the deep cerebellar nuclei. The deep cerebellar nuclei transmit information from the cerebellum primarily through the rostral cerebellar peduncle to the motor nuclei of the brain stem and subcortical region and the motor areas of the cerebral cortex. By this interaction, the cerebellum can correct any mistakes or inaccuracies of muscle movement. Without cerebellar function, voluntary movement can still occur, but such movements are jerky and lack control.

The cerebellum functions in the maintenance of normal posture, along with the vestibular system. The flocculonodular lobe and fastigial nuclei of the cerebellum also play an important role in orientation and balance of the animal (Chap. 12). The rostral lobe of the cerebellum has a profound effect on muscle tone (Chap. 14).

Patient evaluation

Signalment and history

The age and breed of the animal are important to consider when evaluating cere-

bellar disease. Several cerebellar disorders have been described in which the signs become apparent when the animals begin to ambulate or before 6 months of age. Kerry Blue terriers, Labrador Retrievers, Irish Setters, Samoyeds, Gordon Setters, Rough Coated Collies, Border Collies, Bull Mastiffs, Airdale terriers, Golden Retrievers, Cocker Spaniels, Cairn terriers, Great Danes, and Beagles have specific cerebellar disorders. Animals with lysosomal storage disorders may show signs of cerebellar dysfunction during the course of the disease process (Chap. 7). Virus-induced cerebellar malformations in dogs and cats produce signs that are apparent when the animals first begin to ambulate. Cerebellar dysfunction in an adult animal may be due to viral, protozoal, fungal, or bacterial infections and other inflammations such as granulomatous meningoencephalitis (reticulosis), corticosteroid responsive meningoencephalitis, or neoplastic processes.

The onset and course of the disease process is important to ascertain. Virus-induced and miscellaneous forms of cerebellar hypoplasia and degeneration produce cerebellar deficit, evident on ambulation, that does not progress. Cerebellar neuronal abiotrophy and storage diseases usually begin in animals under 6 months of age, and become progressively worse over the following weeks and months. Traumatic and vascular disorders of the cerebellum have an acute onset of signs that do not progress and often regress somewhat, in time. Infections with viral, protozoal, fungal, or bacterial agents and other inflammations are often progressive. Neoplasms of the cerebellum can begin with mild cerebellar signs that progress at various rates, depending on the tumor type.

Questions must be asked concerning systemic illness, infections, trauma, or neoplasia to determine whether involvement of the cerebellum is associated with one of these processes.

Any signs of neurologic dysfunction

unrelated to the cerebellum should also be described.

Physical and neurologic examinations

The physical examination should be used to evaluate the rest of the body for signs of congenital defects, illness, infection, trauma, or neoplasia.

The neurologic examination aids in localizing the lesion to the cerebellum alone or detecting dysfunction related to other parts of the nervous system. The severity of cerebellar dysfunction can be estimated, and serial neurologic examinations can serve to monitor progress.

The neurologic findings associated with cerebellar lesions are described here. The presence of other neurologic signs signifies involvement of other parts of the nervous system and the presence of a multifocal disease process.

The animal is bright and alert, with no history of seizures or endocrine disturbances. No head tilt should be observed unless the flocculonodular lobe of the cerebellum is involved (Chap. 12). Head coordination is obviously abnormal. A fine head tremor is often present, even at rest, and becomes worse when the animal attempts to perform a specific task such as sniffing the floor or beginning to eat, and is called an intention tremor. When the head is lowered to the floor to sniff or to the food bowl to eat, a series of jerky, bobbing movements occurs. The animal is unable to judge distances or control the range of head movements. When drinking water, the animal's nose is often plunged too deeply into the bowl. It quickly withdraws the nose and makes multiple snorting noises to expel the water that has entered the nostrils.

On testing the cranial nerves, the examiner may find the menace-response decreased or absent in severe cerebellar disease. It has been suggested that the cerebellum is necessary for a normal men-ace-response.[9] Ocular movement is present, but can be somewhat jerky, and a fine intention tremor of the eyeballs is seen, owing to the lack of cerebellar control. All other cranial nerves should be normal and reflect only incoordinated muscle movements. Nystagmus is present only if the vestibular components of the cerebellum are affected (Chap. 12).

The only signs to indicate involvement of the nervous system above the level of the foramen magnum should be the incoordinated head and eye movements related to the cerebellar dysfunction. The rest of the neurologic examination, including evaluation of the gait, thoracic, and pelvic limbs, should also show only abnormalities associated with the cerebellar involvement.

The gait is composed of a series of jerky, choppy, uncoordinated movements, referred to as dysmetria. Hypermetria is commonly seen, and consists of exaggerated flexion and extension of the limbs (Fig. 15–2). If severe, the hypermetria and incoordination may cause the animal to lose its orientation and fall. Ataxia of trunk muscles is also seen. A unilateral cerebellar lesion may produce incoordination of the thoracic and pelvic limbs on the same side of the body. The gait of the animal is strong, and no paresis is present.

When the animal stands quietly, the feet are placed widely apart for support (Fig. 15–3). The body often shifts back and forth, with the head bobbing slightly. Animals with cerebellar dysfunction can have difficulty jumping in an arc to get onto furniture. Cats might jump up in the air and come down in the same spot, instead of achieving their goal on the couch.

Hopping and placing response tests on the limbs are performed, but the dysmetria is usually obvious. Proprioceptive positioning (conscious proprioception) is normal, but the movement reflects the incoordination.

Spinal reflexes and sensation are normal. All findings on the neurologic exam-

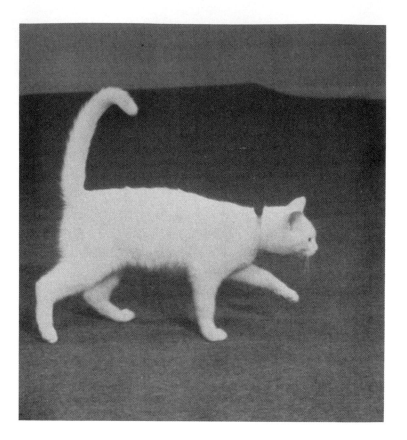

Figure 15–2. Hypermetria in a cat with cerebellar dysfunction.

ination indicate only loss of muscle coordination.

Ancillary diagnostic investigations

Routine clinical laboratory tests are normal or indicate disease processes in other systems. CSF analysis is useful in diagnosing active infections and other inflammations or neoplasia of the cerebellum (Chap. 5).

EEGs are normal in animals that have cerebellar disease alone, without involvement of the cerebral cortex (Chap. 5).

Routine skull radiographs can be helpful in diagnosing fractures of the skull in the region of the posterior fossa and neoplastic processes affecting osseous structures.

MRI and CT scans can outline neoplasms, inflammations, hematomas, and infarcts in the cerebellum (Fig. 15–4).

Exploratory craniotomy of the posterior fossa is a relatively safe and simple technique. A gross examination of the cerebellum and cerebellar biopsy can be the greatest aids to the specific diagnosis of cerebellar disease (Fig. 15–5). The approach to the diagnosis of an animal with ataxia of the head and limbs is summarized in Table 15–1.

Congenital and familial disorders

Panleukopenia virus in kittens

Incidence: Frequent

Signalment and history. Kittens at 3 to 4 weeks of age might demonstrate cerebellar ataxia when they begin to ambulate.[1,2,7,14] One or more kittens in the litter

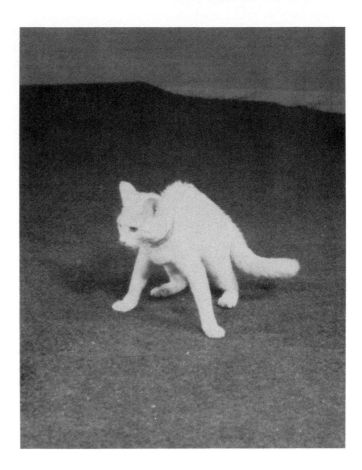

Figure 15–3. A wide-based stance is a typical posture associated with cerebellar dysfunction.

are affected to varying degrees. The queen or kittens usually show no signs of systemic illness associated with panleukopenia virus infection. The cerebellar deficit does not progress.

Physical and neurologic examinations. The physical examination is usually normal. The neurologic deficit ranges from mild ataxia and head tremors in some kittens, to hypermetria, severe tremors, and falling after a few steps in other kittens. The ataxia is generally symmetric, and only signs related to cerebellar dysfunction are present.

Ancillary diagnostic investigations. Clinical laboratory tests are usually normal. The diagnosis is often based on the signalment, history, and neurologic exam-

ination, because this disorder is so common in kittens.

Therapy and prognosis. No therapy will alter the damage that has already been done to the developing cerebellum. However, mildly affected kittens make acceptable pets if kept in a protected environment. Because the neurologic signs do not progress, the animals adapt well as house cats. If the neurologic symptoms are severe, euthanasia is the most humane choice.

Prevention. Proper vaccination of the queen against the panleukopenia virus prior to breeding is the most effective way of preventing in utero infections in the kittens. Affected kittens do carry active vi-

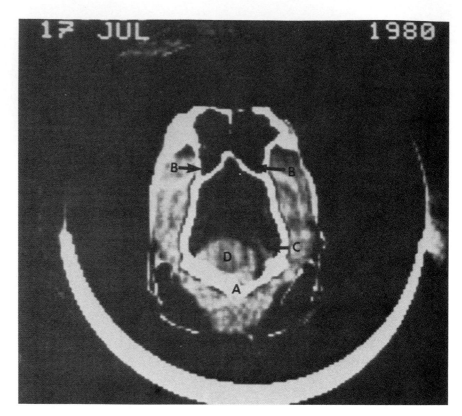

Figure 15–4. A CT scan on a 4-year-old German Shepherd female with a slow progressive cerebellar deficit of 6 months duration. The animal has severe generalized incoordination with hypermetria more severe on the left thoracic limb than the right thoracic limb. Head bobbing, tremor, and a mild left head tilt are present. The brain is viewed from a dorsal section. The tumor is shown in the caudal fossa on the left, eroding through the tentorium cerebelli. (A) occipital protuberance, (B) frontal sinuses, (C) tentorium cerebelli on right, (D) tumor enhanced with intravenous organic iodide contrast media.

rus for weeks to months after birth, as evidenced by kidney biopsy and virus isolation studies.

Pathology. The panleukopenia virus attacks cells of the developing cerebellum in utero or shortly after birth. The cerebellum may have a normal shape, but is usually small (Fig. 15–6). Many cells of the external granular layer of the fetus are destroyed, and this results in a deficiency of cells in the granular cell layer of the adult. Purkinje cells are also destroyed. By a few weeks after birth, the active infection is over and no further degeneration occurs.

Herpesvirus in puppies

Incidence: Rare

Signalment and history. Puppies at 3 to 4 weeks of age can demonstrate cerebellar ataxia following septicemia from a herpes virus infection. Shortly after birth, up to 2 weeks of age, signs of colic, diarrhea, constant crying, and dyspnea are seen. Affected puppies usually die within 1 to 3 days. Puppies that survive the active infection may show signs of cerebellar deficit when ambulation begins.[2,9,14]

Physical and neurologic examinations. Physical examination is often normal, once the systemic disease has passed.

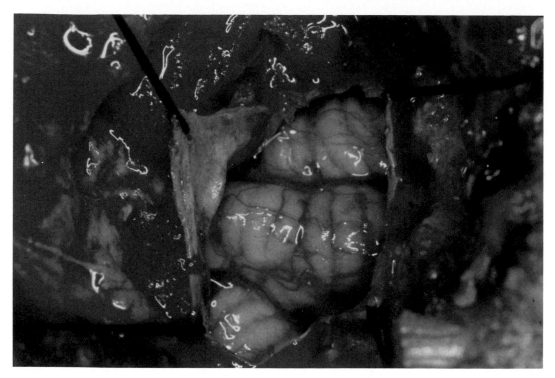

Figure 15–5. Exploratory surgery and examination of the cerebellum. The dura mater has been incised and four sutures are placed in the dura for retraction to visualize the underlying cerebellar follia.

On neurologic examination, varying degrees of ataxia and head tremor may be seen. Neurologic signs that are not related to cerebellar dysfunction can also be seen, as the virus is not specific to the cerebellum.

Ancillary diagnostic investigations. Once the active infection is over, there might be no abnormalities seen on clinical laboratory tests. Diagnosis is often made on the history of a systemic disease, with puppy death among the litter and cerebellar deficit in surviving puppies. The isolation of virus from puppies that died from the systemic disease can help to make a definitive diagnosis.

Therapy and prognosis. There is no specific therapy. By the time the neurologic signs are noted, the active infection has passed. If the cerebellar ataxia is mild,

the puppy might make an acceptable pet in a protected environment.

Prevention. No vaccines are currently available. Herpes virus infections are sporadic and relatively rare.

Pathology. Herpes virus infection in the newborn generally produces encephalitis and necrosis of the cerebellum. Although the herpes virus does not have a specificity for cerebellar tissues, it can produce cerebellar dysplasia and resultant malformation. Lesions may be found in other parts of the nervous system as well.

Miscellaneous cerebellar hypoplasia and degeneration

Incidence: Occasional

Signalment and history. Irish Setters, Wire Haired Fox terriers, Samoyeds,

Table 15–1
Diagnostic approach for the evaluation of ataxia of the head and limbs

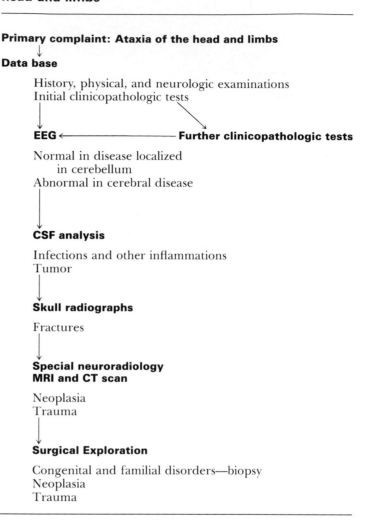

Primary complaint: Ataxia of the head and limbs
↓
Data base

History, physical, and neurologic examinations
Initial clinicopathologic tests

EEG ←———————— **Further clinicopathologic tests**

Normal in disease localized
   in cerebellum
Abnormal in cerebral disease

↓

CSF analysis

Infections and other inflammations
Tumor

↓

Skull radiographs

Fractures

↓

Special neuroradiology
MRI and CT scan

Neoplasia
Trauma

↓

Surgical Exploration

Congenital and familial disorders—biopsy
Neoplasia
Trauma

Chow Chows, Rough-Coated Collies, Border Collies, Bull Mastiffs, Labrador Retrievers, Beagles, and other breeds of dogs and cats have been sporadically reported to have signs of cerebellar dysfunction at 3 to 4 weeks of age, when ambulation begins.[2,5,7,9,12] One or more animals in the litter may be affected with cerebellar deficits in varying degrees. There is no history of systemic illness in the mother or in the litter. The signs are generally nonprogressive.

Physical and neurologic examinations. Head tremors, hypermetria of the limbs, and generalized ataxia are apparent on the neurologic examination. Samoyeds are reported to demonstrate only pelvic limb ataxia with minimal involvement of the head. Bull Mastiffs may have depression and abnormal behavior associated with hydrocephalus as well.[5]

Ancillary diagnostic investigations. Clinical laboratory tests are often normal.

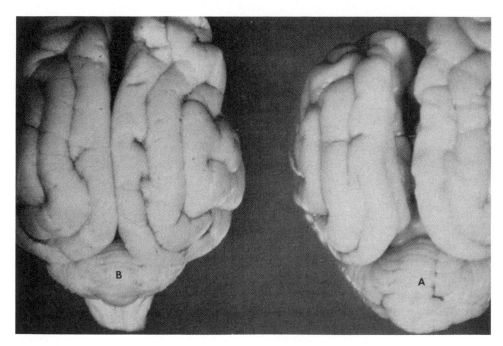

Figure 15–6. A comparison of a normal-sized cerebellum (A) with the cerebellum of a kitten who suffered an in utero infection caused by the panleukopenia virus (B). (Courtesy of Dr. Adalbert Koestner, Dept. of Pathology, The Ohio State University, College of Veterinary Medicine.)

The diagnosis is suspected from the history and neurologic findings. An exploratory craniotomy of the posterior fossa, with histologic examination of a cerebellar biopsy, is the only method of obtaining a definitive diagnosis in the living animal. However, the diagnosis is most often made at necropsy.

Therapy and prognosis. There is no specific therapy for these disorders. If the symptoms do not progress and the cerebellar deficit is minimal, these animals may make acceptable pets.

Prevention. Some of these disorders may have a genetic basis; others may be due to a teratogen. Selective breeding trials aid in the understanding of genetic processes, and in eliminating the problem.

Pathology. A variety of lesions are found during necropsy of these animals.

The entire cerebellum may be small, or only a portion such as the vermis or hemispheres may be underdeveloped (Fig. 15–7). The cerebellum may appear normal on gross examination. A loss of Purkinje cells and some decrease in granule cell neurons may be the only abnormalities found. Beagles and Irish Setters are reported to have lissencephaly along with the cerebellar dysgenesis (Chap. 7). Although these cases represent different pathologic processes, they are grouped together because the clinical presentation, management, and prognosis are the same.

Cerebellar neuronal abiotrophy

Incidence: Occasional

Signalment and history. A cerebellar neuronal abiotrophy is described in Kerry Blue terriers.[6] A cerebellar neuronal abiotrophy has also been suspected in other

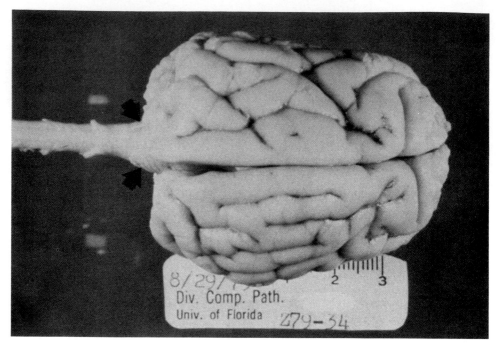

Figure 15–7. An underdeveloped cerebellum (arrows) in a 3-month-old Wire Haired Dachshund that had cerebellar deficit apparent when it began to ambulate.

breeds such as Rough-coated Collies in Australia, Finnish Harriers, Bern Running dogs, Irish Setters, and Gordon Setters.[1,8,17] The affected animals are usually normal when ambulation begins, but at 6 to 16 weeks of age cerebellar deficit appears. The Gordon Setter may not develop signs until 6 to 18 months of age. Although the signs are most often progressive, the progression may occur at different rates. Kerry Blue terriers are severely affected by 1 year of age. Gordon Setters continue to progress very slowly for the next 1 to 2 years or remain static. Other breeds may deteriorate much more rapidly over a period of a few weeks. The age of onset and progression of signs differentiate these disorders from virus-induced and hypoplastic disorders of the cerebellum.

Physical and neurologic examinations. Various degrees of cerebellar deficit are seen on the neurologic examination, ranging from mild ataxia and head tremors to frequent falling and inability to stand because of severe incoordination. No signs of dysfunction of other parts of the nervous system are usually seen.

Ancillary diagnostic investigations. Hematologic studies and CSF analysis of Kerry Blue terriers have been reported to be normal. The diagnosis of a cerebellar neuronal abiotrophy may be suspected on the basis of the signalment, history, and neurologic examination findings. A progressive cerebellar syndrome that begins in a young puppy with no evidence of active infection in the nervous system is suggestive of neuronal abiotrophy. A diagnosis may be made by exploratory craniotomy of the posterior fossa and biopsy of the cerebellum. Examination of biopsy material reveals active degeneration, primarily in the Purkinje cell layer in Kerry Blue terriers.

Therapy and prognosis. No therapy is known to alter the course of the disease. The signs progress until the animal is incapacitated, and the prognosis is grave.

Prevention. An autosomal recessive inheritance is suggested in Kerry Blue terriers. A genetic basis is also suspected in many of the other cases. Selective breeding can prevent this disorder.

Pathology. Histologic examination shows that Kerry Blue terriers have degeneration of neurons in the olivary nuclei, substantia nigra, and caudate nuclei, as well as in the cerebellum. The neurons that degenerate are believed to be lacking some vital material necessary to maintain their health.

Spongiform degeneration

Incidence: Rare

A slow progressive ataxia of head and limbs has been described in Labrador Retrievers at 4 to 6 months of age.[13] Episodes of extensor rigidity and opisthotonus may be seen. A generalized vacuolation of white matter, referred to as spongiform degeneration, occurs in cerebellar and cerebral white matter, as well as other CNS and PNS regions. An inherited problem is suspected.

Egyptian Mau cats develop a cerebellar ataxia at 7 weeks of age from spongiform degeneration.[1] These kittens may improve with age.

Spongiform degeneration has been described in Samoyeds and Silky Terriers as well.[1]

Lysosomal storage diseases

Incidence: Rare

A description of the diagnosis and management of the lysosomal storage diseases is presented in Chapter 7. Signs of cerebellar involvement may be seen at various stages of the disease process, but occur particularly in GM_1 gangliosidosis, sphingomyelinosis, glucocerebrosidosis, and globoid cell leukodystrophy. Portuguese water dogs with GM_1 gangliosidosis develop dysmetria, a wide base stance, and intention tremors at 5 months of age.[15] Nystagmus and pelvic limb weakness may develop as well. The neurologic dysfunction progresses rapidly over the next 1 to 2 months, and most dogs are euthanized.

These storage diseases affect multiple sites within the nervous system, so that signs of dementia, seizures, and quadriplegia or paraparesis are often seen along with the signs of cerebellar deficit. Lysosomal storage diseases can be differentiated from cerebellar neuronal abiotrophy by the presence of signs unrelated to the cerebellar deficit.

Neuroaxonal dystrophy

Incidence: Rare

Neuroaxonal dystrophy has been described in Rottweilers, Collies, and cats. Affected Rottweilers insidiously develop a progressive cerebellar ataxia in the first 1 to 2 years of life.[1,2,4] The ataxia progresses and intention tremors of the head, nystagmus, and a menace deficit occurs. By 6 years of age, most Rottweilers are severely affected. Distal axons swell to form spheroids in many nuclei, including the nucleus of the dorsal spinocerebellar tract and vestibular nuclei. There is also a loss of Purkinje cells. An autosomal recessive inheritance is suspected.

In neuroaxonal dystrophy of Collies, progressive cerebellar ataxia, intention tremors, and balance problems develop at 2 to 4 months of age. Axonal spheroids are present in the cerebellum and vestibular nuclei. An autosomal recessive inheritance is thought to exist.[2]

Neuroaxonal dystrophy of cats begins at 5 to 6 weeks of age with head tremors.

A progressive ataxia then develops. Tricolor cats are affected. Axonal spheroids are present in nuclear groups in the cerebellar vermis as well as other brain stem nuclei. There is a loss of Purkinje and granule cells as well. An autosomal recessive inheritance is suggested.[2]

Infections and other inflammations

Viral, protozoal, fungal, and bacterial infections and granulomatous meningoencephalitis, steroid-responsive meningoencephalitis, and other inflammations

Incidence: Viral infections, frequent; others, rare

Signalment and history. Almost any age, breed, or sex of dog or cat can show cerebellar signs resulting from an inflammatory process.[2,7,9,10,14] The animals may have a history of a systemic illness due to viral, fungal, protozoal, bacterial, or other infection (see Tables 7–6 and 7–7). Distemper virus infection in dogs is common, and can have a predilection for the cerebellar peduncles. Signs of cerebellar deficit can be seen with or without signs of systemic disease. Dementia, seizures, or other signs may also be present and indicate involvement of other parts of the nervous system.

Distemper virus infections should be considered in any adult dog with progressive cerebellar signs. A head tilt or other vestibular signs may also be associated with the head tremor, hypermetria, and ataxia if the flocculonodular lobe is involved (Chap. 12). The diagnosis and management of canine distemper virus and other CNS infections and inflammations are discussed in Chapters 7 and 12.

Physical and neurologic examinations. Evidence of gastrointestinal and respiratory disease may be apparent in animals suffering from distemper virus infections. Other dogs with distemper virus infections may be normal on physical examination. Cats with feline infectious peritonitis (FIP) virus infections can have peritoneal and pleural effusions or may be normal. Evidence of bacterial or fungal infections can be present in other body systems. Neurologic signs such as head tremor, hypermetria of the limbs, and truncal ataxia indicate cerebellar involvement. However, these agents have no specificity for the cerebellum, so other signs, such as dementia, specific cranial nerve abnormalities, paresis, and conscious proprioceptive deficits, can be present.

Ancillary diagnostic investigations. Neutrophilic leukocytosis can be seen on a complete blood count in bacterial infections, with septicemia and resulting cerebellar infection. Lymphopenia can be present in early viral infections. CSF analysis is the greatest aid in diagnosing cerebellar inflammations. In viral infections, the CSF can be normal or contain increased mononuclear cells and protein. In fungal infections, the CSF may contain increased neutrophils, eosinophils, or mononuclear cells and protein. Fungal organisms may be observed in the CSF. In protozoal infections, the CSF might have increased mononuclear cells and protein. In bacterial infections, the predominant cell type is the neutrophil, and the protein is often greatly elevated. The organism can often be cultured from the CSF. In granulomatous meningoencephalitis and corticosteroid-responsive meningoencephalitis there is often a mixture of mononuclear cells and neutrophils and elevated protein. Because CSF changes can be similar with various inflammations, CSF and serum titers may be helpful to determine the cause (see Table 7–8).

The EEG is usually abnormal if the cerebral cortex is also involved in the inflammation.

Skull radiographs are usually normal, unless a bacterial osteomyelitis is present.

Therapy and prognosis. There is no specific therapy for viral infections. Prednisolone, 2 mg/kg divided every 12 hours, can be tried in decreasing doses over a month. However, if the virus causes severe immunosuppression or if an incorrect diagnosis is made and a bacterial, protozoal, or fungal infection is present, the aforementioned treatment will cause the animal's condition to worsen. A viral infection (distemper, FIP) is more common than a protozoal (toxoplasmosis) infection, but it can be difficult to differentiate the two in a live animal. If there is improvement on glucocorticoid therapy, the animal may continue to improve and be an acceptable pet. If the signs progress, the prognosis is poor. Treatment for fungal infections can be attempted as discussed in Chapters 6 and 7, but the prognosis is poor. Bacterial infections can be treated with the appropriate antibiotic, and the prognosis can be fair, depending on the severity of cerebellar involvement. Once the infection is arrested, if the cerebellar signs are mild, the animal may be able to live with the remaining deficit. The prognosis for granulomatous meningoencephalitis is often poor, and a definitive diagnosis is only made at necropsy.

If no organism can be found, a therapeutic trial of prednisone 2 mg/kg orally and then decreasing over the next month should be attempted (Chaps. 6 and 7). Corticosteroid-responsive meningoencephalitis may affect the cerebellum.

Prevention. Because infections are difficult to anticipate, they cannot be easily prevented. Vaccination against the distemper virus can help to prevent CNS infection, but it is not always completely effective.

Pathology. Most infections, regardless of cause, are usually not localized to the cerebellum alone. The pathology of various CNS infections is discussed further in Chapter 7. Canine distemper and feline infectious peritonitis are the most common viral infections. Toxoplasmosis is the most common protozoal infection, but it is rare in both cats and dogs. Cryptococcus infections are the most common fungal infections, but they rarely occur. Bacterial infections are also rare. Granulomatous meningoencephalitis (reticulosis) may also rarely affect the cerebellum.[10]

Trauma and vascular disorders

Traumatic or spontaneous hemorrhage or infarcts

Incidence: Trauma, frequent; spontaneous infarct or hemorrhage, rare

Signalment and history. Any age, breed, or sex of dog or cat is susceptible to cranial trauma. Occipital bone fractures may lead to hemorrhage and compression of the cerebellum.[9,14] Infarcts of the cerebellum rarely occur in adult or older animals. Spontaneous hemorrhages of the cerebellum from bleeding disorders or arteriovenous malformations also are rare. The onset of cerebellar deficit is acute in either trauma or vascular disorders. History of a head injury is often obtained. With no history of injury or infections, acute onset of severe cerebellar signs may be caused by a spontaneous hemorrhage or infarct. In either trauma or vascular disorders, the cerebellar signs may be acute and severe, but do not progress and should improve with time.

Physical and neurologic examinations. The initial evaluation of patients with cranial trauma is discussed in Chapter 10, and the same procedure is followed in all cases. Life-threatening processes are managed and monitored first. Palpable fractures, bruising, lacerations, and other signs of trauma may be found on physical examination. No abnormal physical findings may be found in an animal with a cerebellar infarct or hemorrhage.

The neurologic signs may vary greatly, depending on other sites of the central nervous system that are subjected to trauma. The animal may be presented with opisthotonos from damage to the rostral lobe of the cerebellum (Chap. 14). The opisthotonos initially appears as a severe neurologic deficit, but usually passes in a few weeks to months. Head tremor, truncal ataxia, and hypermetria may be obvious once the animal begins to walk, and the signs may be asymmetric.

Therapy and prognosis. Immediate management of a patient with cranial trauma is discussed in Chapter 10. Corticosteroid therapy is often continued at decreasing doses for 1 week to 10 days. Nursing care is of the utmost importance until the animal can ambulate. Surgical decompression of the cerebellum may be needed if bony fragments are lodged in the nervous tissue. Improvement and compensation is possible with time. Residual cerebellar deficits are often permanent, but animals can be acceptable pets again.

Degeneration

Late-onset cerebellar degeneration

Incidence: Rare

Signalment and history. Adult dogs may develop a slow, progressive cerebellar disorder.[3] The initial signs may begin in the pelvic limbs, and then up to 1 year later, the thoracic limbs and head may be involved with ataxia and tremors.

Physical and neurologic examinations. The physical examination is normal. Only signs of cerebellar dysfunction are present on the neurologic examination. The signs include head bobbing, intention tremor, symmetric hypermetria, and truncal ataxia.

Ancillary diagnostic investigations. A complete blood count and chemistry profile are normal. Findings on CSF analysis and EEG are normal. A CT or MRI scan may show a small cerebellum. Exploratory craniotomy into the posterior fossa can be performed. The cerebellum may be properly shaped, but small. Active degeneration in all three layers of the cerebellum may be found on a cerebellar biopsy. The cause is unknown.

Therapy and prognosis. No therapy is known to alter this type of cerebellar degeneration. The prognosis is grave, if active degeneration is seen on the biopsy specimen. The signs are likely to progress until the animal is completely incapacitated.

Neoplasia

Primary or metastatic neoplasia of the cerebellum

Incidence: Occasional

Signalment and history. Any adult dog, often over 5 years of age, may develop a neoplasm of the cerebellum.[7,9,14] As discussed in Chapter 7, Boston terriers and Boxers commonly develop primary brain tumors, such as astrocytomas and oligodendrogliomas. With a tumor of the cerebellum, signs can begin slowly or progress rapidly, within days to a few weeks in the case of astrocytomas and oligodendrogliomas.[16] Cerebellar signs may progress more slowly over several months with meningiomas. Neoplastic GME (reticulosis) may occur in cerebellar white matter, but is difficult to differentiate clinically from the others. A history of mammary or prostatic adenocarcinoma might indicate cerebellar metastasis of these tumors. Lymphosarcoma may also involve the cerebellum and overlying meninges.

Physical and neurologic examinations. The physical examination may be noncontributory, except in cases of metastatic neoplasia.

On neurologic examination, only signs of cerebellar deficit are seen. Signs are often asymmetric. Ipsilateral hypermetria of the limbs may be present with initially minimal head tremor. The signs then can progress to severe incoordination with both sides involved, but an asymmetry often remains.

Ancillary diagnostic investigations. Elevated CSF pressure and increased protein with no increase in cells are the typical CSF changes of most tumors, except meningiomas, which rarely produce pressure elevation (Chaps. 5 and 7). Routine skull radiographs are often negative, unless a calcified meningioma or sarcoma of the skull is present. Cerebral angiography may demonstrate a tumor blush in the caudal fossa. MRI and CT scans can demonstrate tumors in dogs and cats (see Fig. 15–4).

Therapy and prognosis. A meningioma is the only potentially removable tumor of the cerebellum. Because the cerebellum is easily reached by an exploratory craniotomy of the caudal fossa, gross examination and biopsy of the cerebellum are indicated to obtain a specific diagnosis. Experience with radiation and chemotherapy in brain tumors is increasing and may prove helpful. The prognosis for most brain tumors, except meningiomas, is grave. Glucocorticoid therapy may keep secondary brain swelling suppressed and prolong the animal's life for a short time.

Prevention. No method of preventing brain tumors is currently known.

Pathology. The types of tumors that can affect the cerebellum are meningioma, astrocytoma, oligodendroglioma, medulloblastoma, reticulosis, choroid plexus papilloma, metastatic neoplasia, and sarcoma of the skull.

References

1. Braund, K.G.: Clinical Syndromes. *In* Veterinary Neurology. Baltimore, Williams & Wilkins, 1986.
2. Braund, K.G.: Degenerative and Developmental Diseases in Veterinary Neurology. Edited by J.E. Oliver, B.F. Hoerlein, and I.G. Mayhew. Philadelphia, W.B. Saunders, 1987.
3. Chrisman, C.L., et al.: Late onset cerebellar degeneration in a dog. J. Am. Vet. Med. Assoc., *182*:17, 1983.
4. Chrisman, C.L.: Neuroaxonal dystrophy and leukomyelopathy of Rottweiler dogs. *In* Current Veterinary Therapy IX. Edited by R.W. Kirk. Philadelphia, W.B. Saunders, 1986.
5. Carmichael, S., et al.: Familial cerebellar ataxia with hydrocephalus in Bull Mastiffs. Vet. Rec., *112*:354, 1983.
6. DeLahunta, A. and Averill, D.R., Jr.: Hereditary cerebellar cortical and extrapyramidal nuclear abiotrophy in Kerry blue terriers. J. Am. Vet. Med. Assoc., *168*:1119, 1976.
7. DeLahunta, A.: Disease of the cerebellum. Vet. Clin. North Am., *10*:91, 1980.
8. DeLahunta, A., et al.: Hereditary cerebellar cortical abiotrophy in the Gordon Setter. J. Am. Vet. Med. Assoc., *177*:538, 1980.
9. DeLahunta, A.: Cerebellum. *In* Veterinary Neuroanatomy and Clinical Neurology. Philadelphia, W.B. Saunders, 1983.

10. Gearhart, M.A., et al.: Cerebellar mass in a dog due to granulomatous meningoencephalitis. J. Am. Anim. Hosp. Assoc., 22:683, 1986.
11. Holliday, T.A.: Clinical signs of acute and chronic experimental lesions of the cerebellum. Vet. Sci. Commun., 3:259, 1979/1980.
12. Knecht, C.D., et al.: Cerebellar hypoplasia in Chow Chows. J. Am. Anim. Hosp. Assoc., 15:51, 1979.
13. O'Brien, D.P. and Zachary, J.F.: Clinical features of spongy degeneration of the central nervous system in two Labrador retriever littermates. J. Am. Vet. Med. Assoc., 186:1207, 1985.
14. Palmer, A.C.: Cerebellar disease. *In* Introduction to Animal Neurology. 2nd Ed. Oxford, Blackwell Scientific Publications, 1976.
15. Shell, L.G., et al.: Neuronal-visceral GM_1 gangliosidosis in Portuguese water dogs. J. Vet. Intern. Med., 3:1, 1989.
16. Smith, C.A. and Honhold, N.: Clinical and pathological features of a cerebellar oligodendroglioma in a cat. J. Small Anim. Pract., 29:269, 1988.
17. Steinberg, H.S., et al.: Clinical features of inherited cerebellar degeneration in Gordon Setters. J. Am. Vet. Med. Assoc., 179:886, 1981.

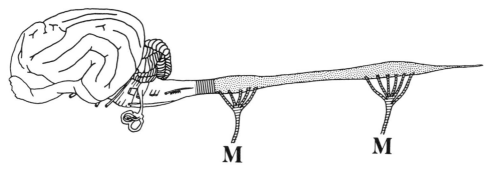

Figure 16–1. Location of lesions producing hemiplegia, hemiparesis, quadriplegia, quadriparesis, and ataxia of all four limbs include focal cervical spinal cord lesion (vertical lines), diffuse or multifocal spinal cord lesions (dots), diffuse peripheral nerve disease (horizontal lines), and polymyopathy (M).

Location of the lesion (Figure 16–1): *focal cervical, diffuse or multifocal spinal cord, diffuse neuromuscular*

Mechanisms of disease and differential diagnosis of spinal cord lesions

Congenital and familial disorders
Lysosomal storage diseases (Chap. 7)
Afghan myelopathy
Leukoencephalomyelopathy of Rottweilers
Hereditary ataxia in Jack Russell and Smooth Haired
 Fox terriers
Cervical vertebral spondylopathy
Atlantoaxial subluxation
Miscellaneous vertebral malformations
Multiple cartilaginous exostoses

Infections and other inflammations
Viral meningomyelitis or myelitis, bacterial, fungal,
 and other meningitis or meningomyelitis
Corticosteriod-responsive meningitis and
 meningomyelitis
Granulomatous meningoencephalomyelitis
Discospondylitis
Parasites (migrating)

Trauma
Spinal cord and vertebral injury
Intervertebral disc disease

Vascular disorders
Fibrocartilaginous infarct
Spontaneous spinal cord hemorrhage
Vascular malformations

Degeneration
Intervertebral disc disease
Spondylosis deformans
Dural ossification

Neoplasia
Extramedullary spinal cord tumors:
 Neurinoma
 Neurofibroma
 Neurofibrosarcoma
 Meningioma
 Meningeal sarcomatosis
Intramedullary spinal cord tumors:
 Astrocytoma
 Ependymoma
 Gliomas
Reticulosis
Metastatic spinal cord tumors
Vertebral neoplasia

Mechanisms of disease and differential diagnosis of diffuse neuromuscular lesions

Congenital and familial disorders
Globoid cell leukodystrophy
Boxer neuropathy
Spinal muscular atrophy—(Brittany spaniels, Swedish
 Lapland, and Rottweilers
Hypomyelinating polyneuropathy (Golden Retrievers)
Hypertrophic polyneuropathy (Mastiffs)
Giant axonal neuropathy (German Shepherds)
Myasthenia gravis

Myotonic myopathy (Chows)
Labrador Retriever myopathy
Golden Retriever myopathy
Irish Terrier myopathy
Nemaline myopathy (cats)
Miscellaneous muscular dystrophy
Myositis ossificans

Location of the lesion (Figure 16–1): *focal cervical, diffuse or multifocal spinal cord, diffuse neuromuscular* (Continued)

Infections

Toxoplasmosis polymyositis/polyneuritis

Inflammatory–immune-mediated disorders

Acute polyradiculoneuritis
Chronic polyradiculoneuritis or polyneuritis
Feline polyneuritis
Brachial plexus neuritis
Myasthenia gravis
Polymyositis

Metabolic disorders

Hyperinsulinism polyneuropathy
Diabetes mellitus polyneuropathy
Hypoadrenocortical neuromuscular disease
Hypothyroid polyneuropathy
Hypothyroid polymyopathy
Hypokalemic polymyopathy (cats)
Hyperadrenocortical and corticosteroid-induced
  polymyopathy

Toxicity

Tick paralysis
Botulism
Snake venom
Organophosphate toxicity
Miscellaneous chemical agents (see Table 16–3)

Nutritional disorders

Nutritional myodegeneration

Neoplasia

Paraneoplastic polyneuropathy—Lymphosarcoma

Idiopathic

Distal axonopathies

Episodic weakness

Congenital and familial disorders

Myasthenia gravis

Inflammatory–immune-mediated disorders

Polymyositis
Myasthenia gravis

Metabolic disorders

Hypoxia—cardiopulmonary disease
Hypoglycemia
Hyperkalemia—hypoadrenocorticism
Hypokalemic polymyopathy
Hyperthyroidism

Chapter 16

Hemiplegia, hemiparesis, quadriplegia, quadriparesis, ataxia of all four limbs, and episodic weakness

When hemiplegia, hemiparesis, quadriplegia, quadriparesis, or ataxia of all four limbs is unaccompanied by signs associated with disease above the foramen magnum (Chaps. 7 through 15), a focal cervical spinal cord disorder, multifocal or diffuse spinal cord disease, or diffuse neuromuscular disease is likely.

A focal cervical spinal cord lesion produced by an extramedullary mass C1 to C6 may produce signs that vary with the spinal cord tracts involved. If the extramedullary mass only irritates the meninges and dorsal root and causes little spinal cord compression, then the main sign will be neck pain with little neurologic deficit.

If mild compression of the spinal cord occurs, the spinocerebellar tracts in the lateral funiculus may be distorted and their blood supply altered, producing ataxia or incoordination of the limbs (Fig. 16–2). If the lesion is mainly unilateral, the signs will be worse on the side of the lesion. If only the spinal cord tracts and not the caudal cervical nerve roots to the brachial plexus (C6 to T2) are affected, the pelvic limbs may appear more ataxic than the thoracic limbs, which may actually appear normal in comparison. The fibers from the pelvic limbs are lateral to the fibers from the thoracic limbs in the spinocerebellar tracts; therefore, pelvic limb fibers are affected

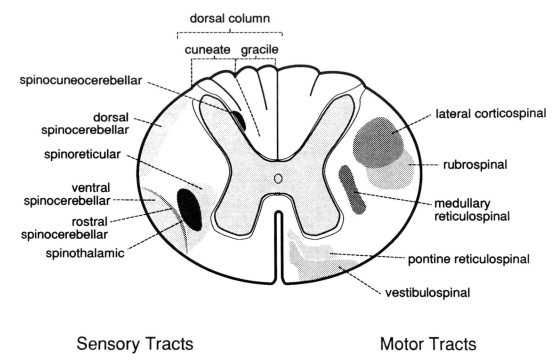

Sensory Tracts   ## Motor Tracts

Figure 16–2. The sensory and motor tracts of the spinal cord in the dog and cat. The position of these tracts is approximate. In the motor tracts, axons to the pelvic limbs are lateral to those to the thoracic limbs. (Adapted from King, A.S.: Physiological and Clinical Anatomy of the Domestic Mammals. Vol 1, Central Nervous System. New York, Oxford University, 1987) The rostral spinocerebellar tract is correctly referred to as the cranial spinocerebellar tract.

first by mild lateral extramedullary compression.

Examination of the thoracic limbs alone may be needed to detect the minimal signs that would place the lesion in the cervical region rather than the thoracolumbar region (Chap. 3). In caudal cervical lesions, C6 to T2, the brachial plexus nerve roots are affected along with the spinal cord, so the thoracic limbs may appear more involved than the pelvic limbs. Mild compressive lesions in the caudal cervical region may not produce detectable depression of the thoracic limb spinal reflexes, as a mild compressive lesion in the caudal lumbar region would depress pelvic limb reflexes. There are several reasons for this. The caudal cervical vertebral canal has more space compared with the lumbar vertebral canal. Also, the tendon reflexes and muscle responses of the thoracic limbs are often more difficult to obtain than those of the pelvic limbs in normal dogs, so the interpretation of a depressed response may be difficult (Chap. 3). The flexor reflex of the thoracic limb is the easiest spinal reflex to test, but is composed of five spinal cord segments and nerve roots (C6–T2) (Fig. 16–3). It takes an extensive lesion three to four vertebral bodies in length for an external compressive lesion to depress or abolish the flexor reflex. Intramedullary spinal cord lesions such as infarction, hemorrhage, or neoplasia are more likely to affect multiple segments and abolish thoracic limb spinal reflexes when they occur in the caudal cervical region.

In cranial cervical lesions such as compression at C1–C2 with an atlantoaxial subluxation, the medial spinal cord tracts seem to be affected most and the thoracic limbs appear worse than the pelvic limbs.

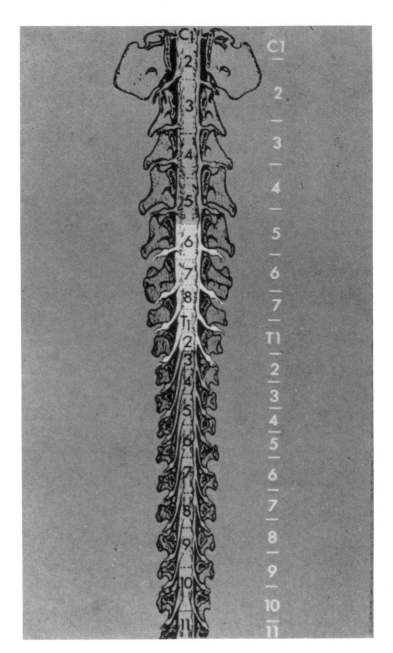

Figure 16-3. The relationship of spinal cord segments and nerve roots to vertebrae in the cervical region. C6–T2 spinal cord segments are displayed in white and are the main contributions to the brachial plexus. (After Miller, 1964)

The spinal reflexes in all four limbs may be normal or hyperactive. It can be difficult, therefore, to differentiate mild compressions of the cranial cervical and caudal cervical region based on spinal reflex changes.

If the dorsolateral funiculus of the spinal cord is affected, conscious proprioception to the limbs is altered and the animal stands knuckled over on the dorsum of the paw.

As tracts in the ventral funiculus are

distorted and their blood supply altered, the animal may have difficulty supporting its weight and standing. This is caused by vestibulospinal and reticulospinal tract dysfunction (see Fig. 16–2). Even if the animal is unable to stand, it may retain some voluntary movement if the reticulospinal, rubrospinal, and corticospinal tracts are still functioning. At this stage, the animal is hemiparetic if one side is involved or quadriparetic if both sides are involved. As the reticulospinal, rubrospinal, and corticospinal tracts become more involved, voluntary movement ceases and the animal is hemiplegic or quadriplegic (see Fig. 16–2). Hemiplegia is usually caused by an intramedullary unilateral spinal cord lesion.

Superficial sensation may be decreased or absent caudal to the lesion in a quadriplegic animal with a cervical spinal cord compression, but deep pain usually remains. The major spinal cord tracts and their function are discussed in Chapter 1. Descending sympathetic fibers in the tectotegmentospinal tract may be disturbed (Chap. 1), and problems associated with sympathetic denervation and temperature regulation may be seen. Respiratory muscle paresis or paralysis is a life-threatening complication of cervical spinal cord lesions. Lesions above C5 spinal cord segments will affect upper motor neurons (UMN) to the phrenic and intercostal nerves. At C5–C7 segments, the lower motor neurons (LMN) of the phrenic nerve are affected. Below C7, only UMN and LMN to intercostal muscles will be affected. Respirations should be carefully monitored on all animals with cervical lesions, especially during anesthesia.

In diffuse or multifocal spinal cord disease, the signs vary with the segmental location of the lesions and the involvement of gray or white matter. If only white matter is involved diffusely, or at several foci, with at least one of the foci in the cervical spinal cord, then ataxia, hemiparesis, quadriparesis, or quadriplegia with normal or hyperactive reflexes will be seen. Gray matter affected at C6 to T2 or L4 to S2 segments of the spinal cord, produces spinal reflexes that are depressed or absent, localizing at least one of the lesions to those particular sites.

There are eight cervical segments and nerve roots in the cervical spinal cord and only seven vertebrae. The nerve roots exit prior to the vertebra of the same number: C1 nerve roots exit between the skull and C1 vertebra, C2 nerve roots exit between C1 and C2 vertebrae, C3 nerve roots exit between C2 and C3 vertebrae, and so on down to T1. The C8 nerve root exits between C7 and T1 vertebrae. Therefore, caudal to T1, the corresponding nerve root exits after the vertebrae of the same number: T1 nerve root exits between T1 and T2, T2 nerve root exits between T2 and T3 and so on through the caudal segments. Eight spinal cord segments are crowded within seven vertebrae (Fig. 16–3). This difference in vertebrae and spinal cord segments and nerve roots must be taken into consideration when localizing an extramedullary lesion to certain segments and nerve roots, and then deciding the vertebral level to which that would correspond. This is of greater clinical significance in the thoracolumbar region than in the cervical region (Chap. 17).

In peripheral neuropathies primarily affecting sensory axons, the animal may show ataxia, conscious proprioceptive deficits, or self-multilation (Chap. 20). If the motor axons or neuromuscular junctions are affected, then quadriparesis (weakness) and quadriplegia are seen. In peripheral neuropathies, the components of the spinal reflexes to the limbs are involved, so spinal reflexes in all four limbs may be depressed or absent. In mild lesions, the patellar reflex may be the only one depressed, but the animal will have quadriparesis.

In myopathies, the animals may have

a stiff, stilted gait, exhibit episodic weakness, or be quadriparetic, but are rarely quadriplegic unless the myopathy is severe and widespread in all muscle groups. The spinal reflexes are usually normal, but in severe lesions may be depressed.

Episodic weakness or a transient quadriparesis or quadriplegia may be produced by several diffuse metabolic, brain, and spinal cord diseases or by diffuse neuromuscular diseases, many of which have been discussed in other sections of this book.

Patient evaluation

Signalment and history

Because there are many mechanisms of disease producing hemiplegia, hemiparesis, quadriplegia, quadriparesis, or ataxia, the clinician must rely heavily on a thorough history to determine possible causes.

As discussed in Chapter 2, young animals are the most likely candidates for congenital and familial disorders. They may have minimal protection against viral infections, and be more likely to chew on foreign objects and become intoxicated. Their lack of experience with moving vehicles makes them more susceptible to injuries. Older animals are most commonly affected by spinal cord neoplasms.

Congenital and familial disorders may also affect certain breeds, such as myelopathy in Afghan hounds and myotonia in Chow Chows, and this information should be considered (see Table 2–2) in the differential diagnosis.

Knowing whether the disease process has been acute nonprogressive, acute progressive, or chronic progressive, as discussed in Chapter 2, greatly aids in deciding which type of mechanism is most likely. Acute hemiplegia is most commonly associated with a fibrocartilaginous infarction of the spinal cord. Acute quadriplegia is most commonly associated with acute polyradiculoneuritis, tick paralysis, botulism, spinal cord injury with or without a vertebral fracture, a herniated intervertebral disc, and a fibrocartilaginous infarct or hemorrhage of the spinal cord (Tables 16–1 and 16–2). Spinal cord injuries are common in cats, but the other disorders are rare.

Chronic progressive ataxia and quadriparesis over a few weeks may be associated with some congenital and familial disorders, such as one of the lysosomal storage disorders, Afghan myelopathy, or cervical vertebral spondylopathy, or be caused by spinal cord infections, chronic polyradiculoneuritis, toxic or metabolic neuromuscular disease, slow protruding intervertebral discs, and some spinal cord tumors (Tables 16–3 and 16–4). Spinal cord infections and tumors occur in cats, but the other diseases are rare.

Chronic progressive ataxia and quadriparesis over several months' duration is most characteristic of chronic polyneuropathies, slow protruding intervertebral discs, and spinal cord tumors (Tables 16–3 and 16–4).

The history of concurrent systemic illness or signs of nervous system involvement above the foramen magnum may support a diagnosis of multifocal disease

Table 16–1
Common disorders producing acute quadriparesis or quadriplegia with normal or exaggerated spinal reflexes in dogs

1. Spinal cord injury
2. Intervertebral disc herniation
3. Fibrocartilaginous infarct (usually hemiplegia)
4. Meningomyelitis
5. Atlantoaxial subluxation

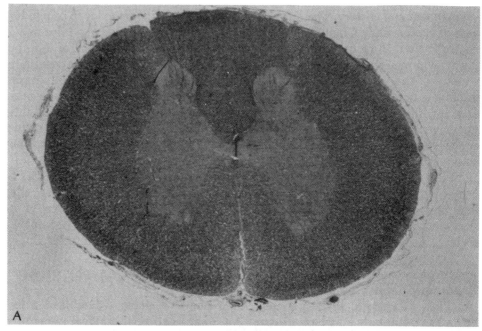

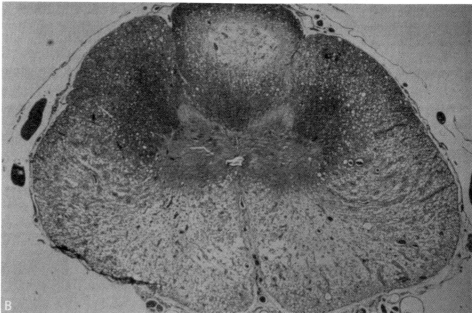

Figure 16–4. *(A)* A cross section of a normal spinal cord. (Courtesy of Dr. Damon Averill, Dept. of Neuropathology, Children's Hospital, Boston, Massachusetts.) *(B)* A cross section of a spinal cord from a quadriplegic Afghan with severe leukodystrophy, especially involving the dorsal and ventral white matter.

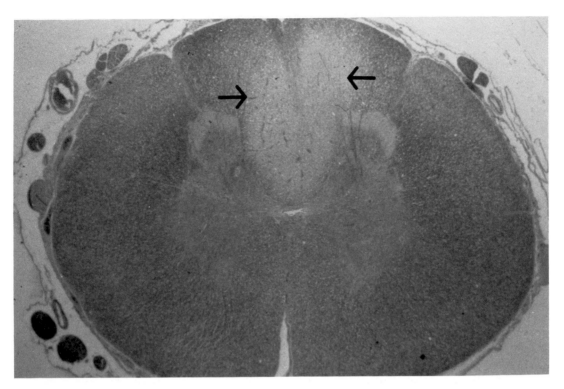

Figure 16–5. Leukomyelopathy in a 3-year-old Rottweiler. Note the light-colored areas of demyelination (arrows) in the dorsal funiculi.

Cervical vertebral spondylopathy

Incidence: Frequent in Great Danes and Doberman Pinschers; occasional in other large breeds

Cervical vertebral spondylopathy and resultant cervical spinal cord compression have been reported primarily in Doberman Pinschers and Great Danes, but also in Afghan hounds, Bull Mastiffs, Bassett hounds, Rhodesian Ridgebacks, Dalmations, and other large breeds of dogs.[79–81,84,94,97] Other names for this disorder include wobbler syndrome, cervical vertebral malformation—malarticulation, spondylolisthesis, and cervical vertebral instability.

Signalment and history. The onset of clinical signs appears before 1 to 2 years of age in many Great Danes, but a few may develop signs at a later age. A few Doberman Pinschers develop clinical signs before 1 year of age, but many develop signs between 3 and 9 years of age. The primary complaint in many of the young Great Danes and Dobermans is ataxia of all four limbs, which is much worse in the pelvic limbs. The pelvic limbs may cross each other when turning, abduct widely, and collapse. The thoracic limbs may appear slightly hypermetric. The spondylopathy is often C3–4 or C4–5. In older Doberman Pinschers and other large breeds of dogs, the lesion is often in the caudal cervical region at C5–6 or C6–7 and the thoracic limbs appear more involved (Fig. 16–6). The thoracic limbs may show a stiff, stilted gait.

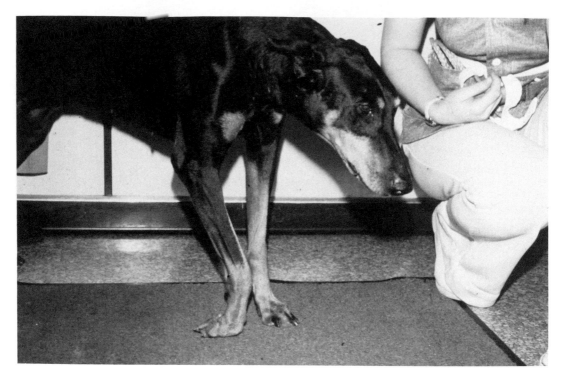

Figure 16–6. An 8-year-old female Doberman Pinscher with cervical vertebral spondylopathy and conscious proprioception deficit of the right thoracic limb.

Physical and neurologic examinations. Spinal reflexes of the thoracic limbs may be normal, but those of the pelvic limbs are usually hyperactive. The patellar reflex often shows clonus, even in mildly affected cases. Usually, there is no associated neck pain. The neck may be stiff on manipulation, or painful if a cervical disc protrusion accompanies the malformed vertebrae in older dogs.

In chronic C5–6 or C6–7 lesions, there may be some atrophy of supraspinatus and infraspinatus muscles.

Ancillary diagnostic investigations. Some positive sharp waves and a few fibrillation potentials may be found on EMG examination of cervical paraspinal muscles and some muscles of the thoracic limbs, depending on the degree of involvement of ventral nerve roots.

Plain radiographs may show an obvious vertebral malformation (Fig. 16–7), but in most cases a myelogram is necessary to demonstrate the location and degree of spinal cord compression (Fig. 16–8). Table 16–8 lists all the plain radiographic and myelographic changes that may occur in the cervical vertebral spondylopathy syndrome. Not every affected dog will have all these changes. Some dogs have spinal cord compression from ventral lesions, others from dorsal lesions, and still others caused by both (Fig. 16–8). On occasion, spinal cord compression will occur laterally, so ventrodorsal views are important to evaluate (Fig. 16–9).

Extreme flexion and extension of the neck is avoided when obvious myelographic changes are seen, because manipulation only further traumatizes the spinal cord. Because of the variability in neck po-

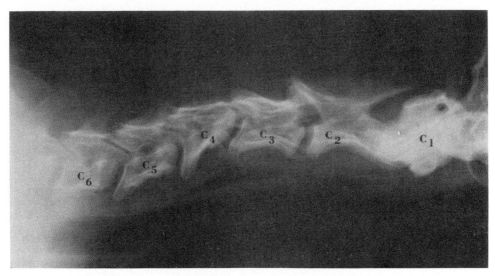

Figure 16–7. Lateral cervical vertebral radiograph of a 5-month-old quadriparetic Doberman Pinscher with a malformed C4 vertebra.

sitioning, a diagnosis of cervical vertebral joint laxity or subluxation (spondylolisthesis) cannot be made from a flexed lateral plain radiograph. Flexion and extension should only be performed during myelography after no obvious lesions are found on the straight lateral or ventrodorsal views. The neurologic deficit in many dogs may be worsened by excessive manipulation while anesthetized during radiography.

Therapy and prognosis. Glucocorticoid therapy may transiently improve the neurologic deficit, but some form of surgical correction is necessary for dogs with progressive signs.[34,79,84,97] In geriatric dogs that are mildly affected, 10 mg prednisone orally every other day may control the ataxia and weakness. If neck pain is present, 5 mg diazepam (Valium) every 8 hours orally controls the discomfort from muscle spasms. Surgery may not be indicated for the elderly dog, and a good quality of life is often maintained with conservative medical therapy. A harness instead of a collar should be used to avoid further neck in-

jury. In younger healthy dogs, surgery is advised because the neurologic deficit progresses. Because Doberman Pinschers have a high incidence of Von Willebrand's disease, hypothyroidism, and cardiomyopathy, these should all be evaluated prior to surgery. A dorsal laminectomy in the caudal cervical region of large breeds of dogs can be difficult. Severe flexion during surgery to improve visualization may compromise the spinal cord blood supply and render an animal that was only ataxic prior to surgery, quadriplegic after surgery. If the canal is stenotic, or the ligamentum flavum is compressing the spinal cord dorsally, decompression with a dorsal laminectomy is indicated. The owner must be well informed about the potential complications with this approach. If the spinal cord is compressed ventrally by a protruded anulus fibrosus, ventral decompression will improve the signs. There are less complications associated with this surgical approach. Details of the surgical approaches are presented elsewhere.[34,79,84,88,94]

In a mildly affected dog with no surgical complications, recovery may occur

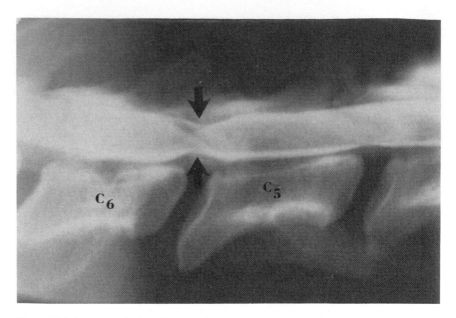

Figure 16–8. Lateral cervical myelogram of a 9-year-old Doberman Pinscher with quadriparesis. Dorsal and ventral spinal cord compression are outlined by the arrows. (C5 and C6 vertebrae are labeled.) The ventral compression was due to a Type II disc protrusion and proliferated dorsal longitudinal ligament. The dorsal compression was due to a proliferated ligamentum flavum.

within 2 to 6 weeks. Even those dogs that are worse after surgery may improve in 3 to 6 months. Most dogs are maintained on prednisone for 2 weeks after surgery to reduce spinal cord swelling. Diazepam (Valium) 5 mg every 8 hours orally will also prevent postoperative muscle spasm pain. The nursing care of large quadri-

plegic dogs can be stressful and tedious for owners, so they must be committed prior to surgery.

Dogs may develop second lesions later in life. Dogs with two lesions at the time of initial evaluation are poor surgical candidates.

The pathophysiology of cervical vertebral spondylopathy is still unknown. It does tend to occur in certain breeds of dogs and is thought to have a familial basis. The remodeling changes that occur in the involved vertebrae may be caused by some malarticulation and joint laxity, which is suspected of also being the cause of ligament, joint capsule, and intervertebral disc degeneration. A nutritional imbalance has been suggested in the pathophysiology. Why it occurs later in life in Doberman Pinschers is unknown. Some older Doberman Pinschers do not have spondylopathy, but only caudal cervical intervertebral disc protrusions, which are discussed later in this chapter.

Table 16–8
Radiographic changes associated with cervical vertebral spondylopathy*

1. Vertebral malformation, vertebral canal stenosis
2. Vertebral instability
3. Spondylosis deformans
4. Osteoarthritis of articular' facets
5. Proliferated ligamentum flavum
6. Proliferated dorsal longitudinal ligament
7. Protruded or herniated intervertebral disc

* Each case may have some of these changes and not others.

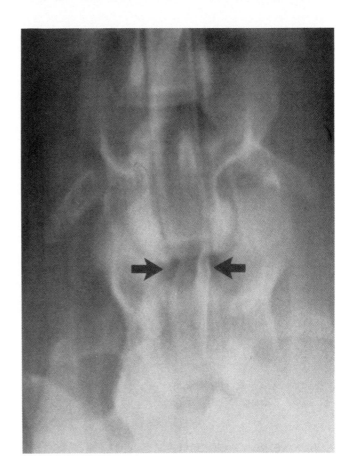

Figure 16–9. Ventrodorsal cervical myelogram of a 2½-year-old Great Dane with ataxia of all four limbs. Lateral spinal cord compression due to cervical vertebral spondylopathy is indicated by the arrows.

Pathology. At necropsy, several vertebral changes are noted. The dorsal articular facets may be asymmetric, which may contribute to malarticulation and osteoarthritic changes. However, asymmetric dorsal articular facets have been found at necropsy of Doberman Pinschers and Great Danes with no evidence of neurologic dysfunction. The ligamentum flavum and dorsal longitudinal ligament may be redundant and proliferated, perhaps from some abnormal joint laxity. Remodeling of the vertebrae can be seen with stenosis of the vertebral canal, particularly in the rostral portion. Most dogs that do not improve after ventral decompressive surgery often have lateral compression still present on necropsy examination. The intervertebral disc may be degenerated and protruded. Microscopic changes in the spinal cord are associated with compression at the affected segments.

Prevention. Not enough is known about the role of genetics and environmental factors, such as diet and oversupplementation, in the development of cervical vertebral spondylopathy, so no recommendations for prevention can be made.

Atlantoaxial subluxation

Incidence: Frequent in toy breeds

A variety of lesions of the atlas and axis produce subluxation and spinal cord compression. One may be caused by an improper development or agenesis or hypoplasia of the dens or lack of proper ligamentous attachment.[20] Traumatic ligamentous rupture or fracture of the dens can also result in atlantoaxial subluxation, and is discussed later in this chapter.

Signalment and history. Toy breeds of dogs, especially Poodles, Yorkshire terriers, Miniature Dachshunds, Chihuahuas, and Pomeranians under 1 year of age, and rarely cats, may be presented with a variety of complaints ranging from neck pain and a mildly ataxic gait of all four limbs to quadriparesis and inability to stand. The signs may wax and wane or be continuous. The thoracic limbs may appear to be more affected than the pelvic limbs. Occasionally, adult toy breed dogs will be presented with a history of several episodes of neck pain, ataxia, or brief collapse, which may or may not have been associated with some mild trauma.

Physical and neurologic examinations. Varying degrees of ataxia of all four limbs and quadriparesis are noted on the neurologic examination. Neck pain may or may not be found, but if the diagnosis is suspected, the neck should be manipulated as little as possible. Spinal reflexes of the thoracic and pelvic limbs are normal or hyperactive. The patellar reflex often has clonus.

Ancillary diagnostic investigations. Lateral plain radiographs show an increased distance between the dorsal arch of the atlas and axis (Fig. 16–10A). Oblique lateral, frontal, open mouth, and ventrodorsal views may show an abnormally developed dens (Fig. 16–10B). The neck must be handled carefully while the animal is anesthetized for radiographs, so that the spinal cord is not further compressed.

Therapy and prognosis. Both dorsal and ventral surgical approaches have been made.[27,62] Dorsally, a wire or heavy suture may be passed under the dorsal lamina of the atlas and then fixed to the dorsal spine of the axis to bring the vertebrae back into alignment. The limiting factor is the life of the wire or suture. The ventral approach involves placing a bone graft between the atlas and axis and securing this with pins or screws until the graft fuses the bones (Figs. 16–11A,B). The dogs must then wear a neck brace for 6 weeks to minimize movement of the bone graft and pins. The prognosis is good if the neurologic deficit is not too severe and surgical stabilization is successful.

Pathology. The abnormality in dens formation and ligamentous attachment and the resultant joint laxity can be seen at necropsy. On rare occasions, a proliferation and abnormal growth of the dens is responsible for the spinal cord compression. Microscopic lesions associated with compression are found at the C1 to C2 spinal cord segments.

Prevention. There is some evidence that this vertebral deformity has a familial basis, but the mode of inheritance is presently unknown.

Miscellaneous vertebral and spinal cord malformations

Occipital dysplasia is a common radiographic finding, but rarely has an associated neurologic deficit. Mild ataxia of all 4 limbs which is responsive to glucocorticoid therapy may be seen. A keyhole shaped foramen magnum is found on radiographic examination but many normal toy breed dogs have this radiographic finding.

Sporadic cases of various vertebral malformations and congenital vertebral fusions may be found in dogs and cats with or without evidence of neurologic deficit (Fig. 16–12).[26,101] Kyphosis, scoliosis, and spinal cord compression may occur. Acquired scoliosis may be associated with sy-

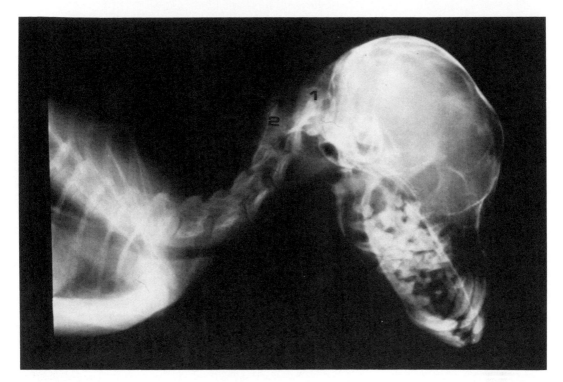

A

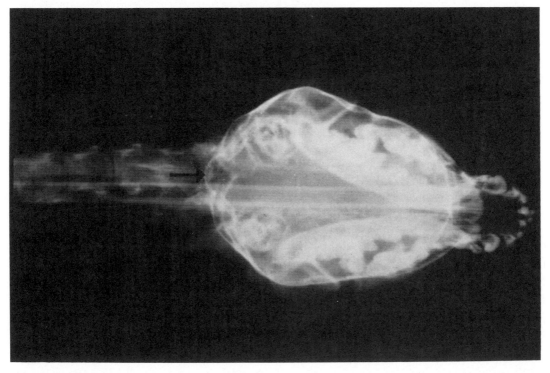

B

Figure 16–10. *(A),* Lateral radiograph of a dog with hypoplasia of the dens and atlantoaxial subluxation. Note the wide separation between the dorsal spinous process of C1 (1) and C2 (2). *(B),* Ventrodorsal radiograph of dog in *A* with atlantoaxial subluxation from a hypoplastic dens.

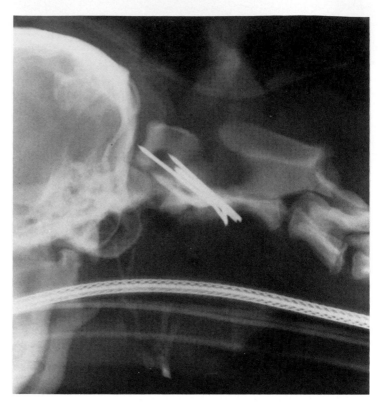

Figure 16–11. Lateral radiograph of a dog with atlantoaxial subluxation from a hypoplastic dens repaired with ventral fusion and pins. *(B)* Ventrodorsal radiography of the dog in *A* showing the pin placement.

A

ringomyelia and hydromyelia.[14] Routine radiography and myelography can demonstrate the lesion, and surgical decompression may be needed to alleviate the signs. Spinal dysraphism may rarely occur in the cervical region and is discussed with thoracolumbar disorders in Chapter 17. Other vertebral and spinal cord malformations are also discussed in Chapter 17.

Multiple cartilaginous exostoses

Incidence: Occasional

Multiple cartilaginous exostoses or osteochondromatosis is a proliferative disease of cartilage and bone. Osteochondromatosis seems to occur in families, may affect any bone of the body, and often occurs at multiple sites. Involvement of cervical vertebrae may result in spinal cord compression, and the animal may have neck pain, ataxia of all four limbs, or quadriparesis.[26] Multiple cartilaginous exostoses have been reported in both young and adult dogs and cats. There seems to be no breed predilection. Bony masses may be palpated on the long bones, digits, and ribs, but radiography may be needed to demonstrate vertebral lesions. Myelography can be used to outline spinal cord compression. Some type of decompressive vertebral surgery may be necessary to alleviate the signs, but will vary with the individual case.

The disorder appears to be inherited

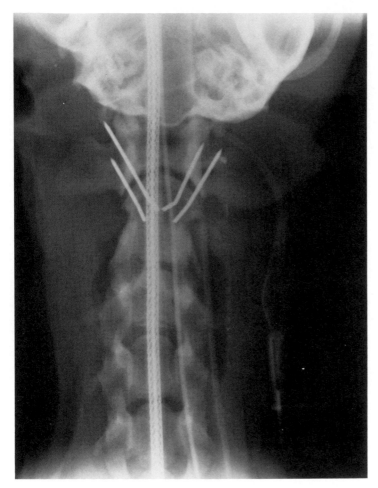

B

in man and is thought to have a familial basis in dogs.

Infections and other inflammations

Infections of the spinal cord, like infections of the brain (Chap. 7), may be caused by a variety of organisms such as bacteria, viruses, fungi, and protozoa or may be from other causes (see Tables 7–6 and 7–7).

Viral meningomyelitis or myelitis

Incidence: Distemper virus myelitis frequent; other causes occasional or rare

Infections of the nervous system produced by canine distemper virus in dogs and feline infectious peritonitis (FIP) virus in cats are discussed in Chapter 7. Both viruses may affect the spinal cord primarily, and the dog or cat may have hemiparesis, ataxia of all four limbs, quadriparesis, or quadriplegia with no other signs.[26] Deficits

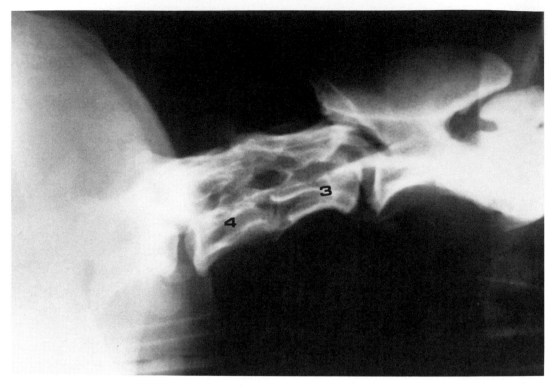

Figure 16–12. Fusion of cervical vertebrae C3 (3) and C-4 (4) may be an incidental finding not producing neurologic problems.

of only the pelvic limbs may also be seen, so these diseases must be considered in the differential diagnosis of paraparesis (Chap. 17). Quadriparesis in these instances is usually spastic with intact or hyperactive spinal reflexes. A diagnosis of myelitis from distemper virus or FIP virus is indicated when CSF contains an increased number of mononuclear cells and protein. CSF and serum titers for distemper and FIP viruses may help confirm the diagnosis. The CSF will have no increased cells and only increased protein if the lesion is primarily demyelination. The prognosis for an animal with viral myelitis is usually grave for recovery from paralysis, as there is often extensive spinal cord white matter damage.

Bacterial, fungal, and other meningitis or meningomyelitis

Bacterial and fungal meningitis are relatively common in man, but comparatively rare in animals.[39,44,70] Pasteurella multocida, Staphylococcus aureus, Staphylococcus epidermidis, and Staphylococcus albus are the most common causative bacteria. Cryptococcus neoformans is the most common fungus. Signs associated with involvement of neuroanatomic structures above the foramen magnum, such as dementia, seizures, and cranial nerve abnormalities, suggest a multifocal CNS disease process. There may or may not be a history or signs of disease in other body systems. An elevated temperature may be evident on the physical examination. The animal may have generalized hyperesthesia and rigidity, particularly of the neck. No weakness of the limbs is present unless spinal cord involvement occurs along with the meningeal disease.

Neutrophilic leukocytosis is often present in the peripheral blood. A massive increase in cells and protein is found in the CSF. The cells consist primarily of neutrophils, but may also include eosinophils, mononuclear cells, and lymphocytes. Bacteria or fungus may be seen in the CSF sediment. Culture and sensitivity of the CSF can yield the bacteria and aid in selecting an appropriate antibiotic. Aerobic and anaerobic cultures should be performed. The treatment of fungal infections is discussed in Chapter 6.

The prognosis in bacterial or fungal meningitis varies with the duration and severity of the infection and the response of the individual animal to therapy. An animal with bacterial meningitis generally has a better prognosis than one with fungal meningitis. Other agents that may produce meningitis or meningomyelitis sporadically include Toxoplasma gondi, Ehrlichia canis, and Prototheca spp. On rare occasions, parasites such as dirofilaria immitis may produce quadriparesis.[3]

A polioencephalomyelitis occurs in cats and may produce paresis and ataxia initially. Later in the course of the disease, tremors of the head, psychomotor seizures, and aggressive behavior occur.[95]

A pyogranulomatous meningoencephalitis occurs in dogs with ataxia and neck pain. The CSF contains increased neutrophils and protein. Affected dogs respond well to antibiotics, but the clinical signs recur when antibiotics are discontinued.[5]

A vasculitis of spinal leptomeningeal arteries may occur in Beagles and Bernese Mountain Dogs and produce generalized hyperesthesia and neck pain.[26,47,69,70] In some cases, an immune-mediated vasculitis may produce these signs.[78] CSF has increased neutrophils and protein. Response to chronic prednisone therapy may be seen.

Corticosteroid-responsive meningitis

Incidence: Frequent

The most common form of meningitis in dogs has no demonstrable organism.[68,70] Affected dogs are usually mature and are presented with hyperesthesia and neck pain. In extreme cases, some weakness in the limbs may be present. A fever may or may not be associated with these signs, and the CBC and chemistry profiles are often normal. Vertebral radiographs of the entire spine are normal. The protein content of CSF is greatly increased. Increased cells within the CSF consist primarily of all neutrophils, all lymphocytes, or a mixture of neutrophils, monocytes, and lymphocytes, and occasionally eosinophils are seen. There is no evidence of bacteria or fungus in the CSF sediment. Aerobic and anerobic bacterial and fungal cultures and CSF titers are negative. The signs respond to oral administration of 1 to 2 mg/kg prednisone within 24 to 72 hours. The prednisone dose may be reduced after 7 to 10 days, and if the signs do not recur, tapered over 1 month. If signs recur as the prednisone dose is reduced, a higher dose should be instituted for 2 to 3 weeks before a dose reduction is again attempted. Some dogs recover within 1 to 3 months. Other dogs have to be maintained on some level of alternate-day prednisone therapy to be free of pain. Necropsies performed on chronic cases showed only inflammation with no organism present. The diagnosis of this form of meningitis is based on the clinical signs, CSF alterations, and response to corticosteroid therapy.

Granulomatous meningoencephalitis (reticulosis)

Incidence: Rare

On rare occasions, granulomatous meningoencephalitis (GME) or the focal form, reticulosis, will produce neck pain and ataxia with no evidence of cerebral or brain stem involvement.[44,70] More frequently, there is evidence of cerebrum and brain stem disease as well as neck pain, generalized hyperesthesia, and ataxia. GME and reticulosis are discussed in Chapters 7 and 12.

Discospondylitis and spondylitis

Incidence: Frequent

Discospondylitis is an infection of the vertebrae and associated intervertebral discs, usually caused by bacteria or a foreign body.[50,56,58] Spirocercosis and fungal infections such as aspergillosis of the vertebrae may also occur occasionally. If only the vertebra is involved, it is called spondylitis. A hematogenous route of infection is thought to exist for bacterial organisms. A correlation between urinary tract infections and discospondylitis has been made. Trauma and a foreign body may be predisposing causes. Discospondylitis can occur as a single lesion or can affect several sites along the vertebral column. Discospondylitis is much more common than spondylitis.

Signalment and history. The age of onset of signs ranges from 5 months to 10 years, with many breeds represented of either sex. The primary complaint is usually either cervical, thoracic, or lumbar pain, depending on the locations of the affected vertebrae. The animal may have difficulty rising and a history of intermittent illness and weight loss. If the cervical vertebrae are involved, cervical pain is evident. The dog may also be depressed and anorexic.

Physical and neurologic examinations. Some dogs may have an associated fever. A heart murmur might suggest concurrent bacterial endocarditis. Neck pain is commonly found when cervical vertebrae are involved, but it is also not uncommon to have several vertebrae affected, and have multiple sites of pain or generalized hyperesthesia. The neurologic deficit varies with the amount of spinal cord involvement, but ataxia, conscious proprioceptive deficits, paresis or paralysis of all four limbs or the pelvic limbs alone may occur, depending on the location of the lesion. The spinal reflex changes also vary with the spinal cord segments affected.

Ancillary diagnostic investigations. Neutrophilic leukocytes may be seen on the CBC. Serum biochemistry profiles are usually normal. A bacterial urinary tract infection may be diagnosed from urinalysis and urine culture. Aspergillus organisms may be found in the urine.

Radiographs are used to confirm the diagnosis of discospondylitis. No radiographic changes may be present for the first couple of weeks after the onset of pain, so repeated evaluations may be necessary to confirm the diagnosis. Lysis of adjacent vertebral endplates with narrowed intervertebral disc spaces is commonly seen (Fig. 16–13). Varying amounts of osteolysis, sclerosis, and ventral spur formation are also seen. Dogs with aspergillosis may have osteolytic lesions of the sternebrae on thoracic radiographs.

Blood cultures are more likely to be positive if the animal is febrile. Bacterial agents isolated from the blood have included hemolytic staphylococci, hemolytic streptococci, Brucella canis, Nocardia, and Staphylococcus epidermidis, but Staphylococcus aureus is the most commonly found.

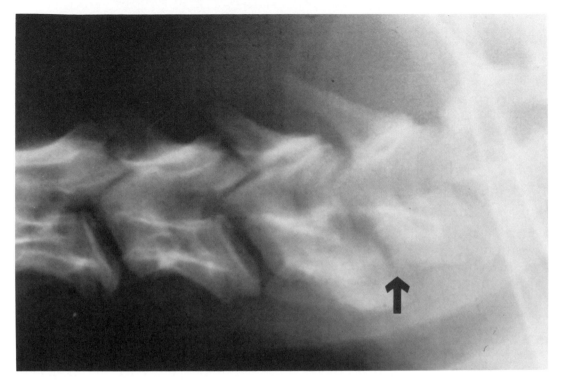

Figure 16–13. Discospondylitis of C6–C7 vertebrae and disc (arrow).

Although rare, serologic testing for Brucella canis should be performed in all discospondylitis cases.

CSF analysis may be normal or may show increased cells (mononuclear type) and increased protein, or increased protein alone. The CSF should be cultured, but cultures are often negative.

Therapy and prognosis. Conservative medical therapy is suggested in animals having only pain with minimal neurologic deficit. The antibiotic may be selected on the basis of the antibiotic sensitivity information from the blood culture if available. If no culture information is available, a combination of trimethoprim sulfadiazine (Tribrissen) 15 mg/kg every 12 hours and cephradine (Velosef) 20 mg/kg every 8 hours, is given orally for 6 to 8 weeks, and most bacterial infections resolve. Oral ac-

etaminophen (Tylenol) 5 mg/kg divided doses daily or buffered acetylsalicylic acid (aspirin) not to exceed 10 mg/kg daily may be used for 1 to 2 weeks if pain is severe. Control of pain is discussed in Chapter 6. Even if signs rapidly improve, antibiotic therapy should be continued. Corticosteroids should not be used even if they initially appear to improve the signs.

If aspergillus is the causative agent, the prognosis is grave. The currently available antifungal agents are not effective in curing the infection.

If neurologic signs are severe and do not respond to medical therapy, a myelogram may show spinal cord compression. A dorsal laminectomy or hemilaminectomy along with systemic antibiotic therapy may be indicated.

The prognosis can vary greatly with the severity of neurologic dysfunction, the type of organism, and sensitivity to therapy. Discospondylitis may affect several vertebrae, and therapy may have to be provided for several months. Recurrences of disease have been seen up to 1 year after the infection was apparently cured, so discospondylitis can be a chronic problem in the dog.

Pathology. Localized meningitis may be associated with the site of discospondylitis. In more severe cases with proliferation of bone and swelling of inflamed perivertebral soft tissue, spinal cord compression may occur. In rare instances, the vertebrae may collapse and compress the spinal cord.

Trauma

Spinal cord and vertebral injury

Incidence: Frequent

Injury to the vertebral column and spinal cord is a common cause of hemiparesis, quadriplegia, quadriparesis, or ataxia of all four limbs.[19,89] A fracture subluxation or luxation of the vertebrae may accompany the spinal cord insult.[86,92] Occasionally, no evidence of vertebral fractures can be found, and only spinal cord hemorrhage and edema are the cause of neurologic deficit. The pathophysiology of spinal cord trauma will be discussed further in Chapter 17.

In the cervical region, injuries are commonly sustained owing to automobile accidents and large dogs picking up small dogs by the back of the neck and shaking them, i.e., "the big dog–little dog" syndrome. Many dogs are presented only with neck pain and minimal neurologic deficit. The neurologic deficit may worsen over the following several days because of vertebral instability. Fractures in the cervical area most often involve the atlas and axis. The wings of the atlas or the dens of the

axis are involved, and atlantoaxial subluxation occurs.

Occasionally a traumatic rupture of an invertebral (IV) disc will produce spinal cord injury. Caudal cervical vertebral fractures are rare. The neck must be handled with great caution to prevent further spinal cord damage produced by manipulation, especially while the animal is anesthetized. Respirations should be carefully monitored while the animal is awake and anesthetized. A fractured vertebra may be seen on plain radiographs, but a myelogram may be necessary to determine the amount of spinal cord compression and whether decompressive or stabilization surgery are necessary (Fig. 16–14A,B). Methylprednisolone sodium succinate (Solu-Medrol) 30 mg/kg is administered intravenously initially then reduced to 15 mg/kg every 6 to 8 hours for 24 to 48 hours. Then, oral prednisone 1 mg/kg is begun for 5 to 7 days. The prednisone dose can be tapered and discontinued over the following 7 days. Mannitol is not used, as most animals with spinal cord injury have hemorrhage in the spinal cord (Chap. 6). Antibiotics may be administered prophylactically for the first 5 to 7 days while on the high glucocorticoid doses. If evidence of melana, anorexia, and vomiting occur from the glucocorticoid therapy, give a combination of cimetidine (Tagamet) 4 mg/kg orally every 6 to 8 hours followed in 2 hours by sucralfate (Carafate) 250 mg to 1 g orally, until these signs resolve. Various surgical techniques are used to decompress the spinal cord and stabilize fractured vertebrae.[86,88,92,93]

The prognosis for recovery is good if the neurologic deficit is minimal and the vertebrae are stabilized.

Intervertebral disc disease

Incidence: Frequent

Intervertebral (IV) disc degeneration in the cervical region can result in protrusion

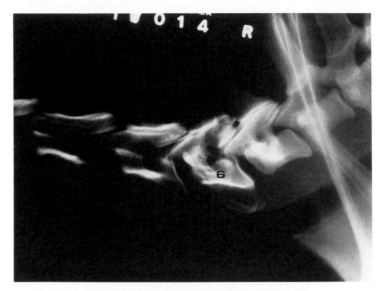

A

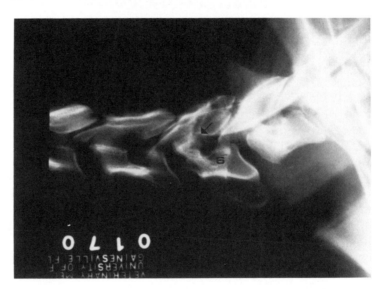

Figure 16–14. *(A)* Fracture of C6 vertebra (6). *(B)* Myelogram of dog in Fig. 16–14A showing the degree of spinal cord compression (arrow).

B

of the anulus fibrosus or extrusion of nucleus pulposus material ventral or lateral into the spinal canal.[6,38,49,76,96] Severe neck pain, lameness of a forelimb, hemiparesis, ataxia of all four limbs, and quadriparesis can result. IV disc degeneration is discussed further in Chapter 17. Intervertebral disc disease often produces signs associated with the thoracolumbar spinal

cord. Special aspects of cervical IV disc degeneration are discussed here.

Cervical IV disc degeneration is common in adult Beagles, Dachshunds, Pekingese, Cocker spaniels, Poodles, and Doberman Pinschers, as well as mixed-breed small dogs and some other large breeds of dogs. Intermittent, continual, acute, or chronic neck pain are common complaints associated with cervical disc disease. The dog may not want to bend its neck or turn from side to side. The head may be held down with the neck rigid and only the eyes moving.

The neurologic examination findings support the complaint of neck pain, but the neck should be manipulated as little as possible. The animal may be lame, or knuckle onto, or carry a front limb. Lifting of the limb has been referred to as a "root signature" indicating disc material is irritating nerve roots to the limb on that side (C4–T1). As spinal cord compression increases, ataxia of all four limbs and quadriparesis occurs. At this stage, spinal reflexes in the forelimbs may still be preserved, even in caudal cervical lesions, and reflexes of the rear limbs will most likely be hyperactive. Quadriplegia may occur in cases of disc herniation with severe spinal cord compression.

Degenerated IV discs may calcify in Beagles, Dachshunds, Cocker spaniels, and Pekingese. The calcified IV discs can easily be seen on radiographs, protruded or extruded into the spinal canal. In Doberman Pinschers and other breeds of smaller dogs, the degenerated disc may not calcify and be readily visible. A narrowed intervertebral disc space may be seen on plain vertebral column radiographs. Myelography is often needed to demonstrate the actual site of spinal cord compression (Fig. 16–15). In small breeds of dogs, C2–3 and C3–4 are commonly affected. In the larger breeds of dogs such as Doberman Pinschers, the lesion is most commonly at C5–6 and C6–7.

Treatment for cervical disc disease is usually some type of surgical correction. The recurrence of problems in dogs medically treated alone is high. Acupuncture may relieve the pain.[54] Several surgical procedures are advocated and vary with the individual patient.[12,13,49] If the major sign is acute pain, and several cervical discs are degenerated and disc material is not herniated into the spinal canal, often a simple ventral fenestration of all cervical vertebrae can be performed, provided that intervertebral disc spaces are not narrowed.[49,63,76] If the intervertebral disc space is narrow and material is extruded into the spinal canal, a ventral slot and removal of disc material may be necessary.

Diazepam (Valium) 2 to 5 mg orally every 8 hours and prednisone 1 mg/kg daily for 3 days, then reduced to 0.5 mg/kg for 3 days, then 0.25 mg/kg for 3 days, then every other day for 3 times may be used with surgical therapy to minimize muscle spasms and meningeal and nerve root inflammation (Chap. 6).

The prognosis for cervical disc disease is often good when treated with surgery early in the course of the disease. Intervertebral disc explosions and ascending and descending secondary myelomalacia rarely occur in the cervical region as compared with the thoracolumbar region, and the prognosis in these cases is grave.

A complete description of the pathophysiology of intervertebral disc disease and surgical techniques is given elsewhere.[49]

Vascular disorders

Fibrocartilaginous infarct

Incidence: Frequent

Fibrocartilaginous embolization of the spinal cord vasculature and focal ischemic myelopathy are causes of acute hemiplegia and quadriplegia of dogs.[21,43,75] Cats are rarely affected. The fibrocartilaginous material is similar to that of nucleus pulposus, so it is suspected of originating from intervertebral discs. The route of entry into the spinal cord vasculature is unknown, but emboli have been found in arteries in some cases, veins in other cases, and both in still other cases. Theories suggesting retrograde arterial blood flow and arterio-

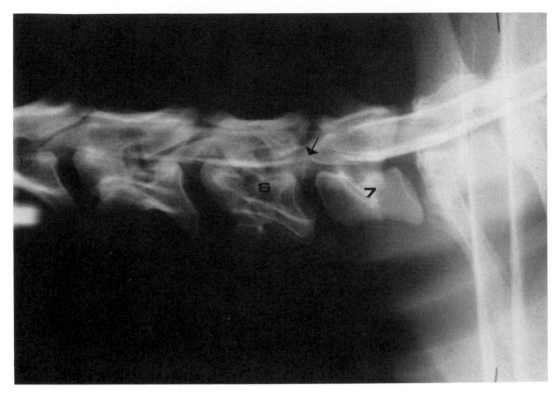

Figure 16–15. A lateral myelogram of a 7-year-old Doberman Pinscher with intervertebral disc protrusion between C6 (6) and C7 (7) vertebrae producing compression of the spinal cord (arrow).

venous anastomosis or anomalous vascularization have been proposed to explain embolization of both arteries and veins. Others have suggested herniation of intervertebral disc material into venous sinuses in the vertebral bone or canal and retrograde flow into the venous supply of the spinal cord. Still others theorize that nucleus pulposus material gains entrance into the vascular supply of the degenerating anulus fibrosus, which then enters the vascular supply of the spinal cord. Some affected dogs have early degeneration and extrusion of intervertebral disc material, and others have no evidence of degenerated intervertebral discs. The dogs that commonly have intervertebral disc disease, i.e., Dachshunds and Beagles, are not the most common dogs presented with fibrocartilaginous infarcts. The origin of the material is still unknown, but the clinical syndrome is common. Fibrocartilaginous infarction can occur anywhere in the spinal cord and is listed in the differential diagnosis of acute hemiplegia, quadriplegia, paraplegia (Chap. 17), and monoplegia (Chap. 18). Findings pertinent to the cervical region are discussed here.

Signalment and history. Adult dogs of large breeds such as Great Danes, Labrador Retrievers, Saint Bernards, and German Shepherds have been reported to be afflicted, as well as small dogs such as Schnauzers, Shetland Sheepdogs, and Wire-haired Fox terriers. As noted, these are not the most common breeds to be affected by intervertebral disc degeneration. Fibrocartilaginous embolism is rare, but occurs, in cats.

The most characteristic presentation for cervical spinal cord fibrocartilaginous infarction is an acute onset of hemiplegia, within 1 to 24 hours (Fig. 16–16). One limb may be affected first, but the other limb on the same side rapidly follows. There is often no known trauma associated with the onset of signs, and the animals do not appear to be in pain once the signs stabilize. A brief episode of pain may occur at the onset of signs.

Physical and neurologic examinations. The neurologic examination findings most often suggest a caudal cervical, primarily unilateral lesion, which would be a rare result of acute IV disc herniations or spinal cord trauma, the other two common causes of acute quadriparesis or quadriplegia. An acute onset of the following neurologic signs supports unilateral vascular spinal cord disease. A unilateral Horner's syndrome may be found on the side of the paralysis. The dogs are usually hemiplegic and may be completely paralyzed on one side, and able to support weight or only mildly paretic on the other side, when hemistanding, hemiwalking, hopping, and placing are attempted. Because gray matter of the caudal cervical spinal cord segments is often affected, the dog may have no reflexes in the thoracic limb and hyperactive reflexes in the pelvic limb on the affected side. The spinal reflexes on the less affected side are often normal. The neck may be stiff, but no obvious pain can be elicited.

Ancillary diagnostic investigations. Initial clinicopathologic tests do not contribute to the diagnosis. Increased protein and, occasionally, increased cells are found

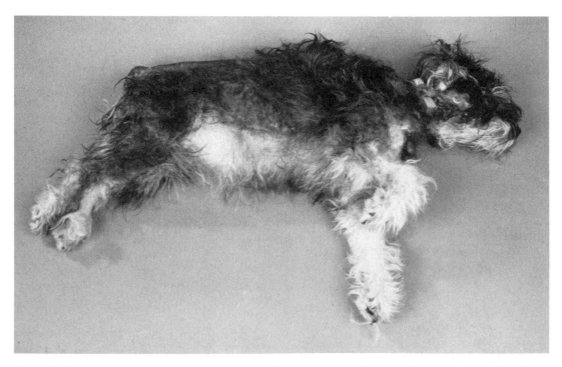

Figure 16–16. A 3-year-old female Miniature Schnauzer with an acute onset of hemiplegia of the left side. Although the dog is in lateral recumbency, note the voluntary movement of the limbs on the right side. A fibrocartilaginous infarct was suspected in the caudal cervical spinal cord on the left.

on CSF analysis. Plain radiographs are usually normal. A myelogram may be normal or show focal cervical spinal cord swelling. The diagnosis is suspected from the acute onset of focal unilateral neurologic deficit unassociated with trauma.

Therapy and prognosis. Oral prednisone can be given as follows: 1 mg/kg for 3 days, then reduced to 0.5 mg/kg for 3 days, then 0.25 mg/kg for 3 days, then 0.25 mg/kg every other day. Many animals will improve rapidly on the less affected side and within a few days to 1 week begin to have movement in the affected limbs. The affected thoracic limb is often the last to recover and may have residual weakness. The animal is often ambulatory within a month. The overall prognosis for functional recovery is very good, although some deficit in one thoracic limb may be permanent.

Pathology. Discoloration of the spinal cord may be seen grossly in hemorrhagic infarction (Fig. 16–17A,B). If arteries are primarily embolized, an ischemic infarction and necrosis of gray and/or white matter occurs. If veins are primarily embolized, a hemorrhagic infarction and necrosis occurs. Often, both arteries and veins are embolized. The lesions seen at necropsy appear severe, but clinically, many dogs recover enough function to be acceptable pets.

Spontaneous spinal cord hemorrhage

Incidence: Rare

Spontaneous spinal cord hemorrhage may occasionally occur associated with congenital and acquired bleeding disorders in dogs and cats. Spontaneous spinal cord hemorrhage, although rare, should be considered in an animal presented with acute quadriplegia. Hemorrhages of other body systems may be found on the physical examination. Whole blood clotting time, partial thromboplastin time, one-stage prothrombin time, bleeding time, platelet count, clot retraction, and platelet adhesiveness are useful tests for the diagnosis of most bleeding disorders.

Vascular malformations

Incidence: Rare

Instances of vascular malformations and hemangiomas of the spinal cord are rare in dogs and cats.

The arteriovenous malformations produce chronic hypoxia, local edema, necrosis, and hemorrhage of the spinal cord. Hemangiomas may produce compressive changes in adjacent spinal cord tissue. Myelography and exploratory decompressive laminectomy may be used to diagnose and treat vascular malformations.

Neoplasia

Tumors of the spinal cord that are primary or metastatic and vertebral tumors that secondarily affect the spinal cord can occur at all levels.[41,64] They may produce cervical pain, ataxia of all four limbs, quadriparesis, hemiparesis, and quadriplegia, as well as ataxia, paresis, or paralysis of pelvic limbs, and urinary incontinence, dilated anus, and drooped tail (Chaps. 17 and 19). Neoplasia of the nervous system is discussed in Chapter 7. Many of the same tumors occur in the spinal cord as well as in the brain.

Extramedullary spinal cord tumors

Incidence: Frequent

Extramedullary neoplasia of nervous tissues includes neurinoma, neurofibroma, neurofibrosarcoma, and meningioma.[7,40] Any breed of adult dog or cat can be af-

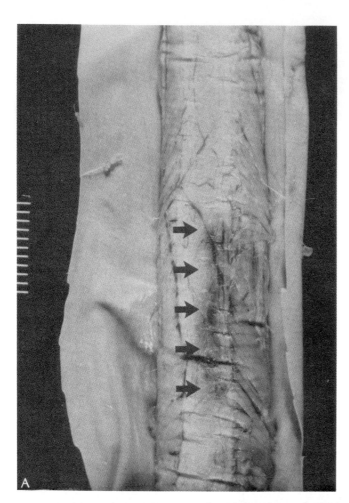

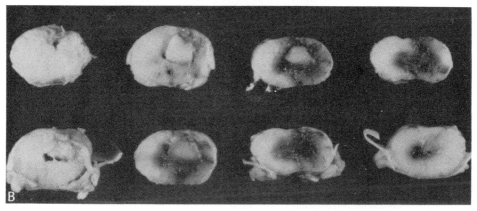

Figure 16–17. (*A*) Gross necropsy findings of a 3-year-old Great Dane with quadriplegia due to a fibrocartilaginous infarct. Note the spinal cord discoloration on the right side of the spinal cord indicated by the arrows. (*B*) Transverse spinal cord sections of the same Great Dane as in Figure *A*. Note the hemorrhagic infarction primarily affecting the right side of the spinal cord at several caudal cervical sections.

fected. The onset of clinical signs can be slow and insidious over several months because of the slow rate of tumor growth. Thoracic limb lameness or "root signature" and neck pain may be the presenting signs. The neurologic deficit becomes more severe as the spinal cord is further compressed. EMG is often abnormal in the affected paraspinal muscles, and supports a diagnosis of focal spinal cord disease. An increase in protein content is found on CSF analysis. Plain radiographs are normal, but a mass may be outlined by myelography and CT or MRI scans (Fig. 16–18A,B). Surgical exploration of the spinal canal and removal of the tumor can produce rapid improvement of clinical signs. Because these are potentially removable tumors, aggressive diagnosis and therapy early in the course of the disease offer the best prognosis. Neurofibromas, neurofibrosarcomas, and neurinomas may occur in multiple nerve roots, so the prognosis is guarded even with surgery (Chap. 18). A diffuse meningeal sarcomatosis may occur and produce multifocal hyperesthesia and ataxia. The diagnosis is usually confirmed after necropsy examination.

Intramedullary spinal cord tumors

Incidence: Occasional

Intramedullary spinal cord tumors of dogs and cats include astrocytomas, ependymomas, and gliomas.[41,64] These tumors can occur in any age dog or cat, but older Boxers and Boston terriers have a tendency to develop primary spinal cord tumors as well as brain tumors. Often, no pain is associated with intramedullary spinal cord tumors. The early signs may be hemiparesis or ataxia of all four limbs. The speed of progression of the neurologic deficit can vary with the tumor type and growth, but the animal may be quadriplegic in a few weeks to a few months. EMG may be used to localize the lesion.

CSF usually contains increased amounts of protein. Myelography and CT and MRI scans can outline the spinal cord mass. Diffuse spinal cord swelling and discoloration may be seen following an exploratory laminectomy to rule out a surgically removable mass. The prognosis is grave, and the final tumor classification is usually made at necropsy.

Metastatic spinal cord tumors

Incidence: Occasional

Lymphosarcoma is the most common metastatic spinal cord tumor in cats and also has been reported in dogs.[24,26] Meningeal lymphocyte infiltration or extradural masses and spinal cord compression occur in many animals. Infiltration of nerve roots and spinal cord also occurs. If the lymphocytic mass is in the epidural space, the tumor may be removed and the spinal cord surgically decompressed. Tumor removal at least temporarily improves the neurologic status of the animal while chemotherapy is administered. The longterm prognosis is grave.

Prostatic, perianal, and mammary adenocarcinomas and hemangiosarcomas are other metastatic neoplasms that affect the spinal cord.

Granulomatous meningoencephalitis (reticulosis)

Incidence: Occasional

Granulomatous meningoencephalitis (GME or reticulosis) is an inflammatory or neoplastic proliferation of adventitial cells around blood vessels in the nervous system. GME may occur as a focal spinal cord lesion, but is usually diagnosed at necropsy. GME is discussed in Chapters 7 and 12.

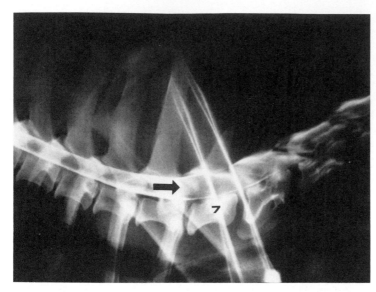

A

Figure 16–18. *(A)* Lateral myelogram of a dog with progressive quadriparesis. Note how the contrast media column thins at vertebrae C7 (7) and the spinal cord appears enlarged (arrow). *(B)* A meningioma (arrow) at the C7–C8 spinal cord segments in the dog whose myelogram appears in Fig. *A.*

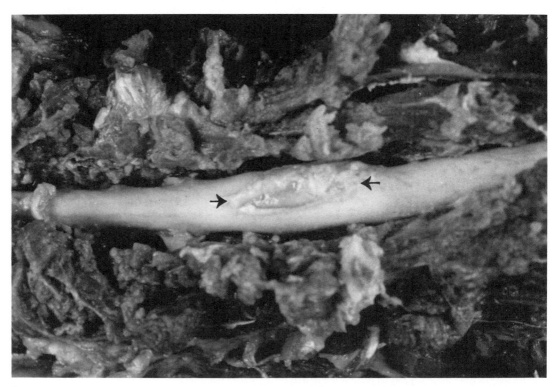

B

Vertebral neoplasia

Incidence: Occasional

Osteosarcoma, fibrosarcoma, and chondrosarcoma are vertebral neoplasms that may secondarily encroach on the cervical spinal cord and produce neck pain, ataxia of all four limbs, quadriparesis, or quadriplegia.[41,72] Other neoplastic processes that metastasize to bone, such as multiple myeloma and adenocarcinomas, can also produce similar signs. Most vertebral neoplasms are readily visualized on plain radiographs of the affected vertebrae. Myelography may be needed to outline the degree of spinal cord compression. The prognosis for bone tumors in general is grave.

Neuromuscular disorders
Congenital and familial disorders

A few congenital and familial neuromuscular disorders have been described in dogs and cats. Most of the disorders are rare and affect specific breeds.

Globoid cell leukodystrophy

Incidence: Rare

Globoid cell leukodystrophy is a congenital disorder of dogs, especially Cairn Terriers, and cats characterized by demyelination throughout the nervous system. Demyelination with some axonal degeneration and accumulation of periodic acid-Schiff (PAS) positive staining globoid-type macrophages are seen on histologic examination of peripheral nerves. Globoid cell leukodystrophy often begins as paraparesis and is further discussed in Chapter 17. A progressive neuronopathy has been described in young Cairn terriers between 5 and 7 months of age. No globoid cells are found at necropsy.[74]

Boxer neuropathy

Incidence: Rare

A disorder of the CNS and PNS neurons has been described in which UMN, LMN, and sensory neurons are demyelinated and degenerated.[46] Affected Boxers are usually less than 6 months of age when signs of slow, progressive pelvic limb ataxia and paresis with depressed or absent patellar reflexes and proprioception develop.[31] Pelvic limbs are more severely involved than thoracic limbs. Motor nerve conduction velocities are normal or slightly reduced. Sensory nerve conduction is absent. Diagnosis is made by sensory nerve biopsy. Prognosis is poor; however, the neurologic deficit progresses so slowly, affected Boxers may be acceptable pets for many months to years; an inherited disorder is suspected.

Spinal muscular atrophy

Incidence: Rare

An autosomal recessive inherited abiotrophy of ventral horn cells, cerebellar Purkinje cells, and other neurons in the brain stem has been described in Swedish Lapland dogs.[8] Clinical signs of generalized weakness begin at 5 to 7 weeks of age and rapidly progress to flaccid quadriplegia with severe atrophy within a few weeks. Needle EMG studies show evidence of denervation in limb musculature. Motor nerve conduction velocities are decreased. The prognosis is grave.

Rottweiler puppies between 4 and 6 weeks of age develop a progressive flaccid quadriparesis with head tremors, dysphagia, and megaesophagus.[82] Degeneration of the lower motor neuron cell bodies in brain stem and spinal cord are found at necropsy. An inherited spinal muscular atrophy is thought to be the cause.

An inherited slow, progressive atrophy and flaccid quadriparesis in Brittany spaniels has also been described.[8] Affected dogs develop severe paraspinal muscle atrophy initially, which progresses to involve limb musculature and produces severe muscle atrophy and loss of spinal reflexes. Sensation is normal. Clinical signs progress over 1 year. The prognosis is grave. Lesions are primarily located in the ventral horns of the spinal cord.

Hypomyelinating polyneuropathy

Incidence: *Rare*

A hypomyelinating polyneuropathy is seen in Golden Retriever puppies at 5 to 7 weeks of age.[11] Affected dogs have pelvic limb weakness. Spinal reflexes of the pelvic and thoracic limbs are depressed. The sciatic–tibial and ulnar motor nerve conduction velocities are reduced. The prognosis for recovery is poor. By 5 months of age, dogs remain affected. An inherited disorder is suspected.

Hypertrophic polyneuropathy

Incidence: *Rare*

A progressive quadriparesis and hyporeflexia has been described in Tibetan mastiff puppies beginning at 7 to 12 weeks of age.[22] The degree of neurologic deficit may vary among litter mates. An inherited metabolic defect of Schwann cells is suspected. A widespread demyelination is found throughout peripheral nerves and nerve roots.

Giant axonal neuropathy

Incidence: *Rare*

Giant axonal neuropathy has been reported in young German Shepherds 14 to 16 months of age.[8,31] Pelvic limb paresis, loss of proprioception, depressed patellar reflexes, and reduced pain perception are found on the neurologic examination. Af-

fected dogs may also develop weak vocalizations and megaesophagus. The prognosis is poor and an autosomal recessive inheritance is thought to be responsible. Axonal swelling at the distal portion of CNS and PNS axons is found on necropsy.

Myasthenia gravis

Incidence: *Rare*

Congenital myasthenia gravis has been described in the Jack Russell terriers, Springer spaniels, and Fox terriers.[71,73] Weakness in all four limbs is usually noticed by 6 to 8 weeks of age, with the pelvic limbs most affected. The weakness may be exacerbated by exercise and alleviated by rest. In severe cases, the animal is unable to stand or lift its head and has swallowing difficulties. Megaesophagus has not been reported. Affected puppies respond to 0.1 to 0.5 mg of edrophonium chloride (Tensilon) intravenously. A decremental response is seen on repetitive nerve stimulation during EMG testing. Pyridostigmine (Mestinon) liquid 10–30 mg orally twice daily is given using the lowest dose that will control the signs. Congenital myasthenia does not appear to have an immune-mediated basis as acquired myasthenia does. There is a congenital deficiency of acetylcholine receptor in the postsynaptic membrane. The condition is thought to be inherited, and affected animals must be maintained continually on some form of therapy. The response to therapy is often poor, as is the prognosis.

Myotonic myopathy

Incidence: *Rare*

Myotonic myopathy has been reported in Chow Chows, Labrador Retrievers, Staffordshire bull terriers, Great Danes, and West Highland White terriers, and is characterized by a generalized muscle stiffness that begins in the first few months of life.[30,36] Myotonia is a continued active contraction and delayed relaxation of a muscle. Myotonia is a result of a hyperexcitable muscle cell membrane and is not a primary neurologic disorder.

Affected dogs have difficulty advancing the thoracic limbs because of a decreased ability to flex the joints because of muscle stiffness, which becomes worse with excitement. A persistent dimple is observed at the site of muscle percussion. EMG confirms the diagnosis of myotonia, with bizarre high-frequency discharges that wax and wane and have a dive-bomber sound. Serum CPK determinations may be elevated, indicating muscle fiber necrosis. No therapy currently has proven effective. Muscle fiber necrosis and increased connective tissue are found on histologic examination of the muscle. Inherited myotonic muscular dystrophy is thought to be responsible.

Labrador retriever myopathy

Incidence: Rare

Affected Labrador Retrievers develop generalized muscle stiffness, especially with exercise or excitement, usually prior to 6 months of age.[65,66] The pelvic limbs are often more affected than the thoracic limbs, and affected dogs may have difficulty lifting their heads. Megaesophagus may occur. Cold weather may aggravate the muscle stiffness. The signs improve with rest. As the dogs mature, the clinical signs stabilize so they may be suitable pets, especially if the signs are mild. Bizarre high frequency discharges and fibrillation potentials are found in the muscles on EMG examination. Serum CPK levels are elevated. Oral diazepam (Valium) 5 mg every 6–8 hours may give them relief from some muscle stiffness. A deficiency of Type II muscle fibers has been found on histochemical examination of muscle. A neurologic component to the disorder may

also be present. A simple autosomal recessive inheritance is thought to be the cause.

Irish terrier myopathy

Incidence: Rare

A recessive X-linked myopathy of Irish terriers is characterized by a stiff gait, difficulty in swallowing, an enlarged tongue, and atrophic muscles.[31] Signs begin at 8 to 12 weeks of age. No sustained dimpling is found on percussion of the muscle, and bizarre high-frequency discharges are seen on EMG examination. Serum CPK, AST, and adolase levels are elevated. Muscle fiber necrosis and phagocytosis are the primary changes found on muscle biopsy.

Golden retriever myopathy

Incidence: Rare

An X-linked myopathy occurs in Golden Retriever puppies.[57] As early as 1 day of age, CPK values are elevated. When affected dogs begin to ambulate, the gait is stiff and stilted. Generalized muscle atrophy, including temporalis muscles, progresses over the next few months. Some dogs develop dysphagia. Severely affected puppies die, but mildly affected dogs may live several years. Cardiac muscle disease is the usual cause of death. CPK levels remain elevated. Bizarre high-frequency discharges are found in muscles diffusely. Myofiber necrosis and mineralized fibers are found on muscle biopsy. Mildly affected dogs may be acceptable pets for a few years, but will never recover.

Nemaline myopathy

Incidence: Rare

Nemaline rods are intramyofiber structures associated with Z bands. Young cats may develop a hypermetric gait and depressed patellar reflexes. CPK may be

tis.[2,15,17,25] This disorder is also referred to as "coonhound paralysis" because of the great number of hounds that developed the ascending flaccid paralysis after contact with a raccoon. There are probably many inciting causes in dogs. The bite of a raccoon is the best known cause, but a similar syndrome may occur following rabies vaccination in animals. Experimental allergic neuritis in dogs appears very similar to naturally occurring cases of acute polyradiculoneuritis. Acute polyradiculoneuritis has been seen in cats, although rarely compared with dogs.

Signalment and history. Any age, breed, or sex of dog or cat could be affected, but most animals are over 6 months of age. The onset of signs is characterized by a weakness of the pelvic limbs, which rapidly ascends over the next 24 to 48 hours until the animal is quadriplegic. On rare occasions, the paralysis begins in the thoracic limbs and descends to involve the pelvic limbs. There may or may not be any history of contact with raccoons, recent vaccination, or systemic illness.

Physical and neurologic examinations. An old bite wound from a raccoon may be noted on physical examination. The animal is often presented in lateral recumbency and little voluntary movement is seen. If presented early in the course of the disease or in a mild form of the disease, the animal may have generalized weakness, with the pelvic limbs weaker than the thoracic limbs. Often no spinal reflexes can be elicited in the limbs, but this may vary with the severity of the paralysis. In severe cases, intercostal and phrenic nerves are significantly affected and respiratory difficulties are seen. The animal may have normal sensation, but is often hyperesthetic, and overreacts to simple manipulation. Pain may often be elicited on direct palpation of the nerves.

The bark may be altered and sound hoarse. Swallowing, chewing difficulties, and facial paralysis may be seen, and indicate cranial nerve involvement (Chap. 11). In severe cases, animals die from respiratory paralysis or aspiration pneumonia, but many animals never become affected that severely. The differential diagnosis for an acute flaccid quadriplegia is listed in Table 16–2.

Ancillary diagnostic investigations. Positive waves and fibrillation potentials are usually seen on needle EMG studies and suggest diffuse denervation. Early in the course of acute disease, the EMG may be normal. Motor nerve conduction velocity studies may be normal or may be slow, depending on the involvement of peripheral axons. Cisternal CSF analysis is usually normal, whereas lumbar CSF may show a mild elevation of protein. The diagnosis is based on the history, physical and neurologic examinations, and EMG findings.

Therapy and prognosis. There is no specific therapy. Some clinicians give dexamethasone 0.05 mg/kg or prednisone 1 mg/kg orally in decreasing doses over the first 10 days of the disease. The animals must be assisted to eat, drink, urinate, and defecate. Respirations and ability to swallow should be closely monitored during the first week. If respiratory paralysis develops, assisted ventilation may be necessary for a few days until the signs regress. After 1 week, the neurologic signs begin to slowly improve. The animal should be placed on an air mattress or water bed and turned every 4 to 6 hours to prevent decubital ulcers and lung congestion. Spinal reflexes and voluntary movements can be monitored to evaluate return of function. With nursing care, the prognosis for recovery in most cases is good. Recovery time may vary from a few weeks to a few months. Some of the muscle atrophy will be permanent, but most animals recover well enough to become functional again.

Once an animal has been affected and recovered, it may be prone to have recurrences of the disease.

Pathology. Extensive demyelination, cellular infiltration and disruption of axons are found primarily in the ventral roots of the spinal cord and peripheral spinal nerves, and to a lesser extent, in the dorsal roots.

Chronic polyradiculoneuritis or polyneuritis

Incidence: Occasional

Chronic forms of polyradiculoneuritis have been described in dogs and cats, but the underlying cause has not often been determined.[26,33,61,85] The neurologic signs may chronically progress or go into remission and relapse.

Signalment and history. Adult dogs and cats are affected. The initial clinical signs may be a lameness in a limb. Over a few to several weeks quadriparesis insidiously occurs. Any possible continuing exposure to chemicals or chronic metabolic or endocrine disorder should be questioned in the history. Polyneuropathies associated with toxic, metabolic, and endocrine disorders are discussed later in this chapter.

Physical and neurologic examinations. Varying degrees of quadriparesis are found on the neurologic examination. The quadriparesis may be asymmetric and more evident in one limb. The pelvic limbs are often more involved than the thoracic limbs. In mild or early disease, spinal reflexes may be intact except for the patellar reflex, which is often depressed or absent. Later in the course of the disease, all spinal reflexes may be depressed or absent. Muscle atrophy may be diffuse. Facial muscle paresis, weak jaw tone, atrophy of the temporalis and masseter muscles, and a depressed swallowing reflex are indicative of cranial nerve involvement.

Ancillary diagnostic investigations. Positive waves and fibrillation potentials seen on EMG examination suggest diffuse denervation. Motor nerve conduction velocity studies are slower than normal, suggesting peripheral nerve disease. Some of the known causes of chronic polyneuropathy in dogs are listed in Table 16–9. These disorders should be considered and ruled out when a polyneuropathy is diagnosed based on the neurologic examination and EMG findings. Some cases have elevated CSF protein. Serum biochemistry profiles should be evaluated to examine for metabolic disorders such as hypoglycemia, hyperglycemia, uremia, electrolyte imbalances, and evidence of hepatopathy. If the chemistry profile is normal, thyroid and adrenal cortex function may be assessed. Serum and CSF protein electrophoresis, antinuclear antibody (ANA), and preparations to detect systemic lupus erythematosus should be evaluated for a possible immune-mediated underlying process. Toxoplasmosis titers and muscle biopsy should be evaluated to rule out Toxoplasmosis infections as described above. Thoracic and abdominal radiographs may be useful in some cases of neoplasia, which might produce secondary polyneuropathy, discussed later in this chapter.

Therapy and prognosis. In many cases, no underlying disease process can be determined, no specific therapy can be instituted, and signs continue to progress. Prednisone 1 mg/kg may be given orally for 5 to 7 days to see if the signs improve. If there is improvement of signs, the dose may be reduced and given alternate days for 1 month. Some animals improve and then go into remissions. Others are not responsive to prednisone therapy.

Table 16–9
Differential diagnosis of chronic polyneuropathy in dogs

1. Chronic immune-mediated polyneuropathy
2. Hyperinsulinism polyneuropathy
3. Diabetes mellitus polyneuropathy
4. Hypothyroid polyneuropathy/polymyopathy
5. Paraneoplastic polyneuropathy
6. Idiopathic distal axonopathy
7. Toxic polyneuropathy (Table 16–11)

Pathology. Many different histologic examination findings have been described that probably represent the many causes of the clinical syndrome. Some cases in the dog and in the cat have lymphocyte and plasma cell infiltration associated with demyelination and axonal necrosis of many peripheral nerves. The lesions in chronic polyneuropathies are in the peripheral nerves mainly, but in some cases affect the nerve roots.

Brachial plexus neuritis

Incidence: Rare

A few cases of brachial plexus neuritis in dogs have been reported.[8,26] Studies on serum neuritis in man suggest that the brachial plexus may be vulnerable to allergic reactions. Neurologic signs may develop 48 hours after an allergic reaction such as generalized urticaria and facial edema. An acute onset of asymmetric weakness of the thoracic limbs is characterized by hyporeflexia and loss of sensation.

Cranial nerve signs of a facial paralysis and dropped jaw may occur. EMG and nerve conduction velocity studies support a diagnosis of bilateral brachial plexus disease with peripheral nerve involvement. Axonal necrosis and wallerian degeneration are the main histologic features seen

on peripheral nerve biopsy. The prognosis is poor for recovery.

Myasthenia gravis

Incidence: Rare

Acquired myasthenia gravis has been reported in adult dogs and cats,[1,15,52] and is an immune-mediated disorder involving acetylcholine receptors in muscle. Circulating serum antibodies to acetylcholine receptors have been found in affected dogs.

Signalment and history. Myasthenia gravis has been reported in several breeds of dogs and cats. German Shepherds approximately 2 years of age are frequently affected. There may be an inciting febrile illness or no known underlying cause. The primary complaint is often episodic weakness and decreased exercise tolerance. Difficulty barking, swallowing, and prehending food may also occur. Regurgitation from megaesophagus has been reported. During a myasthenic crisis, the animal may collapse in lateral or sternal recumbency and be unable to rise or lift its head.

Physical and neurologic examinations. An affected animal may become progressively weaker when exercised, but improves with rest. Mild cases may be difficult to differentiate from polymyositis, which also has associated decreased exercise tolerance, dysphagia, megaesophagus, and regurgitation. Polymyositis is discussed later in this chapter. Affected cats may have quadriparesis that worsens on exercise, and difficulty lifting the head. Table 16–10 lists several disorders that will produce these signs in cats. There may be some degree of bilateral ptosis, facial muscle weakness, decreased jaw tone, and a depressed swallowing response with excessive salivation. These cranial nerve deficits may be the most obvious finding.

Flaccid quadriparesis is commonly seen during a myasthenic crisis (see Table

Table 16–10

Differential diagnosis of quadriparesis and neck weakness in cats

1. Myasthenia gravis
2. Polymyositis
3. Hypokalemic polymyopathy
4. Organophosphate toxicity
5. Hyperthyroidism
6. Diabetic polyneuropathy
7. Thiamine deficiency
8. Hypernatremia

16–2). The animal may be unable to lift its head or move the limbs. All spinal reflexes are depressed or absent, but sensation is preserved.

Ancillary diagnostic investigations. Because subacute organophosphate toxicity can produce episodic weakness and decreased exercise tolerance, serum cholinesterase determinations should be evaluated if there has been exposure to any organophosphates. If edrophonium chloride is given to a dog or cat with organophosphate toxicity, a cholinergic crisis will occur and the neurologic signs will worsen. Edrophonium chloride (Tensilon), a short-acting anticholinesterase drug, given intravenously at a dose of 0.1 to 1 mg, usually produces a dramatic improvement in an animal collapsed in a myasthenic crisis or one who is exercise-intolerant. Within 1 to 2 minutes, the animal is up on its feet walking around with renewed strength. The strength only lasts a few minutes and weakness returns. If an animal is only mildly weak, the Tensilon test may be difficult to interpret, as many mild diffuse neuromuscular disorders may appear slightly improved with edrophonium chloride.

Megaesophagus may be seen on contrast radiographic studies of the upper gastrointestinal tract. The diagnosis of myasthenia gravis is best made with electromyographic studies.

EMG and nerve conduction velocity studies are usually normal. On repetitive nerve stimulation, a decremental response is seen (see Fig. 16–20A) that is most characteristic of myasthenia gravis. The decremental response disappears when Tensilon is given (see Fig. 16–20B).

Neostigmine (Progstigmin) 0.5 to 2.5 mg may be given IM to cats and dogs in a myasthenic crisis. Other animals may begin oral liquid pyridostigmine (Mestinon). The dose will vary depending on the size of the animal and effect. A cat may be maintained on 10 to 15 mg twice daily. A German Shepherd may require 30 to 60 mg twice daily. In severe cases, 2 mg/kg prednisone may be given for 1 week and the dose decreased, and then discontinued when the animal is stable. Thymomas have occurred with myasthenia in dogs and cats.[1]

The prognosis for the control of myasthenia gravis may be good. There may be remissions and relapses, but often the disease can be controlled by medical therapy and may even be self-limiting. The megaesophagus may resolve, but can be a permanent problem.

Polymyositis

Incidence: Occasional

Idiopathic polymyositis is a diffuse inflammation of skeletal muscle and the most common polymyopathy seen in dogs.[17,35,77,83] Polymyositis can occur in cats as well, but is less frequent than in dogs. An autoimmune process is suspected. In several cases, hypergammaglobulinemia, positive serum antinuclear antibody (ANA) and circulating anti-muscle antibody, demonstrable by indirect immunofluorescence studies of affected muscle, have been found. Polymyositis associated with systemic lupus erythematosus in a dog

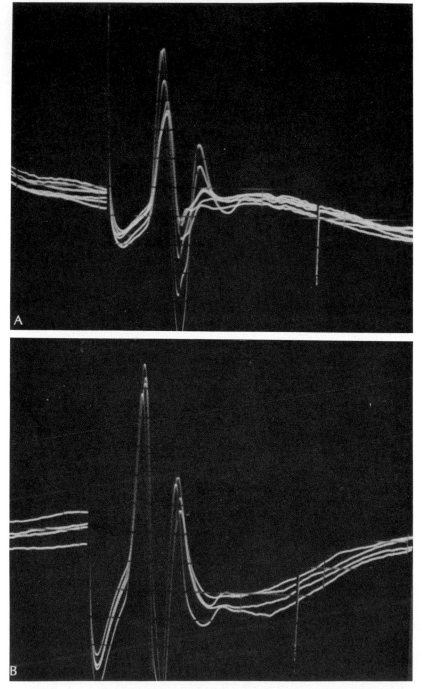

Figure 16–20. *(A)* A decremental evoked response seen on 5/sec nerve stimulation of a 2½-year-old Cairn Terrier with myasthenia gravis. (From Chrisman, C.L.: Electromyography in Animals. *In* Pathophysiology in Small Animal Surgery. Edited by M.J. Bojrab. Philadelphia, Lea & Febiger, 1981.) *(B)* The loss of the decremental evoked response in the same Cairn Terrier as in *A* after the administration of Tensilon. (From Chrisman, C.L.: Electromyography in Animals. *In* Pathophysiology in Small Animal Surgery. Edited by M.J. Bojrab. Philadelphia, Lea & Febiger, 1981.)

has been seen. Dermatomyositis is reported in Shelties and Collies, but affected dogs show no weakness. Inflammation is mainly in temporalis and masseter muscles.[48,60] A familial disorder is probable.

Signalment and history. Adult dogs and cats of either sex are affected with a generalized weakness, which becomes worse with exercise. They may also have a stiff, stilted gait, lameness, and painful muscles. Occasionally, a generalized, non-painful loss of skeletal muscle bulk may be seen. Regurgitation and aspiration pneumonia may be a complaint, as affected animals commonly have megaesophagus. The animal also may have an abnormal voice, difficulty in swallowing, and excessive salivation. The animal may have a history of remission and recurrence of these signs.

Physical and neurologic examinations. Animals with secondary aspiration pneumonia may be depressed, anorexic, and febrile. Regurgitation of food and difficulty swallowing may be seen.

Exercise intolerance and generalized weakness is seen even in those animals without secondary pneumonia (Fig. 16–21). Affected cats may have difficulty raising their heads. In some cases, the gait is stiff, and the animals may appear to have painful muscles on palpatation. The spinal reflexes are usually normal. There may be generalized muscle atrophy, especially of temporalis and masseter muscles if the signs are chronic or recurrent.

Ancillary diagnostic investigations. Elevated muscle enzymes help differentiate polymyositis from myasthenia gravis, in which no serum muscle enzyme elevation is usually present. CPK, AST, aldolase, and LDH should all be evaluated, but only some of them may be elevated. Heavy exercise may cause an increase in serum muscle enzymes in affected dogs. In cats with reduced exercise tolerance and a weak neck, diseases in Table 16–10 should be considered. The CPK may also be elevated in hypokalemic polymyopathy, discussed later in this chapter.

A contrast radiographic study of the upper gastrointestinal tract can be useful to demonstrate the megaesophagus.

Positive sharp waves, fibrillation potentials, and bizarre high-frequency discharges may be found on needle EMG examination of muscles. In mild cases the EMG may be normal. There is no decremental response to repetitive nerve stimulation, which differentiates polymyositis from myasthenia gravis.

The diagnosis of polymyositis is confirmed on histologic examination of a muscle biopsy specimen. Plasma cell and lymphocyte infiltration with muscle fiber necrosis is most often seen. Toxoplasmosis polymyositis should be ruled out by the muscle biopsy and serum titers.

Therapy and prognosis. Prednisolone 2 mg/kg orally in divided doses daily often improves the weakness within a few days. The prednisone dosage can then be reduced to 1 mg/kg for 3 to 5 days, then 0.5 mg/kg for 3 to 5 days, then 0.25 mg/kg for 3 to 5 days, then alternate-day therapy. If the signs recur as the dosage is decreased, the dosage then is increased for 3 to 5 days again before a decrease is again attempted. Serum muscle enzyme determinations can be measured to follow the animal's response to therapy. If the signs resolve and the muscle enzymes are normal, the prednisone can be discontinued after 1 month. Serial CPK evaluations should be performed monthly to see if the condition stays in remission or is going to recur. Some dogs must be on alternate-day prednisone on a longterm basis. Some dogs and cats may have a thymoma associated with their polymyositis.

The prognosis is generally good for recovery if esophageal, pharyngeal, and la-

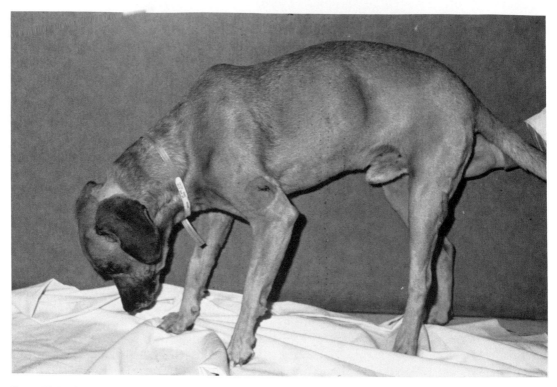

Figure 16–21. Generalized weakness of the limbs and neck in a 3-year-old mixed-breed dog. The serum CPK was 2500 International Units (I.U.) and polymyositis was diagnosed from a muscle biopsy of the left triceps muscle.

ryngeal muscles are not severely damaged. The megaesophagus can recover or may be permanent. Recurrence of the clinical signs is reported, but serial evaluation of serum muscle enzymes may detect recurrence before severe muscle involvement occurs.

Metabolic disorders

There are many polyneuropathies and polymyopathies associated with metabolic disorders in humans, which are now being discovered to also occur in dogs and cats. The cases appear to be sporadic, and the metabolic disorders discussed here do not always produce polyneuropathy or polymyopathy. The polyneuropathies are often characterized by a generalized weakness

with depressed spinal reflexes, which progresses slowly to a flaccid quadriplegia, such as that described in chronic progressive polyneuropathies. EMG changes often include positive waves, fibrillation potentials, bizarre high-frequency discharges, and slowed motor conduction velocities. As discovered earlier in this chapter, when polyneuropathy of unknown cause is diagnosed, then an underlying metabolic or endocrine disorder should be ruled out.

Hyperinsulinism polyneuropathy

Incidence: Rare

Hypoglycemia and hyperinsulinism caused by an islet cell adenocarcinoma of the pancreas can produce polyneuropathy in dogs.[8,17] Affected dogs have quadriparesis with pelvic limbs worse than thoracic limbs. Only the patellar reflex may be depressed, but in severe cases all spinal reflexes are depressed and the quadriplegic animal will be hypoglycemic, and hyperinsulinism is diagnosed as described in Chapter 8. Once the pancreatic tumor is removed, the polyneuropathy resolves over the following 2 weeks.

Diabetes mellitus polyneuropathy

Incidence: Rare

Polyneuropathy associated with diabetes mellitus has been described in dogs and cats.[8,17,59,90] Affected animals may also be quadriparetic with depressed spinal reflexes. Positive waves and fibrillation potentials are found on EMG examination and motor nerve conduction velocity is reduced. Hyperglycemia and glucosuria are found, and therapy for diabetes mellitus should be instituted. Segmental demyelination may be seen on teased nerve biopsy specimens. If the underlying diabetes mellitus can be properly controlled, the prognosis for recovery from the polyneuropathy is usually good.

Hypoadrenocortical neuromuscular disease

Incidence: Rare

Hyperkalemia does produce generalized muscle weakness in dogs and cats. Hypoadrenocorticism with the associated hyperkalemia produces collapse and generalized weakness and should be ruled out in dogs presented with these signs.

Hypothyroid polyneuropathy and polymyopathy

Incidence: Rare

Hypothyroidism can produce polyneuropathy and polymyopathy in dogs.[4,53] Some affected dogs may have paraparesis and others quadriparesis. The patellar reflexes are usually depressed or absent, but all spinal reflexes can be depressed. Positive waves, fibrillation potentials, and bizarre high-frequency discharges may be found on the EMG examination. Motor nerve conduction velocity is reduced. Hypothyroidism is diagnosed using a thyroid-stimulating hormone (TSH) stimulation test. A teased sural nerve biopsy may show segmental demyelination. Type 2 myofiber degeneration may be seen on the muscle biopsy examination. The neuromuscular disorder resolves once thyroid replacement therapy is instituted.

Hypokalemic polymyopathy

Incidence: Occasional

Adult cats are presented for generalized weakness that may worsen on exercise. Often affected cats have a weak neck as well, and the other diseases listed in Table 16–10 must be considered. If serum potassium levels are as low as between 1.5 and 3.5 mEq/l when normal is 4 to 5 mEq/l, then polymyopathy from hypokalemia is probable.[28,29] Most affected cats have renal disease and the serum blood urea nitrogen (BUN) and creatinine are elevated. The hypokalemia is caused by a loss of potassium through the dysfunctional kidneys. The serum CPK is elevated, indicating myofiber necrosis. Myofiber necrosis may be seen on a muscle biopsy examination.

If severe paresis and dyspnea are present, ventilatory support and 0.5 μg/kg/min dopamine may be given intravenously until the crisis has passed. Potassium supplementation of 20 to 80 mEq/l in intravenous fluids is slowly infused. In less severely affected animals, oral potassium gluconate (Kaon) 4 to 8 mEq every 12 hours is given and the potassium level monitored. Dietary supplementation will improve the weakness, and the signs may be controlled. The serum CPK, potassium, and renal

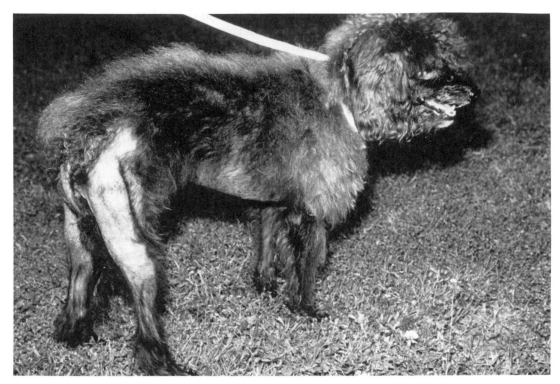

A

Figure 16-22. *(A)* A 10-year-old poodle female with hyperadrenocorticism. Note the thin hair coat. Although the hair on the pelvic limbs was thin, it was shaved to show the muscle atrophy.

tive care should be given. Mildly affected dogs recover in 3 to 4 weeks.

Snake venom neurotoxin

Incidence: Rare

The coral snake produces a neurotoxin that when injected into dogs by a snake bite produces a flaccid quadriparesis.[67] Affected dogs have generalized weakness, with the pelvic limbs more affected than the thoracic limbs, and a depressed patellar reflex early in the course of the disease. Affected dogs can also develop profound quadriparesis and loss of all spinal reflexes, like the other disorders listed in Table 16–2. No needle EMG abnormalities are found, but there are reduced-amplitude evoked potentials on nerve stimulation. If respiratory paralysis does not produce death, affected animals may recover in 2 to 3 weeks.

Organophosphate toxicity

Incidence: Occasional

Subacute organophosphate toxicity may produce only neuromuscular weakness in dogs and cats with no muscarinic signs of salivation, miotic pupils, and gastrointestinal disturbances or seizures (Chap. 8).[18] The onset of signs may be 5 to 7 days after exposure from direct application or home spraying.

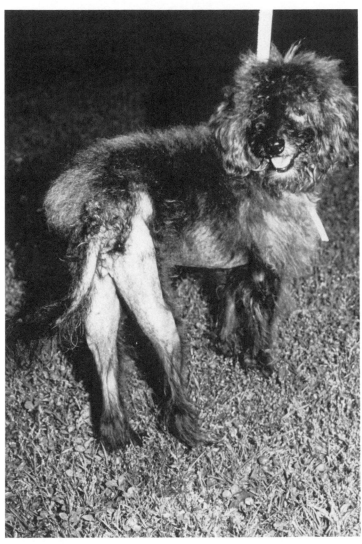

Figure 16–22. *(B)* Another view of the atrophied pelvic limb musculature. All four limbs were stiff, but the pelvic limbs were more stilted during ambulation.

B

Affected animals have weakness that worsens on exercise. Cats also have neck weakness (see Table 16–10). Serum cholinesterase levels are usually below 500 IU. Needle EMG is usually normal, but a decremental response may be seen on repetitive nerve stimulation. Edrophonium chloride (Tensilon) should not be given, as this will worsen the decremental response and the animal will go into crisis.

Diphenhydramine (Benadryl) is given intramuscularly or orally 2 to 4 mg/kg every 8 to 12 hours as needed to control the weakness for 2 to 3 weeks. The serum cholinesterase levels slowly increase over the following 4 to 6 weeks. The cat should be bathed if recently dipped to remove residual toxin. If the environment was recently treated, the animal should be kept out of the environment until recovered. Repeat exposure to organophosphates should be avoided.

Miscellaneous chemical agents

Many chemical agents affect the peripheral nervous system of animals and humans. Polyneuropathy, distal axonopathy, neuromuscular junction malfunction, or polymyopathy may be caused by various toxic agents and produce ataxia of all four limbs, quadriparesis, or quadriplegia. A history of chronic drug therapy or exposure to chemicals should be investigated in all dogs with diffuse neuromuscular disease of unknown origin.

Table 16–11 lists chemical agents that have been reported to produce polyneuropathies in man or animals. There is a variable species-susceptibility to chemicals, which is most likely from variable absorption and metabolism.

Neomycin and muscle relaxants used simultaneously in an animal may produce neuromuscular junction blockage. Streptomycin, kanamycin, gentamicin, polymyxin B, tetracyclines, and sulfonamides also may block the neuromuscular junctions and produce generalized weakness or flaccid quadriparesis.

Table 16–12 lists some of the drug-induced myopathies reported in man that might be considered in polymyopathy of unknown origin in animals.

Nutritional disorders

Nutritional disorders of the neuromuscular system are rare in small animals.

Myodegeneration

Incidence: Occasional

Nutritional myodegeneration from vitamin E deficiency, although uncommon in dogs and cats, is sometimes seen in young animals.[8] Affected animals have a stiff and stilted gait with generalized muscle weakness. Serum muscle enzymes are often elevated. Positive waves, fibrillation po-

Table 16–11
Chemical agents that may produce polyneuropathy

Industrial and cosmetic chemicals

- Acrylamide
- Triorthocresyl phosphate
- Diisopropyl fluorophosphate (DFP)
- Parathion
- Malathion
- Other organophosphorus compounds
- Carbon disulfide
- Trichloroethylene
- n-hexane
- Carbon monoxide
- Methyl bromide
- Chlorophenothane (DDT)
- Lindane
- Polychlorinated biphenyl
- Carbon tetrachloride (CCL_4)
- 2,4-dichlorophenoxyacetic acid (2,4-D)
- Pentachlorophenolate
- Gasoline
- Methyl butyl ketone (MBK)
- Zinc pyridinethione (ZPT)

Heavy metals

- Arsenic
- Lead
- Mercury
- Thallium
- Gold

Drugs

- Chloramphenicol
- Clioquinol
- Diphenylhydantoin
- Disulfiram
- Isoniazid
- Nitrofurantoin
- Thalidomide
- Vincristine
- Vinblastine
- Ampicillin
- Erythromycin
- Tetracycline

tentials, and bizarre, high-frequency discharges may be seen on needle EMG studies. Waxy and hyaline degeneration and necrosis of muscle fibers are seen on mus-

Table 16–12
Chemical agents that may produce polymyopathy

Alcohol
Colchicine
Thiazide
Chlorthalidone
Chlorquine
Heroin
Corticosteroids

cle biopsy. Many necrotic muscle fibers may calcify. If diagnosed and treated early, an animal can have an excellent response to vitamin E therapy. Affected animals may die of involvement of cardiac muscle.

Neoplasia

Diffuse neuromuscular disease secondary to neoplasia elsewhere in the body is well described in humans, but further studies are needed in small animals.

Paraneoplastic polyneuropathy

Incidence: Rare

Neoplastic processes may release substances that alter normal neuromuscular function and produce polyneuropathy and quadriparesis in dogs.[9,87] Spinal reflexes, especially the patellar reflex, is depressed or absent. Positive waves, fibrillation potentials, and bizarre high-frequency discharges are found on EMG examination. Motor nerve conduction velocity is slow. Segmental demyelination and axonal degeneration are found on nerve biopsy examination. All dogs presented with a chronic progressive polyneuropathy (see Table 16–4) should be evaluated for a neoplastic process somewhere in the body. If the underlying cause is irradicated, the polyneuropathy may resolve.

Idiopathic

Some polyneuropathies of dogs and cats are not inflammatory and have no underlying cause that can be determined.

Distal axonopathies

Incidence: Rare

A progressive quadriparesis may occur over a few days to 3 weeks.[31,33] Spinal reflexes are absent and muscle atrophy is severe. Fibrillation potentials and bizarre high-frequency discharges are seen on the EMG examination. Motor nerve conduction velocity may be normal. Distal motor peripheral nerves show axonal degeneration. Distal axonopathies or "dying back" neuropathies may be seen in some toxicities. There may be many different causes, but usually no cause is found. Some animals recover in 4 to 6 weeks. Others never recover.

Sensory neuronopathy

Incidence: Rare

A progressive ataxia and delayed conscious proprioception has been described in dogs with a peripheral sensory neuronopathy.[32,91] The patellar reflex is usually absent. The needle EMG study may be normal. Motor nerve conduction velocity may be mildly reduced. Sensory nerve conduction may be markedly reduced or absent. Degeneration of sensory peripheral nerves or nerve roots may be found. The underlying cause is unknown.

Disorders producing episodic weakness

Myasthenia gravis and polymyositis may produce episodic weakness as well as quadriparesis and ataxia of all four limbs. Episodic weakness may also be produced by several metabolic imbalances that secondarily affect the nervous system.[37]

Congenital and familial disorders

Myasthenia gravis (congenital)

Incidence: Rare

Congenital myasthenia gravis should be considered in the differential diagnosis of a young dog with episodic weakness. The weakness becomes worse with exercise and improves with rest. Congenital myasthenia gravis is discussed earlier in this chapter.

Inflammatory–immune-mediated disorders

Polymyositis

Incidence: Occasional

Polymyositis in dogs and cats may produce weakness that worsens with exercise, improves with rest, and appears episodic. The diagnosis and management of polymyositis are discussed earlier in this chapter.

Myasthenia gravis (acquired)

Incidence: Rare

Myasthenia gravis may also be acquired because of an immune-mediated disorder of muscle endplates. Episodic weakness is a characteristic clinical finding. The diagnosis and management of acquired myasthenia gravis is also discussed earlier in this chapter.

Metabolic disorders

Disease in other systems, which secondarily affects the nervous system, must be ruled out in animals presented with episodic weakness.

Cardiopulmonary disease is a common cause of decreased exercise tolerance and weakness. Auscultation of the heart and lungs, radiographs of the chest, and electrocardiography (ECG) can be useful in the diagnosis of cardiopulmonary disease. Some spontaneous episodic arrhythmias producing episodic weakness can be difficult to diagnose, unless the animal is auscultated and an ECG is obtained during the actual period of weakness. Otherwise, the ECG may appear totally normal between the periods of arrhythmia.

Hypoglycemia is a common cause of generalized weakness that may be episodic in nature. The causes, diagnosis of, and therapy for hypoglycemia are discussed in Chapter 8.

Hypoadrenocorticism and associated hyperkalemia are common causes of generalized weakness, collapse, or episodic weakness. Blood samples should be drawn, preferably during the period of weakness.

Hypokalemia and hyperthyroidism in cats may produce episodic weakness and exercise intolerance. Hypokalemic polymyopathy is discussed earlier in this chapter. All diseases listed in Table 16–10 should be considered in cats presented with episodic weakness. Hyperkalemia may produce episodic weakness in dogs.[55]

References

1. Aronsohn, M.G., et al.: Clinical and pathologic features of thymoma in 15 dogs. J. Am. Vet. Med. Assoc., *184*:1355, 1984.
2. Barsanti, J.A.: Botulism, Tick Paralysis and Acute Polyradiculoneuritis (Coonhound Paralysis). *In* Current Veterinary Therapy VII. Edited by R.W. Kirk. Philadelphia, W.B. Saunders, 1980.
3. Blass, C.E., et al.: Recurring tetraparesis attributable to a heartworm in the epidural space of a dog. J. Am. Vet. Med. Assoc., *194*:787, 1989.
4. Braund, K.G., et al.: Hypothyroid myopathy in two dogs. Vet. Pathol., *18*:589, 1981.

5. Braund, K.G.: Clinical Syndromes in Veterinary Neurology. Baltimore, William & Wilkins, 1986.
6. Braund, K.G.: Intervertebral Disc Disease. *In* Contemporary Issues in Small Animal Practice Neurologic Disorders. Edited by J.N. Kornegay. New York, Churchill Livingstone, 1986.
7. Braund, K.G. and Ribas, J.L.: Central nervous system meningiomas. Compendium on Continuing Education, 8:24, 1986.
8. Braund, K.G.: Diseases of Peripheral Nerves, Cranial Nerves and Muscle. *In* Veterinary Neurology. Edited by J.E. Oliver, B.F. Hoerlein, and I.G. Mayhew. Philadelphia, W.B. Saunders, 1987.
9. Braund, K.G., et al.: Peripheral neuropathy associated with malignant neoplasms in dogs. Vet. Pathol., 24:16, 1987.
10. Braund, K.G., et al.: Toxoplasma polymyositis/polyneuropathy, a new clinical variant in two mature dogs. J. Am. Anim. Hosp. Assoc., 24:93, 1988.
11. Braund, K.G., et al.: Congenital hypomyelinating polyneuropathy in two Golden Retriever littermates. Vet. Pathol., 26:202, 1989.
12. Chambers, J.N., et al.: Ventral decompression for caudal cervical disk herniation in large and giant breed dogs. J. Am. Vet. Med. Assoc., 180:410, 1982.
13. Chambers, J.N., et al.: Update on ventral decompression for caudal cervical disk herniation in Doberman pinschers. J. Am. Anim. Hosp. Assoc., 22:775, 1986.
14. Child, G., et al.: Acquired scoliosis associated with hydromyelia and syringomyelia in two dogs. J. Am. Vet. Med. Assoc., 189:909, 1986.
15. Chrisman, C.L.: Clinical manifestations of multifocal peripheral nerve and muscle disorders of dogs. Compendium on Continuing Education, 7:355, 1985.
16. Chrisman, C.L.: Neuroaxonal dystrophy and leukoencephalomyelopathy of Rottweiler dogs. *In* Current Veterinary Therapy IX. Edited by R.W. Kirk. Philadelphia, W.B. Saunders, 1986.
17. Chrisman, C.L.: Diseases of peripheral nerves. *In* Textbook of Veterinary Internal Medicine. Edited by S.J. Ettinger. Philadelphia, W.B. Saunders, 1989.
18. Clemmons, R.M., et al.: Correction of organophosphate-induced neuromuscular blockade by diphenhydramine. Am J. Vet. Res., 45:2167, 1984.
19. Colter, S. and Rucker, N.C.: Acute injury to the central nervous system. Vet. Clin. North Am., 18:545, 1988.
20. Cook, J.R., and Oliver, L.E.: Atlantoaxial luxation in the dog. Compendium on Continuing Education, 3:242, 1981.
21. Cook, J.R.: Fibrocartilaginous embolism. *In* Common Neurologic Problems. Vet. Clin. North Am., 18:581, 1988.
22. Cooper, B.J., et al.: Canine inherited hypertrophic neuropathy: Clinical and electrodiagnostic studies. Am. J. Vet. Res., 45:1172, 1984.
23. Cornelissen, J.M., et al.: Type C botulism in five dogs. J. Am. Vet. Med. Assoc., 21:401, 1985.
24. Couto, C.G., et al.: Central nervous system lymphosarcoma in the dog. J. Am. Vet. Med. Assoc., 184:809, 1984.
25. Cummings, J.F., et al.: Coonhound paralysis: Further clinical studies and electron microscope observations. Acta Neuropathol. (Berl.), 56:167, 1982.
26. deLahunta, A.: Veterinary Neuroanatomy and Clinical Neurology. Philadelphia, W.B. Saunders, 1983.
27. Denny, H.R., et al.: Atlanto-axial subluxation in the dog. A review of thirty cases and evaluation of treatment by lag screw fixation. J. Small Anim. Pract., 29:37, 1988.
28. Dow, S.W., et al.: Hypokalemia in cats. 186 cases (1984–1987). J. Am. Vet. Med. Assoc., 194:1604, 1989.
29. Dow, S.W. and LeCouteur, R.A.: Hypokalemic polymyopathy of cats. *In* Current Veterinary Therapy X. Edited by R.W. Kirk. Philadelphia, W.B. Saunders, 1989.
30. Duncan, I.D. and Griffiths, I.R.: Myotonia in the dog. *In* Current Veterinary Therapy VIII. Edited by R.W. Kirk. Philadelphia, W.B. Saunders, 1983.
31. Duncan, I.D. and Griffiths, I.R.: Neuromuscular diseases. *In* Contemporary Issues in Small Animal Practice. Edited by J.N. Kornegay. New York, Churchill Livingstone, 1986.
32. Duncan, I.P. and Cudden, P.A.: Sensory

neuropathy. *In* Current Veterinary Therapy X. Edited by R.W. Kirk. Philadelphia, W.B. Saunders, 1989.

33. Dyer, K.R., et al.: Peripheral neuropathy in two dogs: Correlation between clinical, electrophysiological and pathologic findings. J. Small Anim. Pract., *27*:133, 1986.
34. Ellison, G.W., et al.: Distracted cervical spinal fusion for management of caudal cervical spondylomyelopathy in large breed dogs. J. Am. Vet. Med. Asoc., *193*:447, 1988.
35. Farnbach, G.C.: Canine myositis. *In* Current Veterinary Therapy VIII. Edited by R.W. Kirk. Philadelphia, W.B. Saunders, 1983.
36. Farrow, B.R.H. and Malik, R.: Hereditary myotonia in the Chow Chow. J. Small Anim. Pract., *22*:451, 1981.
37. Farrow, B.R.H.: Episodic weakness. *In* Current Veterinary Therapy VIII. Edited by R.W. Kirk. Philadelphia, W.B. Saunders, 1983.
38. Felts, J.R. and Prata, R.G.: Cervical disk disease in the dog: Intraforaminal and lateral extrusions. J. Am. Anim. Hosp. Assoc., *19*:755, 1983.
39. Fenner, W.R.: Meningitis. *In* Current Veterinary Therapy IX. Edited by R.W. Kirk. Philadelphia, W.B. Saunders, 1986.
40. Fingeroth, J.M., et al.: Spinal meningiomas in dogs: 13 cases (1972–1987). J. Am. Vet. Med. Assoc., *191*:720, 1987.
41. Gilmore, D.R.: Neoplasia of the cervical spinal cord and vertebrae in the dog. J. Am. Anim. Hosp. Assoc., *19*:1009, 1983.
42. Gilmore, D.R.: Cervical pain in small animals. Differential diagnosis. Compendium on Continuing Education, *5*:953, 1983.
43. Gilmore, D.R. and deLahunta, A.: Necrotizing myelopathy secondary to presumed or confirmed fibrocartilaginous embolism in 24 dogs. J. Am. Anim. Hosp. Assoc., *23*:373, 1987.
44. Greene, C.E.: Meningitis. *In* Current Veterinary Therapy VIII. Edited by R.W. Kirk. Philadelphia, W.B. Saunders, 1983.
45. Greene, C.E., et al.: Clindamycin for treatment of toxoplasma polymyositis in a dog. J. Am. Vet. Med. Assoc., *187*:631, 1985.
46. Griffiths, I.R.: Progressive axonopathy of boxer dogs. *In* Current Veterinary Ther-

apy X. Edited by R.W. Kirk. Philadelphia, W.B. Saunders, 1989.

47. Harcourt, R.A.: Polyarteritis in a colony of beagles. Vet. Rec., *102*:519, 1978.
48. Haupt, K.H., et al.: Familial canine dermatomyositis: Clinicopathologic, immunologic and serologic studies. Am. J. Vet. Res., *46*:1870, 1985.
49. Hoerlein, B.F.: Intervertebral disc disease. *In* Veterinary Neurology. Edited by J.E. Oliver, B.F. Hoerlein, and I.G. Mayhew. Philadelphia, W.B. Saunders, 1987.
50. Hurov, L., et al.: Diskospondylitis in the dog: 27 cases. J. Am. Vet. Med. Assoc., *173*:275, 1981.
51. Ilkiw, J.E.: Tick paralysis in Australia. *In* Current Veterinary Therapy VIII. Edited by R.W. Kirk. Philadelphia, W.B. Saunders, 1983.
52. Indrieri, R.J., et al.: Myasthenia gravis in two cats. J. Am. Vet. Med. Assoc., *182*:57, 1983.
53. Indrieri, R.J., et al.: Neuromuscular abnormalities associated with hypothyroidism and lymphocytic thyroiditis in three dogs. J. Am. Vet. Med. Assoc., *190*:544, 1987.
54. Janssens, L.A.: Treatment of canine cervical disc disease by acupuncture. A review of thirty two cases. J. Small Anim. Pract., *26*:203, 1986.
55. Jezyk, P.F.: Hyperkalemic periodic paralysis in a dog. J. Am. Anim. Hosp. Assoc., *18*:997, 1982.
56. Johnson, R.G., Prata, R.G.: Intradiskal osteomyelitis: A Conservative approach. J. Am. Anim. Hosp. Assoc., *19*:743, 1983.
57. Kornegay, J.N.: Golden Retriever Myopathy. *In* Current Veterinary Therapy IX. Edited by R.W. Kirk. Philadelphia, W.B. Saunders, 1986.
58. Kornegay, J.N.: Diskospondylitis. *In* Current Veterinary Therapy IX. Edited by R.W. Kirk. Philadelphia, W.B. Saunders, 1986.
59. Kramek, B.A., et al.: Neuropathy associated with diabetes mellitus in the cat. J. Am. Vet. Med. Assoc., *186*:42, 1984.
60. Kunkle, G.A., et al.: Dermatomyositis in Collie dogs. Compendium on Continuing Education, *7*:185, 1985.

61. Lane, J.R. and deLahunta, A.: Polyneuritis in a cat. J. Am. Anim. Hosp. Assoc., 20:1006, 1984.
62. LeCouteur, R.A., et al.: Stabilization of atlantoaxial subluxation in the dog. J. Am. Vet. Med. Assoc., 177:1011, 1980.
63. Lincoln, J.D., Pettit, G.D.: Evaluation of fenestration for treatment of degenerative disc disease in the caudal cervical region of large dogs. Vet. Surg., 14:240, 1985.
64. Luttgen, P.J., et al.: A retrospective study of twenty nine spinal tumors in the dog and cat. J. Small Anim. Pract., 21:213, 1980.
65. McKerrell, R.F. and Braund, K.G.: Hereditary myopathy in Labrador Retrievers: Clinical variations. J. Small Anim. Pract., 28:479, 1987.
66. McKerrell, R.E. and Braund, K.G.: Hereditary myopathy of labrador retrievers. In Current Veterinary Therapy C. Edited by R.W. Kirk. Philadelphia, W.B. Saunders, 1989.
67. Meerdink, G.L.: Bites and stings of venomous animals. In Current Veterinary Therapy VIII. Philadelphia, W.B. Saunders, 1983.
68. Meric, S.M., et al.: Corticosteroid responsive meningitis in ten dogs. J. Am. Anim. Hosp. Assoc., 2:677, 1985.
69. Meric, S.M.: Necrotizing vasculitis of the spinal pachyleptomeningeal arteries in three Bernese mountain dog littermates. J. Am. Anim. Hosp. Assoc., 22:459, 1986.
70. Meric, S.M.: Canine meningitis, a changing emphasis. J. Vet. Intern. Med., 2:26, 1988.
71. Miller, I.M., et al.: Congenital myasthenia gravis in 13 Smooth Fox Terriers. J. Am. Vet. Med. Assoc., 182:694, 1983.
72. Morgan, J.P., et al.: Vertebral tumors in the dog. Clinical, radiographic and pathologic study of 61 primary and secondary lesions. Vet. Radiol., 21:197, 1980.
73. Oda, K., et al.: Congenital canine myasthenia gravis. I. Deficient junctional acetylcholine receptors. Muscle Nerve, 7:705, 1984.
74. Palmer, A.C. and Blakemore, W.F.: A progressive neuropathy in the young Cairn terrier. J. Small Anim. Pract., 30:101, 1989.
75. Penwick, R.C.: Fibrocartilaginous embolism and ischemic myelopathy. Compendium on Continuing Education, 3:287, 1989.
76. Prata, R.G.: Cervical and thoracolumbar disc disease in the dog. In Current Veterinary Therapy VIII. Edited by R.W. Kirk. Philadelphia, W.B. Saunders, 1983.
77. Presthus, J. and Lindboe, C.F.: Polymyositis in two German wirehaired pointer littermates. J. Small Anim. Pract., 29:239, 1988.
78. Randell, M.G. and Hurvitz, A.I.: Immune-mediated vasculitis in five dogs. J. Am. Vet. Med. Assoc., 183:207, 1983.
79. Read, R.A., et al.: Caudal cervical spondylomyelopathy (Wobbler syndrome) in the dog: A review of thirty cases. J. Small Anim. Pract., 24:605, 1983.
80. Seim, H.B. and Withrow, S.J.: Pathophysiology and diagnosis of caudal cervical spondylomyelopathy with emphasis on the Doberman pinscher. J. Am. Anim. Hosp. Assoc., 18:241, 1982.
81. Seim, H.B.: Wobbler Syndrome in the Doberman Pinscher. In Current Veterinary Therapy X. Edited by R.W. Kirk. Philadelphia, W.B. Saunders, 1989.
82. Shell, L.G., et al.: Spinal muscular atrophy in two Rottweiler littermates. J. Am. Vet. Med. Assoc., 190:878. 1987.
83. Shelton, G.D. and Cardinet, G.H.: Pathophysiologic basis of canine muscle disorders. J. Vet. Intern. Med., 1:36, 1987.
84. Shores, A.: Canine cervical vertebral malformation/malarticulation syndrome. Compendium on Continuing Education, 6:326, 1984.
85. Shores, A. and Braund, K.G.: Chronic relapsing polyneuropathy in a cat. J. Am. Anim. Hosp. Assoc., 23:569, 1987.
86. Smith, G.K. and Walton, M.C.: Fractures and luxations of the spine. In Textbook of Small Animal Orthopedics. Edited by C.D. Newton and D.M. Nunmaker. Philadelphia, J.B. Lippincott, 1985.
87. Sorjonen, D.C., et al.: Paraplegia and subclinical neuromyopathy associated with a primary lung tumor in a dog. J. Am. Vet. Med. Assoc., 180:1209, 1982.
88. Sorjonen, D.C.: Vertebral and spinal cord surgery, small animal cervical surgery. In

Veterinary Neurology. Edited by J.E. Oliver, B.F. Hoerlein, and I.G. Mayhew. Philadelphia, W.B. Saunders, 1987.

89. Sorjonen, D.C. and Vaughn, D.M.: Membrane interactions in central nervous system injury. Compendium on Continuing Education, 3:248, 1989.

90. Steiss, J.E., et al.: Electrodiagnostic analysis of a peripheral neuropathy in dogs with diabetes mellitus. Am. J. Vet. Res., 42:2061, 1982.

91. Steiss, J.E.: Sensory neuronopathy in a dog. J. Am. Vet. Med. Assoc., 190:205, 1987.

92. Stone, E.A., Betts, C.W., and Chambers, J.N.: Cervical fractures in the dog. J. Am. Anim. Hosp. Assoc., 15:463, 1979.

93. Tomlinson, J. and Schwink, K.L.: Surgical approaches to the spine. In Textbook of Small Animal Surgery. Vol 1, Edited by D.H. Slatter. Philadelphia, W.B. Saunders, 1985.

94. Trotter, E.J.: Canine wobbler syndrome. In Current Veterinary Therapy IX. Edited by R.W. Kirk. Philadelphia, W.B. Saunders, 1986.

95. Vandevelde, M. And Braund, K.G.: Polioencephalomyelitis in cats. Vet. Pathol., 16:420, 1979.

96. Van Gundy, T.E.: Disc-associated wobbler syndrome in the Doberman Pinscher. In Common Neurologic Problems. Vet. Clin. North Am., 18:667, 1988.

97. Van Gundy, T.E.: Canine wobbler syndrome. Part II. Treatment. Compendium on Continuing Education, 3:269, 1989.

98. Van Nes, J.J., et al.: Electrophysiologic evidence of peripheral nerve dysfunction in 6 dogs with botulism C. Res. Vet. Sci., 40:372, 1986.

99. Waldron, D., et al.: Progressive ossifying myositis in a cat. J. Am. Vet. Med. Assoc., 187:64, 1985.

100. Walvoovt, H.C., et al.: Canine glycogen storage disease type II: A clinical study of four affected lapland dogs. J. Am. Anim. Hosp. Assoc., 20:279, 1984.

101. Watson, A.G., et al.: Congenital occipitoatlantoaxial malformation in a cat. Compendium on Continuing Education, 7:245, 1985.

Chapter 17

Paraplegia, paraparesis, and ataxia of the pelvic limbs

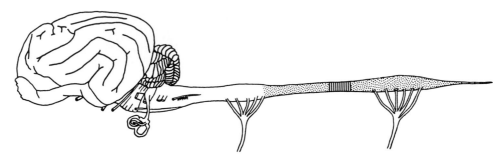

Figure 17–1. Location of lesions that will produce paraplegia, paraparesis, or ataxia of the pelvic limbs are either a focal thoracolumbar spinal cord lesion (vertical lines) or a diffuse or multifocal thoracolumbar spinal cord lesion (dots).

Location of the lesion (Figure 17–1): *focal, multifocal, or diffuse thoracolumbar spinal cord*

Mechanisms of disease and differential diagnosis

Congenital and familial disorders

Lysosomal storage diseases (Chap. 7)
Afghan myelopathy (Chap. 16)
Spinal dysraphia
Demyelination of Miniature Poodles
Miscellaneous meningeal and spinal cord
  malformations
Thoracolumbar vertebral malformations
Multiple cartilaginous exostoses (Chap. 16)

Infections and other inflammations

Meningomyelitis or myelitis—bacterial, viral,
  protozoal, fungal, and parasitic (Chap. 16)
Discospondylitis (Chap. 16)
Spondylitis
Granulomatous meningoencephalitis (reticulosis)
Corticosteroid-responsive meningoencephalitis

Trauma

Spinal cord and vertebral injury
Intervertebral disc disease

Vascular disorders

Fibrocartilaginous infarct (Chap. 16)
Spontaneous spinal cord hemorrhage (Chap. 16)
Vascular malformations (Chap. 16)
Ischemic neuromyopathy—aortic embolism

Degeneration

Degenerative myelopathy of German Shepherds
Spondylosis deformans
Dural ossification
Intervertebral disc disease

Neoplasia (Chap. 16)

Extramedullary spinal cord tumors
Neurinoma,
Neurofibroma,
Neurofibrosarcoma
Meningioma
Meningeal sarcomatosis
Intramedullary spinal cord tumors
Astrocytoma
Ependymoma
Glioma
Reticulosis
Metastatic spinal cord tumors
Vertebral neoplasia

Chapter 17

Paraplegia, paraparesis, and ataxia of the pelvic limbs

When paraplegia, paraparesis, or ataxia of the pelvic limbs is unaccompanied by signs associated with disease above the foramen magnum or disease of the cervical spinal cord (Chaps. 7 through 16), a focal, multifocal, or diffuse thoracolumbar spinal cord disease is the likely cause (Fig. 17–1).

As in the cervical region, a focal thoracolumbar extramedullary spinal cord mass, such as a protruded or herniated intervertebral disc, produces signs that vary with the spinal cord pathways involved. If the extramedullary mass only irritates the meninges and dorsal root and causes little spinal cord compression, the main sign is back pain with little neurologic deficit.

Mild compression of the spinal cord from T2 to L3 distorts the spinocerebellar tracts in the lateral funiculus, alters their blood supply, and results in ataxia of the pelvic limbs. Involvement of the dorsolateral funiculus of the spinal cord may decrease conscious proprioception. When the reticulospinal and vestibulospinal tracts in the ventral funiculus become involved, the animal has difficulty supporting weight, but continues to have voluntary movements. When the rubrospinal, corticospinal, and reticulospinal tracts, which lie deep to spinocerebellar tracts in the lateral funiculus, become involved there is little or no voluntary movement.

Paraparesis is weakness with some voluntary movement still present. Paraplegia is the loss of voluntary movement. At this stage, superficial sensation is usually lost because the large myelinated fibers that carry superficial sensation are more susceptible to the effects of distortion and compression than the small nonmyelinated fibers that carry deep pain.

Deep pain is usually the last modality to be affected in spinal cord compression. When deep pain is lost, a severe bilateral spinal cord lesion is thought to be present. The ascending and descending spinal cord pathways are discussed in Chapters 1 and 16.

No nerve roots from T2 to L3 spinal cord segments contribute to the sensory and motor supply of the pelvic limbs and tail. In the dog, the spinal cord segments from the fourth lumbar (L4) segments through all the caudal segments are housed in vertebrae L3 to L6 (Fig. 17–2). The nerve roots from the various segments, however, continue caudally and exit after the vertebra of the same number (Fig. 17–2). Therefore, below L6 the vertebral canal contains no spinal cord, only nerve roots L7 to Cd, referred to as the cauda equina.

When extradural masses compress the spinal cord and nerve roots below L3, the weakness and alterations of sensation are not from involvement of spinal cord tracts alone, but are also caused by involvement of dorsal (sensory) and ventral (motor) nerve roots that supply the pelvic limbs, anus, bladder, and tail. The lesion may be localized to the region above or below L3 by the alterations in spinal reflexes seen on the neurologic examination, which is discussed later in this section. Even mild compressive lesions below L3 spinal cord segments often depress reflexes in pelvic limbs, anus, or tail.

In the cat, the spinal cord continues through the vertebral canal to the sacrum, and the nerve roots of each segment exit after the vertebra of the same number, so that a focal compressive lesion may not affect as many spinal cord segments and nerve roots at one time as it can in the dog.

Patient evaluation

Signalment and history

As with all problems of the nervous system, the history aids greatly in determining the mechanism of the disease process (Chap. 2). Young animals with paraplegia, paraparesis, and ataxia of the pelvic limbs are likely to have congenital spinal cord and vertebral abnormalities, myelitis, and spinal cord or vertebral trauma. Old dogs are likely to have degenerative and neoplastic processes.

Many breeds of dogs commonly have specific neurologic disorders (see Table 2–2). Afghans have a myelopathy that begins with pelvic limb weakness. Weimaraners have spinal dysraphia. West Highland White terriers and Cairn terriers have globoid cell leukodystrophy that begins with pelvic limb weakness. Dachshunds, Beagles, Cocker spaniels, and several other breeds commonly have degenerative intervertebral disc disease of the thoracolumbar vertebral column. Great Danes and other large breeds of dogs may have fibrocartilaginous embolization of the thoracolumbar spinal cord. German Shepherds over 5 years of age commonly have degenerative myelopathy. Boxers have spinal cord tumors.

The course and progression of the disease process may be characteristic for a certain mechanism of disease. Acute nonprogressive paraplegia is commonly associated with trauma, intervertebral (IV) disc herniation, and fibrocartilaginous infarction of the spinal cord, spontaneous spinal cord hemorrhage, or iliac artery thrombosis (Table 17–1).

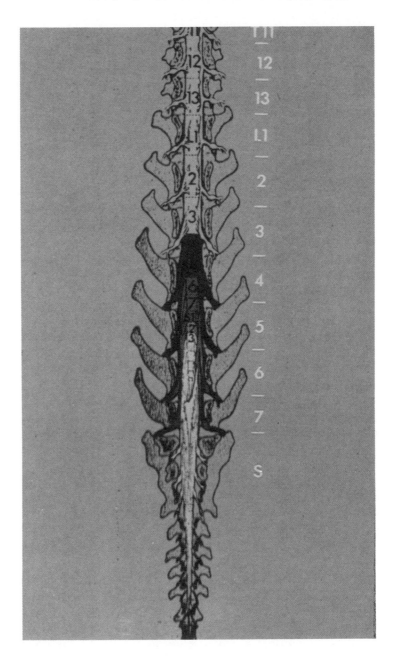

Figure 17–2. The relationship of spinal cord segments and nerve roots to vertebrae in the dog. Note: L4 to L5 are the spinal cord segments for the patellar reflex; L6 to S2 are the spinal cord segments for the gastrocnemius and cranial tibial muscle responses and the flexor reflex; and S1 to S3 are the spinal cord segments for the anal reflex. Only nerve roots are in the spinal canal after the L6 vertebra and they are referred to as the cauda equina. (After Miller, 1964)

A chronic progressive paresis of the pelvic limbs is seen in degenerative myelopathy, type II intervertebral disc protrusion, and spinal cord tumors (Table 17–2).

A progressive paresis of the pelvic limbs that over a few weeks produces paresis of the thoracic limbs could be caused by a focal cervical lesion in which the mild thoracic limb signs were overlooked. It could also be caused by a multifocal or diffuse spinal cord problem such as a ly-

Table 17-1
Common disorders producing acute paraparesis and paraplegia in dogs and cats over 1 year of age

1. IV disc herniation
2. Spinal cord trauma
3. Meningomyelitis
4. Fibrocartilaginous infarct (rare cats)
5. Aortic thromboembolism (rare dogs)

Table 17-3
Common disorders producing acute thoracolumbar vertebral column pain in dogs and cats over 1 year of age

1. IV disc protrusion/herniation
2. Discospondylitis
3. Fractured vertebra
4. Meningitis
5. Meningioma, neurofibrosarcoma, or lymphosarcoma
6. Vertebral neoplasia

sosomal storage disorder, Afghan myelopathy, discospondylitis, myelitis, or a diffuse neuromuscular disorder (Chap. 16). Polyneuropathies may produce more severe signs in the pelvic limbs than in the thoracic limbs.

Back pain is usually indicated in the history when the animal refuses to go up and down stairs and no longer sits up and begs for food or jumps on and off furniture. Sometimes the animal also becomes reluctant to move, and cries out when the owner lifts it. If back pain is a complaint, discospondylitis, meningitis, intervertebral disc protrusion, vertebral injury, or extramedullary spinal cord, nerve root, or vertebral tumor might be considered for the differential diagnosis (Table 17–3).

A history of concurrent systemic illness or signs of involvement above the foramen magnum may support a multifocal disease process such as infection, other inflam-

mations, trauma, metabolic disorder, or toxicity. Many metabolic and toxic disorders that produce behavior alterations or seizures may also produce some pelvic limb weakness.

Physical and neurologic examinations

The physical examination findings may provide information to support the diagnosis of an infection, other inflammations, metabolic or toxic disorder, trauma, or metastatic neoplasia as a mechanism for the paraplegia, paraparesis, or ataxia of the pelvic limbs (Chap. 3).

The neurologic examination is used to rule out disease in the nervous system above T2, to localize the lesion within the thoracolumbar spinal cord, and to determine the severity of spinal cord and nerve root involvement. The neurologic examination is discussed in Chapter 3. The head and thoracic limbs should be thoroughly evaluated, and if considered normal, the lesion is most likely below T2 spinal cord segments and vertebrae. The spinal reflexes are useful to further localize the lesion to specific segments. The spinal reflexes are normal or hyperactive in focal spinal cord lesions from T2 to L3. Lesions below L3 may depress or abolish the spinal reflexes of the pelvic limbs or anus. Table

Table 17-2
Common disorders producing chronic progressive paraparesis in dogs and cats over 5 years of age

1. IV disc protrusion
2. Degenerative myelopathy (German Shepherds)
3. Myelitis/meningomyelitis
4. Spinal cord neoplasia

17–4 outlines the spinal reflexes of the pelvic limbs and anus, the nerve roots, and spinal cord segments they travel through, and the vertebral level in the dog that could alter the reflex.

Superficial sensation can also be helpful in localizing the lesion. An area that is hyperesthetic to light pin-pricking or an area that is painful on palpation can localize a lesion to that site Fig. 17–3. In a paraplegic animal pinching the skin with hemostat forceps and observing for a behavioral response or the cutaneous trunci (panniculus) response may produce no response from the cranial extent of the lesion caudally. This is called the sensory level (Fig. 17–4).

In acute spinal cord trauma from external injuries or intervertebral disc herniations, ascending and descending myelomalacia may occur and have a grave prognosis, and is discussed later in this chapter. A dog with ascending and descending myelomalacia may for example have a loss of spinal reflexes of the pelvic limbs, which suggests a lesion below L3, and a sensory level at T8, which suggests the cranial aspect of the lesion is around T8. The sensory level may be monitored and may continue rostrally through the thoracic segments as the myelomalacia ascends.

In acute trauma to the spinal cord at T2 to L3, *the Schiff-Sherrington syndrome* may occur. The pelvic limbs are paralyzed and the thoracic limbs have extensor rigidity. If severe, the animal may be in lateral recumbency with the thoracic limbs extended. The vertebral column should be manipulated as little as possible until radiography has been used to rule out unstable fractured vertebrae, because the *Schiff-Sherrington syndrome* is most commonly associated with trauma. Once vertebral fracture or instability is ruled out, the animal may be examined further. When held in the proper position, the animal may wheelbarrow and place and hop on the thoracic limbs, although the increase in extensor tone may inhibit the normal range of flexion.

The pelvic limbs are usually paralyzed. If no spinal reflexes are present immediately following the paralysis, spinal shock is likely. Spinal shock often lasts only 1 to 3 hours. After that time, the spinal reflexes return and are most likely hyperactive. It takes a severe insult to the spinal cord to produce spinal shock; therefore, the prognosis is often grave in these animals, but serial neurologic examinations should be performed over several days to give an accurate prognosis. The prognosis is better for an animal that has *Schiff-Sherrington syndrome* with normal or hyperactive spinal reflexes in the pelvic limbs and preserved

Table 17–4

Lesions of spinal cord segments, nerve roots, or vertebrae that can depress or abolish spinal reflexes in the dog

Spinal reflex	Spinal cord segments and nerve roots	Vertebrae
Patellar reflex	L4 to 5	L3 to L5
Gastrocnemius	L6 to S2	L4 to sacrum
Cranial tibial	L6 to S2	L4 to sacrum
Flexor reflex	L6 to S2	L4 to sacrum
Anal reflex	S1 to S3	L5 to sacrum
Tail	Cd1 to Cd5	L6 to sacrum

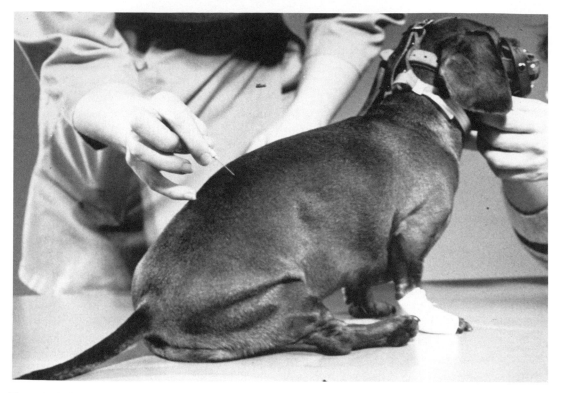

Figure 17–3. An excessive cutaneous trunci (panniculus) or behavioral response to light pin pricking can mean the area is hyperesthetic. The thoracolumbar junction is slightly more responsive than the rest of the region from T1–L6. The cutaneous trunci (panniculus) response is normally lost around the L4–5 region.

deep pain. A normal cutaneous trunci (panniculus) response also indicates that the spinal cord white matter is intact between the site tested and T2.

The *Schiff-Sherrington syndrome* is thought to occur because of the release of ascending inhibition on the extensors of the thoracic limbs from the lumbar spinal cord. These impulses pass through the fasciculus proprius or propriospinal tract, which is a tract surrounding the gray matter deep in the spinal cord and is affected only by acute deep spinal cord lesions.

In any acute spinal cord insult, deep pain may be lost for the first 24 to 72 hours, but its continued absence after that period in an animal that does not appear to be in pain from the lesion indicates that the prognosis is grave, although not hopeless in every case. If deep pain remains absent from the toes of the pelvic limbs 30 days after the insult, the prognosis for recovery from paraplegia is hopeless (Fig. 17–5).

If S1 to S3 spinal cord segments or nerve roots are affected, the bladder has no reflex emptying (Chap. 19). It enlarges, overflows, and dribbles urine. The bladder in these cases is easy to express. Lesions above S1 spinal cord segments and nerve roots may produce a reflex bladder that spurts out urine whenever the animal is handled or when the bladder fills to a certain size (Chap. 19). The bladder in lesions above S1 may be more difficult to express initially until reflex contraction occurs.

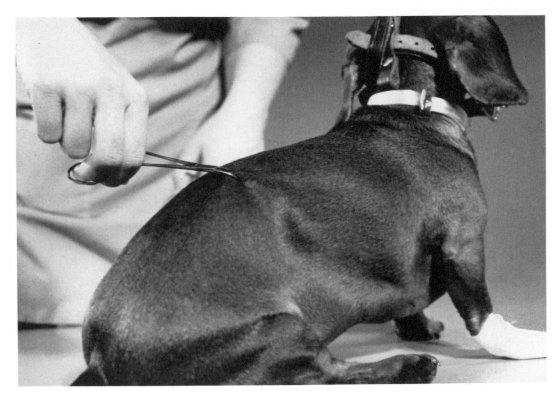

Figure 17–4. A loss of panniculus or behavioral response to hemostat forceps clamping on the skin indicates the sensory level or rostral aspect of a lesion. Asymmetry between left and right paravertebral regions may be helpful to determine which side is most affected.

Ancillary diagnostic investigations

As discussed in Chapter 5, initial clinico-pathologic tests are useful in detecting infections, other inflammations, metabolic disorders, and toxicities and disease in any other body systems that might be life-threatening. A urinalysis should be obtained on all paraplegic animals, as cystitis is common and should be treated to prevent an ascending infection and pyelonephritis. If the animal is stable in other systems, it is anesthetized for EMG, CSF collection and analysis, routine vertebral radiographs, and myelography, if needed.

Needle EMG examination of paraspinal muscles can be useful for localization of the lesion to certain segments. If nerve roots L4 to Cd are involved, EMG abnormalities may be found in pelvic limb muscles, the anal sphincter, or the tail.

Lumbar cerebrospinal fluid should be collected and analyzed. Infections and inflammations such as myelitis and discospondylitis may increase cells and protein in the CSF. Xanthochromia may be found following hemorrhage. Intervertebral disc protrusion, spinal cord or nerve root tumors, and degenerative myelopathy usually have increased protein with no increase in cells. In some cases of spinal cord tumors or intervertebral disc herniation, a mild pleocytosis may occur. The CSF collected at the cisterna magna is often normal or shows less change than lumbar CSF in thoracolumbar spinal cord disease.

Routine vertebral radiographs are useful for the diagnosis of vertebral mal-

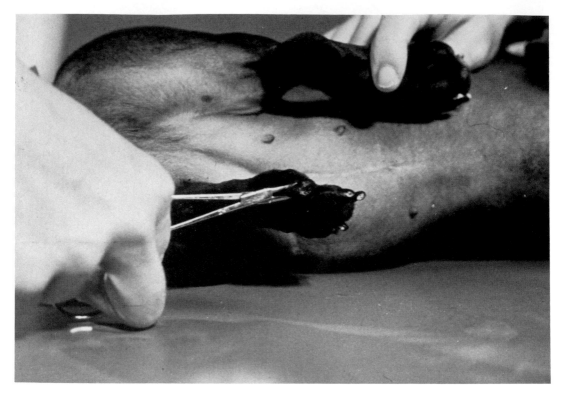

Figure 17–5. Deep pain is tested by clamping hemostatic forceps on the digits and observing a behavioral response such as crying or aggression. Deep pain is declared absent when there is no response from all digits and the tail.

formations, discospondylitis, vertebral fractures, intervertebral disc disease, spondylosis deformans, dural ossification, and vertebral neoplasia. If a focal spinal cord disorder is suspected and the CSF has no increase in cells, a myelogram may be indicated. Spinal cord and meningeal malformations, spinal cord swelling from an intramedullary tumor, edema, hemorrhage, or infarction, and spinal cord compression from an intervertebral disc or extramedullary tumor may be visualized using myelography. Computerized axial tomography and magnetic resonance imaging scans may be used to visualize lesions as well.

Once a focal spinal cord lesion such as a tumor is localized, an exploratory laminectomy should be performed to deter-mine whether or not the mass is removable.

The approach to the evaluation of an animal with paraplegia is outlined in Table 17–5.

Congenital and familial disorders

Lysosomal storage disorders— globoid cell leukodystrophy

Incidence: Rare

GM$_1$ gangliosidosis, sphingomyelinosis, glucocerebrosidosis, and globoid cell leukodystrophy produce pelvic limb ataxia early in the course of disease; but globoid

Table 17-5
Diagnostic approach for the evaluation of paraplegia, paraparesis, and ataxia of the pelvic limbs

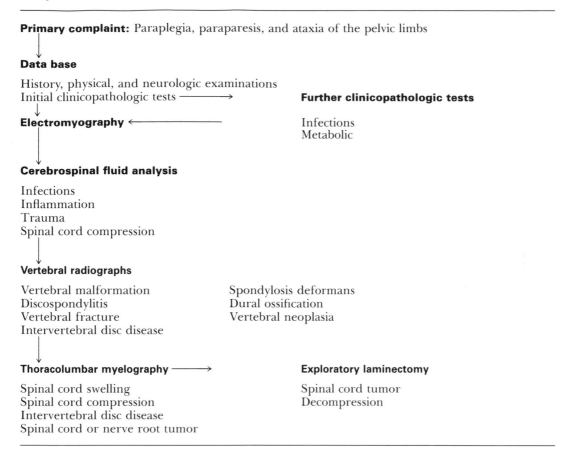

Primary complaint: Paraplegia, paraparesis, and ataxia of the pelvic limbs

↓

Data base

History, physical, and neurologic examinations
Initial clinicopathologic tests ⟶   **Further clinicopathologic tests**

↓

Electromyography ⟵   Infections
                                            Metabolic

↓

Cerebrospinal fluid analysis

Infections
Inflammation
Trauma
Spinal cord compression

↓

Vertebral radiographs

Vertebral malformation   Spondylosis deformans
Discospondylitis   Dural ossification
Vertebral fracture   Vertebral neoplasia
Intervertebral disc disease

↓

Thoracolumbar myelography ⟶   **Exploratory laminectomy**

Spinal cord swelling   Spinal cord tumor
Spinal cord compression   Decompression
Intervertebral disc disease
Spinal cord or nerve root tumor

cell leukodystrophy may initially have only signs related to the pelvic limb weakness, whereas the others often also have head tremors.[1,11] Mucopolysaccharidosis may produce chronic progressive paraparesis in Siamese and other cats.[16]

Signalment and history. Globoid cell leukodystrophy may begin with ataxia or paresis of the pelvic limbs, and has been reported in West Highland White terriers, Cairn terriers, Beagles, Bassetts, Blue Tick Hounds, Poodles, and cats 6 to 12 months of age. There may be no history of asso-

ciated illness. Other litter mates may or may not be affected. The weakness progresses to involve the thoracic limbs.

Physical and neurologic examinations. The animal with pelvic limb signs only may have ataxia, dysmetria, conscious proprioceptive deficits, and weakness. Spinal reflexes may be normal or hyperactive if the myelin of the spinal cord is primarily affected. Later in the course of the disease, peripheral myelin may be affected and the spinal reflexes may be depressed, associated with the peripheral neuropathy (Chap. 16).

Ancillary diagnostic investigations. Initial clinicopathologic tests are normal. Other congenital and familial disorders and myelitis associated with distemper virus infections should be considered.

Large macrophages filled with myelin (globoid cells) may be seen on lumbar CSF analysis, and protein will be elevated.

Definitive diagnosis antemortem can be made by analysis of leukocytes for β-galactocerebrosidase levels. Globoid cells may be seen on examination of tissues from a lymph node biopsy on an affected dog. If peripheral nerves are affected, a peripheral nerve biopsy and examination can be used to support the diagnosis.

Therapy and prognosis. There is no therapy, and the prognosis at present is hopeless.

Pathology. Large phagocytic cells with foamy-appearing cytoplasm called globoid cells are found along blood vessels throughout areas of affected white matter in the CNS. The globoid cells contain non-metachromatic, nonsudanophilic and PAS-positive material.

Prevention. Globoid cell leukodystrophy appears to have an autosomal recessive inheritance. Carrier animals can be detected by assay of leukocytes for β-galactocerebrosidase. The enzyme level is intermediate between affected and normal dogs. Carrier dogs then are culled from future breeding programs.

Afghan myelopathy

Incidence: Occasional

A familial myelopathy of Afghan hounds begins as pelvic limb ataxia and weakness and progresses to quadriparesis. The clinical course and diagnosis of this myelopathy is discussed in Chapter 16.

Spinal dysraphia

Incidence: Occasional in Weimaraners; rare in other breeds

Spinal dysraphia is a malformation of the spinal cord caused by arrested development before complete differentiation of gray and white matter has occurred.

Signalment and history. Spinal dysraphia is seen primarily in Weimaraners, but has been reported sporadically in a few other breeds of dogs as well as in cats.[1,11,24] The neurologic deficit is most obvious when the affected animals begin to walk at 3 to 4 weeks of age. The complaint is often that the animal hops like a rabbit, using the pelvic limbs together. There is no progression or regression of signs.

Physical and neurologic examinations. The neurologic examination findings may vary greatly in severity. The head and thoracic limbs are normal. Mild cases may show little deficit when walking slowly, but when the pace increases to a trot, the pelvic limbs are no longer used separately but are simultaneously flexed and extended. More severely affected animals have a crouched posture, conscious proprioceptive deficits, can only flex and extend the pelvic limbs simultaneously, and may fall to either side. The flexor reflex is bilateral, and when initiated on one side, both limbs flex together. The scratch reflex induced on one side will also cause the limbs on both sides to scratch.

Shortly after birth, affected puppies can be detected by observing simultaneous flexion and extension of the pelvic limbs as they crawl and by the presence of a bilateral flexor reflex.

Ancillary diagnostic investigations. Ancillary diagnostic investigations including EMG, CSF, spinal radiographs, and myelography are often normal. Diagnosis is based on the signalment, history, and characteristic gait and lack of other findings.

Therapy and prognosis. There is no therapy and the dog will not improve. If mildly affected, the animal may make an acceptable pet.

Pathology. A variety of microscopic lesions that may be seen with spinal dysraphia occur primarily in the thoracic spinal cord and become more obvious as the dog ages, even when the neurologic deficit does not progress. Anomalies of the dorsal septum and central canal are seen. Hydromyelia, syringomyelia, and duplication or absence of the central canal can occur. Anomalies of the dorsal gray horns and the ventral median fissure are reported.

Prevention. Spinal dysraphism appears to be an inherited disorder in Weimaraners.

Demyelination of miniature poodles

Incidence: Rare

Miniature Poodles between 2 and 4 months of age may develop a pelvic limb weakness that progresses to paraplegia and later quadriplegia. Spinal reflexes are hyperactive and sensation is normal. No cranial nerve deficits or evidence of cerebral disease are found. The lesions are restricted to white matter and consist of diffuse demyelination and sparing of axons in all funiculi of the spinal cord. A hereditary disorder is suspected.

Miscellaneous meningeal and spinal cord malformations

Spinal dysraphia, myeloceles, meningomyeloceles, and meningoceles are all congenital abnormalities of the spinal cord and meninges that may be associated with vertebral spina bifida in dogs and cats.

Spina bifida is a defect in the closure of the dorsal lamina of the vertebrae. A meningocele is a protrusion of a meningeal pouch containing CSF. A meningomyelocele is a protrusion of a pouch of meninges containing spinal cord and nerve roots. In Bulldogs and Manx cats, spina bifida, sacrocaudal agenesis, and meningomyelocele may produce flaccid pelvic limb paresis or paralysis with a dilated anus, drooped tail, and flaccid paralysis of the bladder (Chap. 19). The vertebral defect can be seen radiographically, but the animal is abnormal from the underlying spinal cord malformations.

Spina bifida can also occur in thoracic vertebrae. If only a meningocele is present, the animal may not have neurologic deficit, but the meningocele may make the portion of the spinal cord more susceptible to injury. Myelography may be useful in outlining the meningocele (Fig. 17–6). No reports of surgical therapy are in the veterinary literature.

Acquired scoliosis may be associated with syringomyelia in the dog.[5]

Thoracolumbar vertebral malformations

Incidence: Occasional

Spina bifida occulta is a vertebral malformation with no associated anomaly of the meninges or spinal cord and usually no neurologic deficit.

Many other vertebral malformations may be found on radiographic evaluation of the vertebral column that have no underlying spinal cord disease or neurologic deficit associated with them. Fusion of two or more vertebrae, called block vertebrae, may occur. Vertebral abnormalities at the cervicothoracic, thoracolumbar, lumbosacral, and sacrocaudal junctions include cervical ribs, lumbarization of T13 to L1, sacralization of L7, and fusion of S3 and Cd1. The total number of vertebrae may vary from the normal amount.

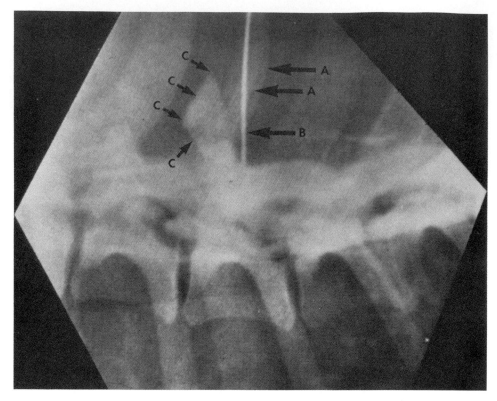

Figure 17–6. Spina bifida of a thoracic vertebra with a meningocele filled with contrast media. The double dorsal spinous processes of the vertebrae are indicated by (A). (B) is the spinal needle inserted between the two vertebral spinous processes used to inject the contrast media. (C) is the meningocele outlined by the contrast media.

Hemivertebra. Hemivertebra, also called butterfly vertebra, is a congenital vertebral malformation produced by a failure of fusion of the left and right ossification centers of the vertebral bodies.[11,24] Scoliosis of the spine may be seen. Hemivertebra is common in Boston terriers and English Bulldogs and is seen occasionally in other breeds. It may have no associated neurologic deficit or may produce ataxia of the pelvic limbs, paraparesis, or paraplegia, depending on the degree of spinal cord compression. The neurologic deficit begins in the young dog and progresses slowly as the animal grows. The vertebral deformity may be seen on plain vertebral radiographs (Fig 17–7) but myelography may be needed to demonstrate the degree of spinal cord compression. Surgical de-compression and stabilization improves the neurologic deficit if performed early.

Miscellaneous vertebral malformations. Congenital stenosis of the vertebral canal unassociated with hemivertebra is seen in English Bulldogs. Myelography is needed to outline the spinal cord compression. Decompression of the spinal cord may improve the neurologic deficit.

Lumbosacral malformations and malarticulations are described in dogs, but usually only cause a drooped tail, dysuria, and fecal incontinence (Chap. 19).

Multiple cartilaginous exostoses

Multiple cartilaginous exostoses are multiple, partially ossified protuberances aris-

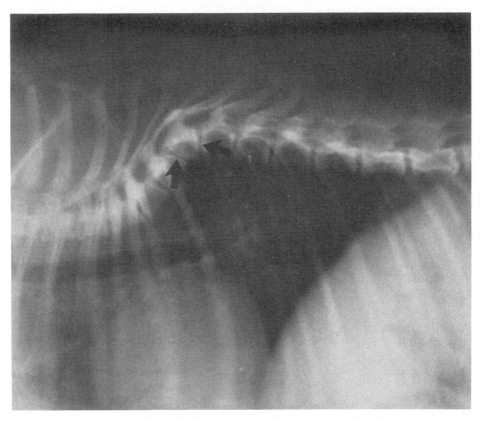

Figure 17–7. A lateral plain radiograph of the thoracic vertebral column showing a hemivertebra (arrows) that is not producing a neurologic deficit in this dog.

ing from the cortex of bones in dogs and cats.[11] If an exostosis from a thoracic or lumbar vertebra protrudes into the spinal canal, spinal cord compression and pelvic limb paresis or paralysis may occur. Surgical decompression of the spinal cord may improve the neurologic deficit. The diagnosis of multiple cartilaginous exostoses is discussed in Chapter 16.

Infections and other inflammations

Meningomyelitis or myelitis

Incidence: Frequent

A common cause of myelitis and paresis or paraplegia of the pelvic limbs in dogs is canine distemper virus infection.[11,24] The diagnosis of and prognosis for distemper infections are discussed in Chapters 7 and 16. Other forms of myelitis, rare in comparison with distemper infections, are also discussed in Chapter 16.

Toxoplasmosis may produce paraplegia in young dogs owing to a radiculitis and myositis.[8] The effected limbs are usually hyperextended. The diagnosis is confirmed on necropsy examination of the spinal cord, nerve roots, and muscles.

Granulomatous meningoencephalomyelitis (reticulosis) may produce signs of paraparesis from thoracolumbar spinal cord involvement.[24]

On rare occasions other granulomas are found compressing the spinal cord, producing paraparesis.[22] Epidural dirofilariasis is another rare cause of paraparesis in dogs.[26,37]

Discospondylitis

Incidence: Frequent

Discospondylitis is an infection of the intervertebral disc with osteomyelitis of the associated vertebrae.[15,21,45] It is a common cause of back pain and an animal's reluctance to move, and may have ataxia or paresis of the pelvic limbs associated with it. Discospondylitis may occur at multiple sites along the vertebral column, and the signs vary with the amount of meningeal and spinal cord involvement (Fig. 17–8A,B). The diagnosis and management of discospondylitis is discussed in Chapter 16. Spondylitis can also occur, but is less frequent than discospondylitis.

Trauma

Spinal cord injury may be produced by vertebral fractures, luxations, and subluxations, or by dorsal protrusion or extrusion of intervertebral disc material.

Spinal cord and vertebral injury

Incidence: Frequent

Vertebral fractures, luxations, subluxations, and traumatic spinal cord injury are common causes of paraplegia, paraparesis, and ataxia of the pelvic limbs in dogs and cats.[4,7,23,40]

Initial spinal cord damage is caused by the mechanical pressure and distortion from the injury, but a secondary chain of events occurs in the spinal cord that produces additional damage. Because the secondary events seem to be preventable in part, much research has been done on spinal cord pathophysiology associated with trauma.

The acute microvascular response to spinal cord trauma is decreased blood flow in the central gray matter within 15 minutes after the injury.[42] This leads to progressive ischemia with extravasation of red blood cells and central hemorrhagic necrosis of the gray matter. Substances released during this process may travel along the central canal of the spinal cord and produce ascending and descending myelomalacia beyond the original site of injury.[42] The amount of hemorrhagic necrosis may vary with the traumatic force applied to the spinal cord. A transient decrease in the blood flow in peripheral white matter occurs, but necrosis and hemorrhage are usually the direct results of the trauma.

Along with the physical trauma and ischemia, edema of the spinal cord results in further functional impairment and parenchymal damage. The amount of edema varies with the severity of the lesion. Vasogenic edema may be caused by extravasated fluid containing plasma proteins that leak into surrounding tissue and attract fluid accumulation. The vascular leakage is greatest during the first hour following injury, but the blood CNS barrier may be altered for up to 14 days.

Much of the current experimental therapy for spinal cord injuries is aimed at preventing alterations in the microvasculature and secondary spinal cord necrosis.

Signalment and history. Any age, breed, or sex of dog or cat may receive an injury to the thoracolumbar vertebral column. If the spinal cord is initially injured, the onset of paraplegia or paraparesis is acute. If vertebrae are fractured and unstable, the neurologic deficit may become worse after manipulation or movement of the vertebrae because of increased impingement on the spinal cord and nerve roots. Pain may be associated with vertebral fractures if meninges and nerve roots are irritated. If a vertebral column injury is suspected, the owner should be instructed to gently place the animal on a

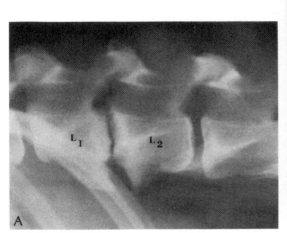
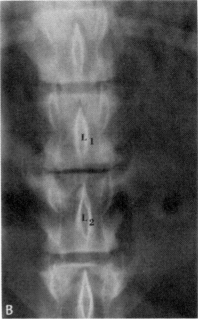

Figure 17–8. *(A)* A lateral plain radiograph of the lumbar vertebral column showing discospondylitis between the first and second lumbar vertebrae (L1 and L2) in a 6-year-old female Rhodesian Ridgeback with back pain. *(B)* A ventrodorsal view of the vertebral column of the same dog as in *A,* showing discospondylitis at L1 to 2.

door or other flat, sturdy structure to carry it to the hospital.

Physical and neurologic examinations. Other life-threatening problems associated with trauma such as shock, hemorrhage, or airway obstruction are initially managed with minimal manipulation of the vertebral column. The animal often has lacerations, abrasions, and bruising of the skin.

The neurologic examination is performed with minimal movement of the animal. The mentation, head posture, and cranial nerves are assessed to evaluate concurrent head injury (Chap. 10). Voluntary movements of the limbs are noted, but the animal is discouraged from moving or attempting to walk, and no postural reactions are tested at this time. A deviation of the vertebral column may be gently palpated, especially with thoracolumbar fractures. Spinal reflexes, superficial sensation, and deep sensation are all evaluated.

Acute diagnosis and management. The therapy for acute spinal cord trauma is methylprednisolone sodium succinate (Solu-Medrol) 30 mg/kg administered intravenously then reduced to 15 mg/kg every 6 to 8 hours for the first 24 to 48 hours; then oral prednisone 1 mg/kg is begun for 5 to 7 days. The dose of prednisone then is reduced over the next 5 to 7 days and discontinued. Mannitol is not used because of associated spinal cord hemorrhage. The animal is monitored for melena, anorexia, or vomiting because of the problems of gastrointestinal ulcers in paraplegic dogs on glucocorticoids.[30,41,46] Antibiotics may be administered prophylactically for the first 5 to 7 days on the high glucocorticoid doses. If signs of gastrointestinal irritation occur, a combination cimetidine (Tagamet) 4 mg/kg orally every 8 hours followed by sucralfate (Carafate) 250 mg to 1 g orally 2 hours later may be given until the signs resolve. A 10% solution of dimethyl sulfoxide (DMSO) in 5% dextrose and' water may be administered intravenously at a dose of 0.5 to 1 g/ kg every 12 hours. If the solution is stronger than 10%, hemolysis may occur. The efficacy of DMSO is controversial.

Once the initial neurologic examination has been performed and therapy begun, the vertebral column is radiographed to further localize the lesion. Fractures, luxations, and subluxations of vertebrae may be seen on routine radiographs. T11 to 12 and T12 to 13 are the areas of greatest mobility in the vertebral column and are common sites for fractures to occur. T11 is usually the anticlinal vertebra or the vertebra that marks the transition from backward-to forward-sloping spinous processes. Fractures may occur at any site and may also occur at multiple sites, so radiographs of the entire vertebral column should be examined. The radiographic examination should never be used to assess the severity of the neurologic deficit, but is helpful in determining an accurate prognosis when used in conjunction with the neurologic examination. (Fig. 17–9A) With no vertebral lesions, myelography may be needed to localize the site of spinal cord involvement. Because of the acute nature of the injury, the needle EMG is normal for 5 to 7 days.

The prognosis varies with the degree of neurologic deficit and the location of the lesion. A paraplegic dog with hyperactive reflexes and a lesion above L3 often has a better prognosis than a paralegic dog with absent spinal reflexes and a lesion below L3. Central hemorrhagic necrosis of gray matter from T2 to L3 only affects lower motor neuron cell bodies to epaxial muscles. Central hemorrhagic necrosis of the gray matter below L3 affects lower motor neuron cell bodies to the pelvic limbs,

anus, and bladder and is usually permanent. Dogs and cats may have an acute loss of superficial and deep pain that may return in 72 hours.

Most clinicians advocate laminectomy and decompression of the spinal cord as soon as possible.[40,43,44] An accurate prognosis often cannot be made prior to surgery. Although a laminectomy will probably not alter the hemorrhagic necrosis of the central gray matter, it will prevent further damage to the white matter from compression. Fractured vertebrae are stabilized by various means and detailed descriptions are found elsewhere. (Fig. 17–9B,C) Duratomy, piatomy, or myelotomy have been suggested to further decompress the spinal cord. Perfusion of the subarachnoid space with hypothermic, normothermic, hypertonic, and isotonic slushes and solutions for varying amounts of time have all been advocated by different surgeons.

Later management and prognosis. Once acute medical and surgical therapeutic measures are performed, the animal is usually continued on glucocorticoids for several days or up to 2 weeks, depending on the neurologic signs. Serial neurologic examinations may be performed to determine a prognosis. If deep pain returns with lesions between T2 to L3, the prognosis may be good for eventual recovery and the animal may be an acceptable pet. No return of deep pain after several days is a poor prognostic sign and is grave if it remains absent after 30 days. Somatosensory spinal cord and cortical-evoked responses can be used to determine spinal cord integrity and be a prognostic guide in spinal cord trauma (Chap. 5).

Nursing care is important to prevent cystitis, decubital ulcers, and dermatitis. If the owner can manage the nursing care, the animal usually does better in the home environment. The bladder may have to be expressed every 6 to 8 hours to ensure proper voiding (Chap. 19). The animal can be returned to the clinic for periodic neurologic examinations. Animals can continue to improve for 6 to 12 months following spinal cord injuries, if the spinal cord is not severely damaged. Animals with severe spinal cord injuries from T2 to L3 may show evidence of spinal walking after a few weeks to months and may appear to be improving when actually the spinal reflexes are only becoming more hyperactive (Chap. 1).

Intervertebral disc disease

Incidence: Frequent

The intervertebral (IV) discs are elastic cushions between the vertebral bodies from C2 and C3 through the caudal vertebrae. They absorb shock and facilitate movement of the vertebral column. The IV discs are composed of an outer fibrous portion, the anulus fibrosus, and an inner gelatinous substance, the nucleus pulposus.

Degeneration of the intervertebral disc may occur at an early age in chondrodystrophoid breeds, such as the Dachshund, Pekingese, Beagle, and Basset hounds, or at a later age in nonchondrodystrophoid breeds.[2,18,35]

In chondrodystrophoid breeds, a chondroid metaplasia of the IV disc occurs. These degenerated IV discs often calcify and can be visualized readily on radiographs of the vertebral column. IV discs that have undergone a chondroid metaplasia are more likely to have a Han-

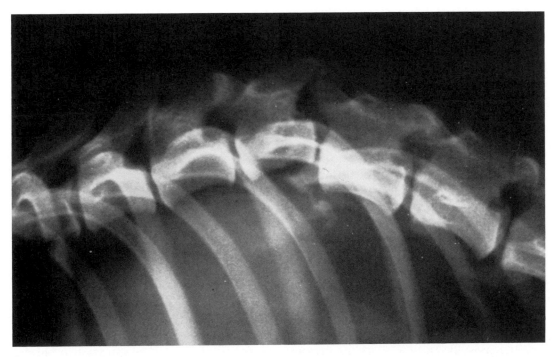

A

Figure 17–9. *(A)* A lateral radiograph of a traumatic T12–13 luxation. Both lateral and ventrodorsal view radiographs should be taken to evaluate the degree of displacement, but the degree of deficit must be determined by the neurologic examination.

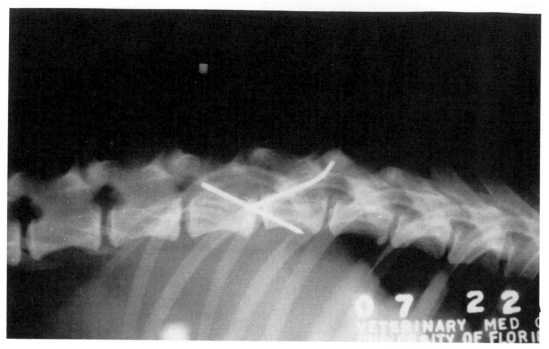

B

Figure 17–9. *(B)* A lateral radiograph of the surgical repair of the luxation in *A*. The vertebral column was realigned and pins were placed in the bodies of the T12–13.

sen's Type I extrusion, which is a complete rupture of the anulus with an extrusion of the nucleus pulposus into the vertebral canal. A type I disc extrusion can result in an explosion of nuclear material against the spinal cord and, therefore, acute paralysis (Fig. 17–10). The severe traumatic spinal cord insult may lead to secondary vascular alterations and ascending and descending myelomalacia. A Type I disc extrusion can also produce a slower periodic extrusion of nuclear material that may produce paresis that becomes more severe over several days or has a waxing and waning course, in which the paresis worsens, then improves, and then worsens again. (Fig. 17–11) In chondrodystrophoid breeds, most of the discs are in various stages of degeneration, so a recurrence of problems from different cervical and thoracolumbar IV discs is common.

In older, nonchondrodystrophoid breeds especially large breed dogs like German Shepherds, fibrous metaplasia of the IV disc occurs. IV discs that have undergone fibrous metaplasia rarely calcify and may not be seen on routine radiographic examination of the vertebrae. These IV discs most often have a Hansen's Type II protrusion, which is a partial rupture of the anulus fibrosus leading to a small, dome-shaped protrusion that compresses the spinal cord. A Type II disc protrusion characteristically produces slow, progressive paresis over several weeks or months.

In both chondroid and fibrous metaplasia of the IV disc, degeneration and protrusion occur that can lead to paraparesis, but the signalment and progression of neurologic signs and the radiographic findings may be very different.

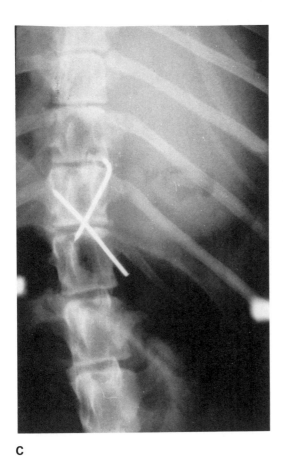

C

Figure 17–9. *(C)* A ventrodorsal radiograph of the surgical repair seen in *A* and *B*.

The anulus fibrosus is thinner dorsally than ventrally, and when it degenerates, it usually ruptures dorsally into the vertebral canal (Fig. 17–12). The dorsal longitudinal ligament passes over the top of the IV disc spaces on the floor of the vertebral canal (Fig. 17–12). In slow Type I disc protrusions, the nuclear material often goes to either side of the dorsal longitudinal ligament and the animal may have a greater deficit in one pelvic limb than the other. The IV disc material is often located on the most affected side. The conjugal ligament, from T2 to T10, runs between the heads of the ribs and over the dorsal surface of the IV disc (Fig. 17–12). The con-

jugal ligament provides a barrier against dorsal IV disc protrusions, and they rarely occur between T2 to T10. The epidural space contains fat. When extruded IV disc material or a protruded anulus fibrosus puts pressure on the spinal cord, the fat becomes necrotic. When surgery is being performed, the absence of white, glistening fat deposits in the epidural space can indicate to the surgeon that the correct region is being explored.

Signalment and history. Lumbar intervertebral disc disease is most common in Dachshunds, Pekingese, Beagles, Cocker spaniels, and Poodles between 3 and 7 years of age, but is also seen in other breeds of dogs. Intervertebral disc disease can occur in older cats.[18,36] The older animals in this group often have a history of previous bouts of pain or paresis, suggestive of past problems with IV disc protrusions. A few animals have clinical signs prior to 3 years of age.

Older, nonchondrodystrophoid breeds of dogs or cats over 5 years of age may suffer from degenerative IV disc disease. German Shepherds 7 to 9 years of age commonly have thoracolumbar disc disease and Doberman Pinschers 5 to 10 years of age commonly have cervical disc disease and on rare occasions thorocolumbar disc herniation or protrusion (Chap. 16).

Young chondrodystrophoid breeds and other dogs may show minimal signs of back pain evidenced by an unwillingness to sit up and beg for treats, go up and down stairs or jump on and off furniture. The owner may report that this has occurred previously, but with rest the animal improved. In these cases, there may be a slight extrusion of nucleus pulposus material or protrusion of the anulus fibrosus, producing compression, irritation, or a local inflammatory reaction of the meninges and dorsal root, with resulting pain. Some of the pain may come from the disc itself. The owner may also complain of varying

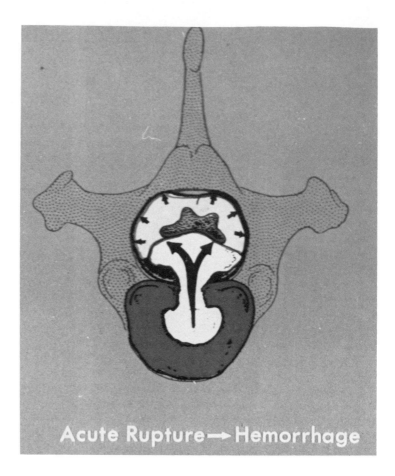

Figure 17–10. Acute Type I intervertebral disc herniation can produce severe spinal cord injury, including hemorrhage, secondary vascular spasms, and necrosis, as well as ascending and descending myelomalacia.

degrees of ataxia and paresis with or without pain. The signs may worsen and improve alternately. The extrusion of nucleus pulposus material may initially compress and irritate the nerve roots and meninges, then later spread along the floor of the vertebral canal. The body tries to wall off and absorb the foreign material from the nucleus, the signs may again worsen. Rupture of the anulus fibrosus and explosion of nucleus pulposus material against the spinal cord may cause acute paralysis of the pelvic limbs, with many of the secondary vascular changes associated with spinal cord trauma described earlier in this chapter. Secondary ascending and descending myelomalacia may occur over the next several days. The animal may be in lateral recumbency and die in respiratory failure caused by intercostal muscle and diaphragm paralysis.

In older, nonchondrodystrophoid breeds with a type II protrusion, the recurrent partial rupture of the anulus fibrosus results in a dome-shaped mass that slowly increases in size and produces progressive compression of the nerve roots and spinal cord. The clinical signs are often pain, ataxia, and paresis that progresses over several weeks', and in some cases, a few months' duration. Rarely is paraparesis acute.

Physical and neurologic examinations. The physical examination may be normal in uncomplicated intervertebral

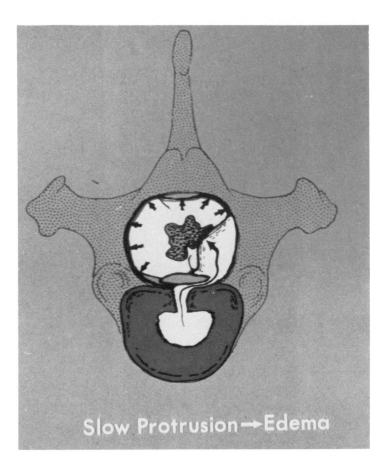

Slow Protrusion→Edema

Figure 17–11. A slow protrusion or extrusion of nucleus pulposus material from Type I intervertebral disc herniation produces spinal cord compression and edema, which rapidly responds to glucocorticoid therapy or decompressive laminectomy.

disc protrusion. The animal may be anxious, in pain, and have severe muscle spasms, which often respond to 2 to 5 mg of diazepam (Valium) given slowly intravenously. If the animal is depressed, anorexic, and febrile, ascending and descending myelomalacia may be occurring and the prognosis is grave. As the spinal cord segments of the intercostal and phrenic nerves become affected, respiratory paralysis occurs.

Muscle spasms and pain may be the only abnormality noted on the neurologic examination in mild lesions. An area of hyperesthesia may help to outline the site of the lesion. The loss of the cutaneous trunci (panniculus) response in one section on one side may further localize the lesion to that area. Varying degrees of ataxia, paresis, or paralysis of the pelvic limbs also may occur. The spinal reflexes of the pelvic limbs are usually normal or hyperactive in focal disc protrusions from T10 to L3. Table 17–6 summarizes the spinal reflex changes most commonly associated with herniated lumbar intervertebral discs in dogs, when the lesion remains focal (see Fig. 17–4). The level at which superficial sensation is lost indicates the cranial aspect of the lesion. If no spinal reflexes are presented in the pelvic limbs and the sensory level is at T10, the disc may have protruded somewhere in between and ascending and descending myelomalacia probably has occurred. Myelomalacia does not always ascend through all thoracic

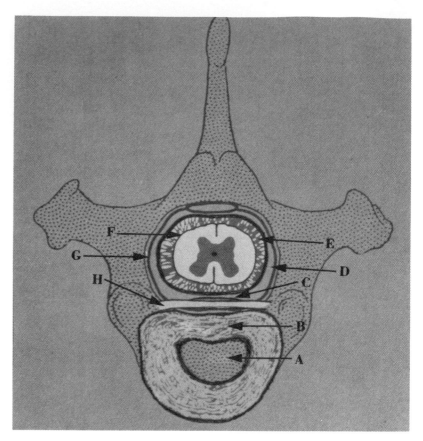

Figure 17–12. A cross section of the vertebra, vertebral canal, and spinal cord showing the nucleus pulposus (A) and anulus fibrosus (B) of the IV disc, the dorsal longitudinal ligament (C), the epidural space (D), the subarachnoid space (E), the spinal cord (F), the vertebral canal (G), and the conjugal ligament (H).

spinal cord segments and produce death. The prognosis is poor in this case if deep pain is also lost. Deep pain may be absent in acute paralysis for 24 to 72 hours, which indicates a poor but not hopeless prognosis. If deep pain is absent after 72 hours, the prognosis worsens. If deep pain is still absent after 30 days, the prognosis for recovery is hopeless. A laminectomy produces best results if performed as soon as possible in an animal with acute paralysis, even if deep pain is not present. If deep pain is present, it has been over 72 hours, and spinal cord compression is seen on the myelogram, a laminectomy may still improve the clinical signs. However it is *not* recommended that the clinician wait 72 hours to see if there is a response to medical management before referral for surgery.

Ancillary diagnostic investigations. Routine clinicopathologic tests usually contribute little to the diagnosis of intervertebral disc disease. A urinalysis should be performed on all animals, as cystitis is a common complication of urinary incontinence (Chap. 19).

EMG may be useful as an aid in localizing the involvement to specific spinal cord segments and nerve roots. For the EMG to be abnormal, the problem has to

Table 17–6
Spinal reflex alterations associated with focal lesions produced by herniated IV discs in the dog

Site of IV disc	Reflex alterations
T10 to L3	All reflexes normal or hyperactive
L3 to 4	Patellar reflex depressed or absent; all other reflexes normal or hyperactive
L4 to 5	Patellar reflex depressed or absent; gastrocnemius, cranial tibial muscle, and flexor reflexes depressed or absent; anal reflex normal
L5 to 6	All reflexes depressed or absent
L6 to 7	Patellar reflex normal or slightly hyperactive (unopposed extensors); gastrocnemius, cranial tibial muscle, and flexor reflexes depressed or absent; anal reflex depressed or absent

have existed for longer than 5 to 7 days. When multiple disc protrusions have occurred in an animal, it might be difficult to differentiate old, nonactive lesions from a new lesion that is causing the current problem.

Routine radiographic findings can vary greatly in IV disc disease. Chondroid degeneration is easily seen as multiple calcified IV discs. If the IV discs are still within their space between the vertebrae, they are probably causing few problems, but pose a threat for the future. Calcified extruded material may be seen in the vertebral canal and the intervertebral disc space may be narrowed. If there are multiple sites that appear narrowed or have calcified material in the vertebral canal, myelography must be performed to outline the present site of involvement, especially when surgical therapy is anticipated. The most common location for intervertebral disc protrusion to occur is just caudal to the anticlinal vertebra at T12 to 13. IV discs that have undergone fibroid degeneration are not readily seen on radiographic examination because they rarely

calcify. A narrowed IV disc space may be the only indication that a disc extrusion has occurred (Fig. 17–13). Myelography is often necessary to obtain a definite diagnosis of IV disc disease, when surgical decompression is contemplated. In acute Type I IV disc herniations, a myelogram is needed to determine the extent of spinal cord swelling (Fig. 17–14). If a hemilaminectomy is to be performed, the myelogram can be used to determine the side the disc material is on.

A myelogram may be necessary to outline a Type II IV disc compression in large breed dogs, as plain radiographs rarely show the lesion (Fig. 17–15).

Therapy and prognosis. The therapy of intervertebral disc disease varies with the experience of different veterinarians.

In an animal having its first bout of back pain with no neurologic deficit, absolute confinement and rest for 2 to 3 weeks is very important. As we discussed earlier, the extruded IV disc material may spread out and cause minimal problems that eventually subside. If the animal has

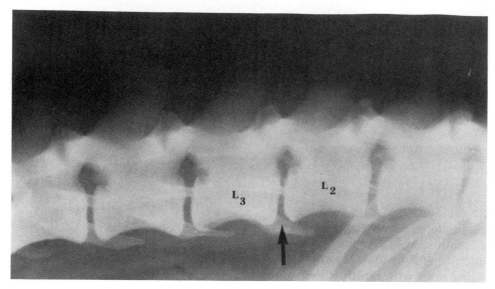

Figure 17–13. A lateral routine radiograph of the vertebral column showing a narrowed IV disc space (arrow) at L2 to 3 from herniation of IV disc material into the spinal canal.

a great deal of discomfort, oral diazepam (Valium) 1 to 5 mg every 6 to 8 hours may be administered. Acupuncture may produce relief from pain and be useful in treatment.[19] Glucocorticoids are contraindicated if the dog has no neurologic deficit, only because they often relieve all of the pain and the animal no longer restricts its own activity. The animal may feel so well that it will dive off the furniture and explode the degenerating disc into the spinal cord, producing ascending and descending myelomalacia and permanent paraplegia or death (see Fig. 17–10). Acetylsalicylic acid (aspirin) is not given if later surgery is contemplated, as platelet function will be altered and excessive bleeding during surgery will occur. In young dogs with multiple degenerating discs and recurrent episodes of pain, dorsolateral fenestration of all discs from T11–T12 through L3–4 is performed to prevent future problems. Although the anesthesia and surgery can be risky, if all goes well, the owner will have an animal that can lead a normal life, free from worry about future disc problems. The recurrence of IV disc problems associated with protrusion of other degenerating discs is common.[25] Some animals, however, do not have further problems and many owners would rather play the odds that their animal will not have future problems, than to spend the money or risk possible anesthetic or surgical complications.[34,35]

When ataxia and paraparesis occur, more aggressive therapy with glucocorticoids and possibly decompressive surgery are indicated. If the neurologic deficit is primarily caused by edema of the spinal cord, the animal may improve greatly 24 hours after glucocorticoid therapy has been begun or the spinal cord is surgically decompressed with a hemilaminectomy or dorsal laminectomy (see Fig. 17–11). If decompressive surgery is performed and recovery is rapid, glucocorticoids usually do not need to be continued. If decompressive surgery is not performed, then oral prednisone 1 gm/kg is given for 3 to 5 days, then reduced to 0.25 mg/kg for 3 to 5 days, then alternate days for 3 times,

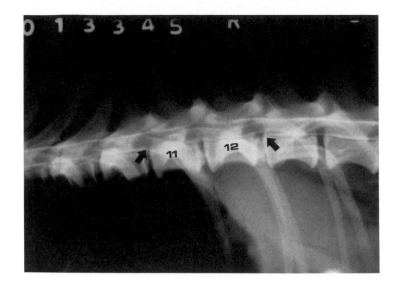

Figure 17–14. A lateral view of a myelogram following herniation of the IV disc between T11 (11) and T12 (12). Spinal cord swelling is present from the cranial aspect of T11 to the caudal part of T12 (arrows). Prophylactic fenestration of the calcified disc between T12–13, as well as others, were performed at the same time as the hemilaminectomy.

then discontinued, and the animal's activity completely restricted. Oral diazepam (Valium) 1 to 5 mg every 8 hours may help control pain and aid bladder expression if necessary. Animals with paresis that improve slightly with glucocorticoids might improve faster with decompressive surgery and glucocorticoids. Prophylactic fen-

estration of the other IV discs from T11–12 through L3–4 is often performed at the same time as the decompressive surgery to prevent recurrences (Fig. 17–14).

Many clinicians believe that acute paralysis is a surgical emergency and the animal should be decompressed within 24 hours.[7,18,38] The animal is given 30 mg/kg

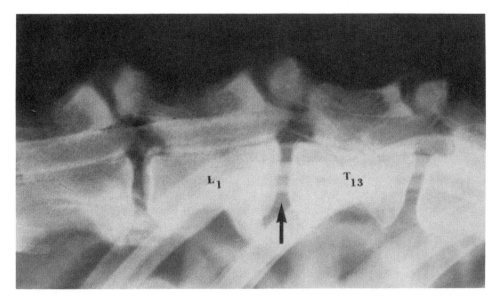

Figure 17–15. A lateral myelogram showing a Type II disc protrusion (arrow) between T13 and L1 vertebrae in a 7-year-old German Shepherd male with pelvic limb weakness.

methylprednisolone sodium succinate (Solu-Medrol) initially, then reduced to 15 mg/kg and placed on oral prednisone as discussed above in spinal cord injuries. If deep pain is absent, the prognosis is poor, but nonetheless not hopeless. When a laminectomy is performed, the spinal cord may be visualized for hemorrhages, the dura may be opened and the spinal cord integrity assessed. If the spinal cord bulges from the durotomy site but holds its shape, then the prognosis is fair. If the spinal cord pours out of the durotomy site, indicating necrosis, the prognosis is grave. Many surgeons bathe the traumatized cord with normothermic or hypothermic saline solutions.[7]

Old dogs with Type II IV disc protrusions often respond well to decompressive surgery. The age of the dog and the presence of problems in other body systems should be assessed, because many of these animals also do well with conservative therapy and can live out their lives comfortably on alternate-day oral prednisone therapy. Often as little as 5 mg prednisone every other day may improve the symptoms in a 5 to 15-kg dog. A dosage of 10 mg prednisone every other day may be needed for larger dogs. Diazepam (Valium) 2 to 5 mg orally every 8 hours may provide further relief of symptoms of discomfort. German Shepherds can have Type II IV disc protrusions and degenerative myelopathy at the same time, producing similar signs. The owner must be informed of this. If spinal cord compression is seen, decompression will at least temporarily improve the neurologic deficit. Degenerative myelopathy is discussed later in this chapter.

The decision to operate on an animal with intervertebral disc disease depends on the availability of an experienced surgeon and the willingness of the owner to take the animal to a surgeon, pay the required fee, take the risk of surgery worsening the condition, and provide nursing care to the animal over the following weeks or months. The risk of an experienced surgeon worsening the condition in thoracolumbar disc disease is minimal. The techniques of intervertebral disc surgery are well described elsewhere.[18]

General supportive care is given as for all paraplegic animals. Prednisone may be continued at reducing dosages for several days to 2 weeks, depending on the clinical improvement. The animal is observed for vomiting and blood in the feces, which might be a complication of treatment. In dogs with intervertebral disc disease, duodenal and colonic ulcers are common problems associated with dexamethasone and prednisone therapy.[30,41,46] Nonsteroidal anti-inflammatory drugs such as flunixin meglumine (Banamine) should *never* be combined with glucocorticoids, as ulcers and perforation are likely. The animal should be monitored for anorexia, vomiting, and melena. If these symptoms occur, the glucocorticoid dose should be reduced and a combination of cimetidine (Tagamet) 4 mg/kg orally every 6–8 hours followed in 2 hours by sucralfate (Carafate) 4 mg/kg orally should be administered until the signs resolve. The bladder may have to be expressed 3 times daily and the urine periodically evaluated for evidence of cystitis. Defecation may occur involuntarily, but if constipation occurs, glycerin suppositories or warm water enemas may be needed to aid defecation. The animal should be kept on a balanced diet, but affected animals are often overweight and their food intake should be restricted. Water intake is often increased because of the prednisone. The animal should be kept on padding to prevent decubital sores around the hips and pelvis. The skin around the perineum and abdomen should be kept free of urine and feces to prevent dermatitis.

A few days to 1 week after surgery, a paraplegic animal can begin physical therapy. Fifteen minutes once or twice daily in a whirlpool can aid circulation in the limb muscles and promote movement. When some voluntary movement is seen, the animal may be exercised with a towel under the abdomen to provide some support to the pelvic limbs. If an animal has not had surgery and there is a possibility of further extrusion of IV disc materal, physical therapy should be mild and occur only after a 2- to 3-week rest period.

Many dogs eventually recover from paralysis caused by IV disc disease; some in only a few days and others in several months. Serial neurologic examinations are the best guide for an accurate prognosis. Many severely affected dogs will continue to improve for 6 to 9 months or longer after the spinal cord insult. Some small dogs with permanent paraplegia may be kept as acceptable pets with a little extra daily care. A special cart can be made for them to prevent dragging of the pelvic limbs.*

Prevention. Recurrence of IV disc problems is common in young chondrodystrophoid dogs. The chance of recurrent problems may be decreased if the animal is kept thin and not allowed to jump on and off furniture, sit up and beg for food, or run up and down stairs. This is often difficult in a young, active dog. Prophylactic surgical fenestration of all discs from T11–12 through L3–4 is the method of choice to minimize the recurrence of future problems in the thoracolumbar area. The owner must be advised that the dog could still have problems from low lumbar or cervical disc protrusion or herniation but a separate surgery may be needed.

In older large breed dogs recurrence of IV disc problems is not as common.

Decreasing the weight of obese animals may help. Older animals often restrict their own activity. Prophylactic fenestration is usually not performed in large breed dogs.

Pathology. Type I disc extrusions produce epidural hemorrhage and local inflammation. The extruded nuclear material may be voluminous, gritty, cheeselike, hemorrhagic, or slate gray and be adhered to the dura of the spinal cord or spread along the vertebral canal.

Type II disc protrusions are focally protruded mounds of hardened disc material that remain primarily over the intervertebral disc space and compress the spinal cord. The spinal cord in the affected area shows degenerative changes associated with compression and alteration of the blood supply.

Acute IV disc protrusions produce varying degrees of edema, hemorrhage, and necrosis. Ascending and descending myelomalacia or hemorrhagic necrosis may occur. The pathology associated with IV disc disease is discussed in detail elsewhere.[18]

Vascular disorders

Vascular disorders of the spinal cord are discussed in Chapter 16. Fibrocartilaginous emboli, spontaneous spinal cord hemorrhage, and vascular malformations may all occur in the thoracolumbar spinal cord as well as the cervical spinal cord. Only fibrocartilaginous infarction of the thoracolumbar spinal cord is discussed in this section, as the other conditions are rare.

Thrombosis of the iliac arteries is a common cause of pelvic limb paresis or paralysis in cats. Thrombosis and embolism of iliac arteries and pelvic limb paralysis is rare in dogs.

---

* K-9 Carts, 532 Newtown Road, Berwyn, PA 19312 (Phone [215] 644-6624).

Fibrocartilaginous infarct

Incidence: Frequent

Infarction of the cervical spinal cord by fibrocartilaginous material is described in Chapter 16. Fibrocartilaginous infarction of the spinal cord also occurs in the thoracolumbar spinal cord.[9,32]

A venous infarction in the caudal lumbar segments in Great Danes from 3 to 5 years of age produces flaccid paralysis. The animals may initially appear to have back pain, which shortly leads to paresis or paralysis of one limb, which can then lead to an asymmetric paraplegia within 2 to 3 hours. Other large breeds such as Saint Bernards, Labrador Retrievers, and German Shepherds have been similarly affected, as have smaller breeds of dogs and cats. The infarction can be caused by emboli in arteries, veins, or both. If the site of infarction is in the spinal cord from T2 to L3, asymmetric spastic paraplegia is often seen.

The degree of spinal cord infarction can vary, as can the severity of clinical signs. Most often, the animals are paraplegic.

Routine spinal radiographs are normal. A focal spinal cord swelling is seen on a myelogram. Lumbar CSF often contains increased amounts of protein.

Oral prednisone can be given as follows: 1 mg/kg for 3 days, then reduced to 0.5 mg/kg for 3 days, then 0.25 mg/kg for 3 days, then 0.25 mg/kg for every other day 3 times. After a few days to a week some improvement begins. The prognosis is better for T2 to L3 spinal cord lesions than for L4 to S2 lesions, because in the latter case there is infarction of gray matter containing the cell bodies for the nerves to the pelvic limbs, bladder, and anus. Serial neurologic examinations are needed to form an accurate prognosis in individual cases. Many animals recover after several weeks to months, but may retain a residual weakness in one limb.

Spontaneous spinal cord hemorrhage

Incidence: Rare

Spontaneous hemorrhage of the spinal cord can occur in animals with coagulation defects. These are rare, but are considered in the differential diagnosis of acute paraplegia in animals. When suspected, clinicopathologic tests for clotting function are performed (Chap. 16).

Vascular malformations

Incidence: Rare

Vascular malformations of the spinal cord may lead to progressive paraparesis, but are rare in animals as compared with man (Chap. 16).

Ischemic neuromyopathy—aortic embolism

Incidence: Frequent in cats

Endocardiac thrombus fragmentation in cats with cardiomyopathy can lead to embolization of the caudal aorta at the bifurcation of the iliac arteries. The embolization leads to a series of events that disrupts the entire blood supply to the pelvic limbs producing ischemic neuromyopathy and paraplegia (Fig. 17–16).[13,24,33]

Ischemic neuromyopathy cannot be experimentally reproduced by ligation of the caudal aorta, but can be recreated when the aorta is double ligated and 5-hydroxytryptamine (5-HT) is injected between the ligatures. It is theorized that 5-HT is released from the platelets that aggregate in the thrombus formation. The 5-HT produces contraction of the smooth muscle of remaining, nonthrombosed small blood vessels, and ischemia of all the nerves and muscles to the pelvic limbs occurs.

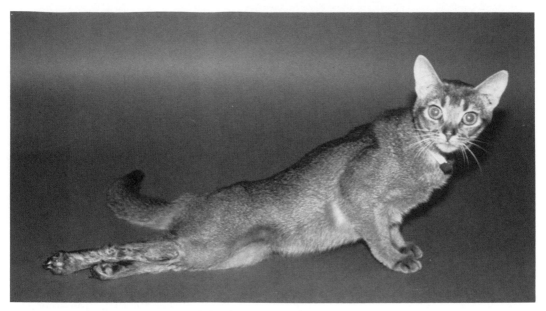

Figure 17–16. A cat with paraplegia from ischemic neuromyopathy.

Signalment and history. Adult cats of any breed can have an acute onset of symmetric or asymmetric paraparesis or paraplegia. The limbs may also be painful.

Physical and neurologic examinations. The animal may be depressed. The pelvic limbs are often painful and cold on palpation. No femoral pulse can be palpated and a holosystolic heart murmur may be auscultated. If the cat is in heart failure, the lung sounds will also be decreased.

Flexion of the hip and stifle are often retained, but there is little movement distal to the hocks. Spinal reflexes are usually absent. Later in the course of the disease, deep and superficial sensations are absent, especially below the hock.

Ancillary diagnostic investigations. Clinicopathologic tests may not contribute to the diagnosis. Thoracic radiographs, ECG, and echocardiography may be useful in evaluating the underlying cardiac

problem. Generalized cardiomegaly and pleural effusion are the characteristic radiographic findings. Normal sinus rhythm, bradycardia, ventricular premature complexes, anterior fascicular block, and changes compatible with left side heart enlargement may be seen on the ECG. The echocardiogram is useful to evaluate cardiac function.

Needle EMG studies show evidence of denervation. Motor nerve conduction velocities of the sciatic-tibial nerve vary with the degree of ischemia, but often are decreased or absent.

The diagnosis is based on the cardiac changes and the lack of circulation to the pelvic limbs.

Therapy and prognosis. The cardiomyopathy is stabilized with therapeutic administration of digitalis, diuretics, and bronchodilators. The specific therapy is well described elsewhere.[13,33] When the blood supply to the pelvic limbs is only partially blocked, heparin therapy may prevent further thrombin formation. Acetylsalicylic acid (Aspirin) 25 mg/kg is given every 3 days to reduce prostaglandin-enhanced platelet aggregation. Early medical therapy gives the best results, but the prognosis is poor or grave in many cases. Recurrence of thromboembolism is seen in recovered cats.

Pathology. Both peripheral nerves and muscles have ischemic necrosis. The lesions begin in the mid-thigh and involve the distal pelvic limbs.

Degeneration

Sporadic cases are seen of spinal cord degeneration producing pelvic limb paresis and paralysis in dogs and cats.[29] The underlying cause is usually unknown. Degenerative myelopathy of German Shepherds is the most commonly seen condition of this type.

Degenerative myelopathy of German Shepherds

Incidence: Frequent in German Shepherds

A slow, progressive pelvic limb paresis is commonly seen in aging German Shepherds.[6,20,24,39] A diffuse degeneration of spinal cord myelin and axons occurs in all funiculi, especially in the thoracic spinal cord.

The underlying cause is unknown, but it is thought to be caused by immune-mediated disorder, as affected dogs also have a T cell malfunction.

Signalment and history. German Shepherd dogs between 6 and 11 years of age are presented for an insidiously progressive pelvic limb weakness. Initially, the weakness is manifested by difficulty rising. This is often attributed to discomfort from hip dysplasia, which is also common in the breed. However, the ataxia and weakness progress, and it becomes more obvious that a neurologic, not an orthopedic, problem exists. The animals do not show back pain. The paresis continues to progress over many months, and fecal and urinary incontinence eventually occur.

Physical and neurologic examinations. The muscles of the pelvic region are often smaller than in normal German Shepherds from disuse atrophy, but otherwise the dog may appear to be in good health.

Spastic paraparesis is most commonly seen. Early in the course of the disease, proprioceptive positioning is abnormal, and this may be the first indication of a spinal cord disease. Spinal reflexes are normal or hyperactive. Crossed extensor reflexes and a positive Babinski sign may be present. Later in the course of disease, the patellar reflexes may become depressed, but the other spinal reflexes remain hyperactive. Superficial and deep sensation are preserved and there is no evidence of hyperesthesia. Late in the course of the disease, bowel and bladder incontinence develops.

Ancillary diagnostic investigations. Routine clinicopathologic tests do not contribute to the diagnosis. EMG examination is usually normal.

An elevated protein content is often found in CSF collected from the lumbar region, but is usually normal in the cisternal CSF.

Spondylosis deformans and/or dural ossification are often seen in vertebral column radiographs, but they rarely produce any degree of neurologic deficit. A Type II intervertebral (IV) disc protrusion might have a similar course to degenerative myelopathy in the early stages. A myelogram is usually needed to rule out an IV disc protrusion. In degenerative myelopathy, the myelogram is normal. A diagnosis of degenerative myelopathy in the live animal is suspected from the signalment, history, neurologic examination findings, and from ruling out other disease processes.

Therapy and prognosis. No therapy currently exists that alters the ultimate progression of spinal cord degeneration. Mild exercise and 5 mg/kg acetaminophen (Tylenol) orally will reduce discomfort from concurrent hip dysplasia and spondylosis deformans. There is some clinical evidence that oral therapy with epsilon amino caproic acid (Amicar) 500 mg every 8 hours may slow the progression of degenerative myelopathy in dogs with mild neurologic deficits. Most affected German Shepherds progress over months or years and are eventually euthanized.

Pathology. The lesions associated with degenerative myelopathy are most extensive in the middle to lower middle thoracic spinal cord and involve all funiculi. Both axons and myelin are lost, and an associated astrocytosis of the white matter is found on histologic examination. In some cases, degeneration occurs in dorsal nerve roots, which may account for a depressed or absent patellar reflex.

Spondylosis deformans

Incidence: Frequent

Spondylosis deformans is a ventral and lateral exostosis of vertebrae, which may be associated with ventral herniation of disc material or vertebral instability. Spondylosis deformans is a common radiographic finding in aged large breed dogs[20,47] (Fig. 17–17A,B). Spondylosis deformans rarely produces neurologic deficit, but may produce some back pain and morning stiffness. Pain from spondylosis deformans may be treated as needed in dogs with oral

acetaminophen (Tylenol) not to exceed 5 mg/kg daily.

On rare occasions, proliferation of bone may occur dorsally into the spinal canal, but this is usually at the lumbosacral region with compression of seventh lumbar, sacral, and caudal nerve roots, and urinary and fecal incontinence develops (Chap. 19).

Dural ossification

Incidence: Frequent

Another common finding on radiographs of large breeds of dogs is dural ossification.[47] It used to be referred to as ossifying pachymeningitis, and was thought to be the cause of paraparesis in older, large breed dogs, especially German Shepherds. However, dural ossification rarely produces neurologic deficit and the disease of German Shepherds was found to be degenerative myelopathy, discussed earlier in this chapter.

Neoplasia

Extramedullary spinal cord tumors

Incidence: Occasional

Neurinomas, neurofibromas, neurofibrosarcomas, and meningiomas all produce slow, progressive ataxia and paresis of the pelvic limbs over a period of several months.[3,12,27] Pain and self-mutilation may be associated with these tumors. The neurologic deficit may be asymmetric, as the tumor may grow on one side. The diagnosis is made with myelography. Surgical removal of these tumors when they are single and located above L3 can give good results. Disseminated meningeal tumors may occur, but are usually diagnosed after a necropsy examination.[17]

Extramedullary spinal cord tumors are discussed further in Chapter 16.

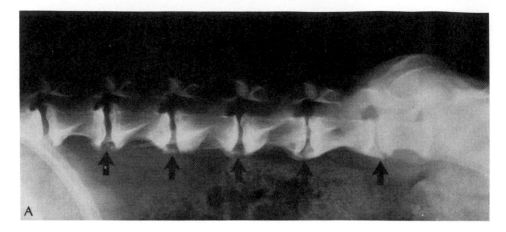

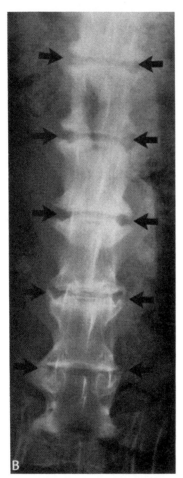

Figure 17–17. *(A)* A lateral radiograph of the lumbar vertebral column showing spondylosis deformans ventrally on the vertebral bodies (arrows). This dog has no neurologic deficit. *(B)* A ventrodorsal radiograph of the lumbar vertebral column showing spondylosis deformans laterally (arrows).

Intramedullary spinal cord tumors

Incidence: Occasional

Astrocytomas, ependymomas, and gliomas are intramedullary spinal cord tumors that occur occasionally, but are less common than neurofibrosarcomas or meningiomas.[14,27] The deficit caused by them is often progressive over several weeks, sometimes months, and there is usually little hyperesthesia. Diagnosis is made with myelography. A removable tumor is ruled out with exploratory surgery, and the final diagnosis is often made at necropsy. Intramedullary spinal cord tumors are discussed in Chapter 16.

Granulomatous meningoencephalitis (reticulosis)

Incidence: Rare

Granulomatous meningoencephalitis (GME—Reticulosis) may also become neoplastic and produce progressive paraparesis. GME is discussed in Chapters 7 and 12.

Metastatic spinal cord tumors

Incidence: Lymphosarcoma, occasional; prostatic, perianal, and mammary adenocarcinoma, occasional

Lymphosarcoma can occur as extradural masses or can infiltrate the meninges and spinal nerves in both dogs and cats.[10] Neoplastic cells may also be found in dura mater and paravertebral tissues such as the vertebrae and paravertebral musculature. Other neoplasms may also metastasize to the spinal cord.

Vertebral neoplasia

Incidence: Occasional

Primary and metastatic vertebral neoplasia can produce secondary compression of the spinal cord, from the growth of the tumor, or a fracture and collapse of the vertebrae.[31] Many vertebral tumors are diagnosed readily on routine radiographs, biopsy, and histologic examination of affected bone.

References

1. Braund, K.G.: Clinical Syndromes in Veterinary Neurology. Baltimore, Williams & Wilkins, 1986.
2. Braund, K.G.: Intervertebral disk disease. In Contemporary Issues in Small Animal Practice. Neurologic Disorders. Edited by J.N. Kornegay. New York, Churchill Livingstone, 1986.
3. Braund, K.G. and Ribas, J.L.: Central nervous system meningiomas. Compendium on Continuing Education, 8:241, 1986.
4. Carberry, C.A.: Nonsurgical management of thoracic and lumbar spinal fractures and fracture/luxations in the dog and cat. A review of 17 cases. J. Am. Hosp. Assoc., 25:43, 1989.
5. Child, C., et al.: Acquired scoliosis associated with hydromyelia and syringomyelia in two dogs. J. Am. Vet. Med. Assoc., 189:909, 1986.
6. Clemmons, R.M.: Degenerative myelopathy. In Current Veterinary Therapy X. Edited by R.W. Kirk. Philadelphia, W.B. Saunders, 1989.
7. Colter, S. and Rucker, N.C.: Acute injury to the central nervous system. In Common Neurology Problems. Vet. Clin. North Am., 18:545,1988.
8. Cone, D.M., et al.: Hindlimb hyperextension as a result of Toxoplasma gondii polyradiculoneuritis. J. Am. Anim. Hosp. Assoc., 19:713, 1983.
9. Cook, J.R.: Fibrocartilaginous embolism. In Common Neurologic Problems. Vet. Clin. North Am., 18:581, 1988.
10. Couto, C.G., et al.: Central nervous system lymphosarcoma in the dog. J. Am. Vet. Med. Asoc., 184:809, 1984.
11. deLahunta, A.: Spinal cord disease. In Veterinary Neuroanatomy and Clinical Neurology. Philadelphia, W.B. Saunders, 1983.
12. Fingeroth, J.M., et al.: Spinal meningiomas

in dogs: 13 cases (1972–1987). J. Am. Vet. Med. Assoc., *191*:720, 1987.

13. Fox, P.R.: Myocardial diseases. *In* Textbook of Veterinary Internal Medicine. Edited by S.J. Ettinger. Philadelphia, W.B. Saunders, 1989.

14. Gilmore, D.R.: Intraspinal tumors in the dog. Compendium on Continuing Education, *5*:55, 1983.

15. Gilmore, D.R.: Lumbosacral diskospondylitis in 21 dogs. J. Am. Anim. Hosp. Assoc., *23*:57, 1987.

16. Haskins, M.E., et al.: Spinal cord compression and hindlimb paresis in cats with mucopolysaccharidosis VI. J. Am. Vet. Med. Assoc., *182*:983, 1983.

17. Hay, W.H., et al.: Disseminated meningeal tumor in a dog. J. Am. Vet. Med. Assoc., *191*:692, 1987.

18. Hoerlein, B.F.: Intervertebral disc disease. *In* Veterinary Neurology. Edited by J.E. Oliver, B.F. Hoerlein, and I.G. Mayhew. Philadelphia, W.B. Saunders, 1987.

19. Janssens, L.A. and DePrins, E.M.: Treatment of thoracolumbar disc disease in dogs by means of acupuncture: A comparison of two techniques. J. Am. Anim. Hosp. Assoc., *25*:169, 1989.

20. Kornegay, J.N.: Congenital and degenerative diseases of the central nervous system. *In* Contemporary Issues in Small Animal Practice. Neurologic Disorders. Edited by J.N. Kornegay. New York, Churchill Livingstone, 1986.

21. Kornegay, J.N.: Diskospondylitis. *In* Current Veterinary Therapy IX. Edited by R.W. Kirk. Philadelphia, W.B. Saunders, 1986.

22. Kraus, K.H., et al.: Paraparesis caused by epidural granuloma in a cat. J. Am. Vet. Med. Assoc., *194*:789, 1989.

23. LeCouteur, R.A.: Central nervous system trauma. *In* Contemporary Issues in Small Animal Practice, Neurologic Disorders. Edited by J.N. Kornegay. New York, Churchill Livingstone, 1986.

24. LeCouteur, R.A. and Child, G.: Diseases of the spinal cord. *In* Veterinary Internal Medicine. Edited by S.J. Ettinger. Philadelphia, W.B. Saunders, 1989.

25. Levine, S.H. and Caywood, D.D.: Recurrence of neurologic deficits in dogs treated for thoracolumbar disc disease. J. Am. Vet. Med. Assoc., *20*:889, 1984.

26. Luttgen, P.J., et al.: Posterior paralysis caused by epidural dirofilariasis in a dog. J. Am. Vet. Med. Assoc., *17*:57, 1981.

27. Luttgen, P.J., et al. A retrospective study of twenty nine spinal tumors in the dog and cat. J. Small Anim. Pract., *21*:213, 1980.

28. Matthiesen, D.T.: Thoracolumbar spinal fractures/luxations: Surgical management. Compendium on Continuing Education, *5*:867, 1983.

29. Mesfin, G.M., et al.: Degenerative myelopathy in a cat. J. Am. Vet. Med. Assoc., *176*:62, 1980.

30. More, R.W., Withrow, S.J.: Gastrointestinal hemorrhage and pancreatitis associated with intervertebral disk disease in the dog. J. Am. Vet. Med. Assoc., *180*:1443, 1982.

31. Morgan, J.P., et al.: Vertebral tumors in the dog. Clinical, radiographic and pathologic study of 61 primary and secondary lesions. Vet. Radiol., *21*:197, 1980.

32. Penwick, R.C.: Fibrocartilaginous embolism and ischemic myelopathy. Compendium on Continuing Education, *3*:287, 1989.

33. Pion, P.D. and Kittleson, M.D.: Therapy for feline aortic thromboembolism. *In* Current Veterinary Therapy X. Edited by R.W. Kirk. Philadelphia, W.B. Saunders, 1989.

34. Prata, R.G.: Neurosurgical treatment of thoracolumbar disks. The rationale, and value of laminectomy with concomitant disc removal. J. Am. Anim. Hosp. Assoc., *17*:17, 1981.

35. Prata, R.G.: Cervical and thoracolumbar disc disease in the dog. *In* Current Veterinary Therapy VIII. Edited by R.W. Kirk. Philadelphia, W.B. Saunders, 1983.

36. Seim, H.B. and Nafe, L.A.: Spontaneous intervertebral disk extrusion with associated myelopathy in a cat. J. Am. Vet. Med. Assoc., *17*:201, 1981.

37. Shires, P.K., et al.: Epidural dirofilariasis causing paraparesis in a dog. J. Am. Vet. Med. Assoc., *180*:1340, 1982.

38. Shores, A.: Intervertebral disc syndrome in the dog. Part III. Thoracolumbar disk surgery. Compendium on Continuing Education, *4*:24, 1982.

39. Shores, A.: The differential diagnosis of ataxia, paresis or paralysis in large breed

dogs. J. Am. Anim. Hosp. Assoc., *20*:265, 1984.

40. Smith, G.K. and Walton, M.C.: Fractures and luxations of the spine. *In* Textbook of Small Animal Orthopedics. Edited by C.D. Newton and D.M. Nunamaker. Philadelphia, J.B. Lippincott, 1985.

41. Sorjonen, D.C., et al.: Effects of dexamethasone and surgical hypotension on the stomach of dogs: Clinical, endoscopic and pathologic evaluations. Am. J. Vet. Res., *44*:1233, 1983.

42. Sorjonen, D.C. and Vaughn, D.M.: Membrane interactions in central nervous system injury. Compendium on Continuing Education, *3*:248, 1989.

43. Swaim, S.F.: Small animal thoracolumbar, lumbosacral and sacrocaudal surgery. *In* Veterinary Neurology. Edited by J.F. Oliver, B.F. Hoerlein, and I.G. Mayhew. Philadelphia, W.B. Saunders, 1987.

44. Turner, W.D.: Fractures and fracture luxations of the lumbar spine: A retrospective study in the dog. J. Am. Vet. Med. Assoc., *23*:459, 1987.

45. Turnwald, G.H., et al.: Diskospondylitis in a kennel of dogs: Clinicopathologic findings. J. Am. Vet. Med. Assoc., *188*:178, 1986.

46. Toombs, J.P., et al.: Colonic perforation in corticosteroid-treated dogs. J. Am. Vet. Med. Assoc., *188*:145, 1986.

47. Walker, T.L., et al.: Disorders of the spinal cord and spine of the geriatric patient. Vet. Clin. North Am., *11*:777, 1981.

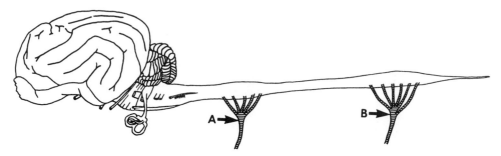

Figure 18–1. Locations of lesions producing paresis or paralysis of one limb include nerves of the brachial plexus (A) and lumbosacral plexus (B).

Location of the lesion (Figure 18–1): *Nerve roots or peripheral nerves of the brachial and lumbosacral plexus*

Infections and other inflammations

Distemper (Chaps. 7 and 16)
Rabies (Chap. 7)
Focal abscesses

Trauma

Injury of peripheral nerves
Intervertebral disc disease lateral herniation
   (Chapter 17)
Infraspinatus muscle contracture
Semitendinosus muscle contracture
Quadriceps muscle contracture

Vascular disorders

Fibrocartilaginous infarct of the spinal cord (Chapters
   16 and 17)

Neoplasia

Neurofibrosarcoma
Neurinoma, neurolemmoma, schwannoma
Lymphosarcoma
Miscellaneous neoplasia compressing or entrapping
   peripheral nerves

Chapter 18

Paresis or paralysis of one limb

Paresis or paralysis of a thoracic limb with no other neurologic abnormalities is caused by an ipsilateral disease process of C6 to T2 nerve roots, the brachial plexus, or individual nerves of the thoracic limb. Paresis or paralysis of a pelvic limb is caused by an ipsilateral disease process of L4 to S2 nerve roots, the lumbosacral plexus, or the individual nerves to the pelvic limb (Fig. 18–1). Paralysis of one limb is called monoplegia.

The peripheral nerves from the brachial plexus that contribute to proper movement of the thoracic limb are the suprascapular, musculocutaneous, axillary, radial, median, and ulnar.[9] The suprascapular nerve is formed from C6 to 7 spinal cord segments and nerve roots and innervates the infraspinatus and supraspinatus muscles that extend the shoulder. The musculocutaneous nerve is formed from C6 to 8 spinal cord segments and nerve roots and innervates the biceps brachii, brachialis, and coracobrachialis muscles that produce flexion of the elbow. The axillary nerve is formed from C7 to 8 spinal cord segments and nerve roots and innervates the deltoid, teres major, and teres minor muscles that flex the shoulder. The radial nerve is critical for supporting weight on the forelimb. Spinal cord segments and nerve roots C7 to T1 contribute mainly to the radial nerve that innervates the triceps brachii, extensor carpi radialis, ulnaris lateralis, common digital extensor and lateral digital extensor muscles that produce extension of the elbow, carpus, and digits. The median nerve is formed from spinal cord segments and nerve roots C8 to T1 and innervates the flexor carpi radialis and superficial digital flexor muscles. The ulnar nerve is also formed from spinal cord and nerve roots C8 to T1 and innervates the flexor carpi ulnaris and deep digital flexor muscles. Together, the median and ulnar nerves produce flexion of the carpus and digits.

The peripheral nerves from the lumbosacral plexus that contribute to proper movement of the pelvic limb are the femoral, obturator, cranial gluteal, caudal gluteal, sciatic, common peroneal, and tibial nerves.[9] The femoral nerve is formed by spinal cord segments and nerve roots L4 to 5 and is the critical nerve for bearing weight on the pelvic limb. The femoral nerve innervates the iliopsoas, quadriceps, and sartorius muscles that produce extension and fixation of the stifle to support weight. The obturator nerve is formed by spinal cord segments and nerve roots L5 to 6 and innervates the obturator, pectineus, gracilis, and adductor muscles that contribute to adduction of the hip. The cranial gluteal nerve is formed by spinal cord segments and nerve roots L6 to 7 and innervates the middle and deep gluteal muscles and tensor fascia lata. The middle and deep gluteal muscles extend the hip joint and tensor fascia lata flexes the hip joint and extends the stifle. The caudal gluteal nerve is formed primarily by nerve roots L7 and innervates the superficial gluteal and piriformis muscles which extend the hip joint. The sciatic nerve is formed by spinal cord segments and nerve roots L6 to S2 and innervates the biceps femoris, semimembranosus, and semitendinosus muscles that produce flexion of the stifle. The sciatic nerve divides at the stifle into the peroneal (fibular) and tibial nerves. The peroneal nerve innervates the peroneus longus, lateral digital extensor, long digital extensor, and cranial tibial muscles and produces flexion of the hock and extension of the digits. The tibial nerve innervates the gastrocnemius, popliteus, and superficial and deep digital flexor muscles and produces extension of the hock and flexion of the digits.

As discussed in Chapter 16, the nerve roots exit rostral to the vertebra of the same number from C1 to C7, then from the T1 level they exit caudally, because there are eight cervical segments and only seven cervical vertebrae.

Patient evaluation

Signalment and history

The most common mechanisms of disease producing paralysis of one limb are trauma and neoplasia, although occasionally, infections, spinal cord infarction, and a lateral herniation of an intervertebral disc may produce similar deficits. The neurologic deficits associated with these disorders may be the same, but the history is different. Any age, breed, or sex of animal may have a peripheral nerve injury. The neurologic deficit is most often immediate following the injury, and usually stays the same or improves over time. In rare instances, fibrosis of surrounding tissues may entrap the nerve and produce progressive signs.

Peripheral nerve neoplasia can affect various ages and breeds of animals. The course of disease is slow and progressive. A lateral herniation of a caudal cervical disc may produce acute thoracic limb lameness or paresis, as well as chronic progressive paresis. Because the prognosis for treatment and recovery is better than for neoplasia, an intervertebral disc problem should always be considered (Chap. 17).

Physical and neurologic examinations

Fractures of the bones of the limb may accompany peripheral nerve damage, but often there is no evidence of fractures or outward signs of trauma. When neoplasms directly affect the nerves, there may be no palpable mass early in the course of the disease.

In nerve trauma, there is no immediate decrease in size of the denervated muscle, but after 1 to 2 weeks the atrophy is easily observed and palpated. The muscles that are atrophied indicate which nerves have been injured.

The neurologic examination is approached systematically as described in Chapter 3, even though the obvious deficit is in one limb. A lesion of C8 to T2 nerve roots may produce Horner's syndrome or decreased sympathetic tone in the eye on the same side (Chap. 11).

The gait and separate thoracic limb and pelvic limb examinations should be carefully performed to determine whether both limbs on one side, the limb on the opposite side, or all four limbs are affected by a disease, localizing the lesion to the cervical spinal cord or the neuromuscular system (Chap. 16) or the thoracolumbar spinal cord (Chap. 17) instead of one peripheral nerve or plexus. If the other three limbs are normal, a critical evaluation of the affected limb can be made.

The neurologic examination findings with lesions of the nerves of the thoracic limb are outlined in Table 18–1. Radial nerve dysfunction is most obvious because the animal is unable to bear weight on the thoracic limb. The elbow is dropped down from the body and the carpus is knuckled, so the animal stands on the dorsum of the paw. Musculocutaneous nerve dysfunction is manifested by inability to flex the elbow during walking or placing. Median and ulnar nerve dysfunction result in a loss of flexion of the carpus and digits. The spinal reflex changes and distribution of superficial skin sensation deficits also outline the nerves involved (Table 18–1).

The neurologic examination findings with lesions of the various nerves of the pelvic limb are outlined in Table 18–2. If the femoral nerve is nonfunctional, the animal is unable to support weight on the pelvic limb. The limb collapses with each step because the inability to extend and fix the stifle. If the sciatic nerve is affected, the animal is able to support weight on the limb, but stands knuckled over onto the dorsum of the paw with a dropped hock because of inability to actively extend or flex the toes and extend or flex the hock. If only the peroneal nerve is affected, the animal knuckles onto the dorsum of the digits. If only the tibial nerve is affected, the animal has extreme flexion of the hock. The spinal reflex alterations and distribution of superficial sensory loss over the skin also outline which nerves are involved.

Once it has been established which nerves are involved, serial neurologic examinations will aid in evaluating any regression or progression of neurologic dysfunction. Weekly, bimonthly, or monthly reevaluations are made to determine an accurate prognosis for each case.

Ancillary diagnostic investigations

Electromyography is the most helpful diagnostic aid in evaluating peripheral nerve function (Chap. 5).[13] The needle EMG study can be used to determine which muscles are denervated and confirm the neurologic examination findings. Following nerve injury, serial nerve stimulation studies can be used to evaluate the integrity and function of the nerve and aid in providing an accurate prognosis for recovery.

When the evidence is conclusive that the nerve is not intact and the injury site

Table 18–1
Lesions of nerves of the thoracic limb and neurologic examination findings

Roots	Nerve	Muscle atrophy	Gait and posture deficit	Spinal reflex alterations	Distribution of sensory loss
C6 to 7	Suprascapular	Supraspinatus Infraspinatus	None	None	None
C7 to 8	Axillary	Deltoid	None	None	Small area of sensory loss on dorsolateral aspect of brachium
C6 to 8	Musculocutaneous	Biceps brachii	No flexion of elbow during gait evaluation or placing	No flexion of elbow during flexor reflex No biceps reflex	Some sensory loss on medial aspect of forearm
C7 to T2	Radial	Triceps brachii Extensor carpi radialis Ulnaris lateralis Common and lateral digital extensors	No extension of elbow No extension of carpus and digits Unable to support weight on limb	No triceps reflex No extensor carpi radialis response	No sensation on the cranial aspect of the limb from toes to elbow
C8 to T1	Median and ulnar	Flexor carpi radialis Superficial digital flexor Flexor carpi ulnaris Deep digital flexor	No flexion of carpus No flexion of digits	No flexion of carpus and digits during flexor reflex	Loss of sensation on caudal aspect of the limb from toes to elbow Loss of sensation from fifth digit (ulnar nerve)

Table 18-2
Lesions of nerves of the pelvic limb and neurologic examination findings

Roots	Nerve	Muscle atrophy	Gait and posture deficit	Spinal reflex alterations	Distribution of sensory loss
L5 to 6	Obturator	Pectineus Gracilis	Slight abduction of hip	None	None
L4 to 5	Femoral	Quadriceps femoris	Inability to extend stifle Limb collapses with weight	No patellar reflex	No sensation on medial surface of thigh, stifle, leg, and paw
L6 to S2	Sciatic	Caudal gluteal Semimembranosus Semitendinosus All muscles of peroneal and tibial nerves	Inability to actively flex stifle Hock flexes and extends passively Hock dropped Knuckled onto digits Caudal gluteal muscle involvement produces adduction of hip	No flexor reflex No cranial tibial reflex No gastrocnemius reflex	No sensation below the stifle to the toes except medial surface
L6 to S1	Tibial	Gastrocnemius Superficial and deep digital flexors	Dropped hock and tarsus Overflexion of hock and overextension of digits	No gastrocnemius reflex	No sensation on caudal and plantar surface of limb from stifle to paw
L6 to S1	Peroneal (fibular)	Peroneus longus Cranial tibial Lateral and long digital extensor	Stands knuckled onto digits Overextension of hock and overflexion of digits	No cranial tibial reflex	No sensation on cranial and dorsal surface of limb from stifle to paw

from the spinal cord or the plexus itself stretched, bruised, or torn. The syndrome has been referred to as radial-brachial paralysis or just radial paralysis, but is usually a mixture of involvement of several nerves of the brachial plexus. The radial, median, and ulnar nerves are most commonly affected, but suprascapular, axillary, and musculocutaneous nerves are often injured as well.

If the musculocutaneous nerve is affected along with the radial, median, and ulnar nerves, the limb drags on the ground with no active flexion or extension of the elbow, carpus, or digits (Fig. 18–2). If the musculocutaneous nerve is spared, the limb may be carried flexed at the elbow with no active extension of the elbow nor extension or flexion of the carpus and digits. Superficial sensation is absent on the limb distal to the elbow.[1] If the suprascapular nerve is affected, atrophy of supraspinatus and infraspinatus muscles is seen (Fig. 18–3).

Damage to nerve roots of the phrenic nerve produces paralysis of the ipsilateral side of the diaphragm that may be seen on fluoroscopic examination of the thorax.

The needle EMG can be used to outline which nerves of the brachial plexus have been injured. Direct stimulation of the suprascapular, radial, and ulnar nerves

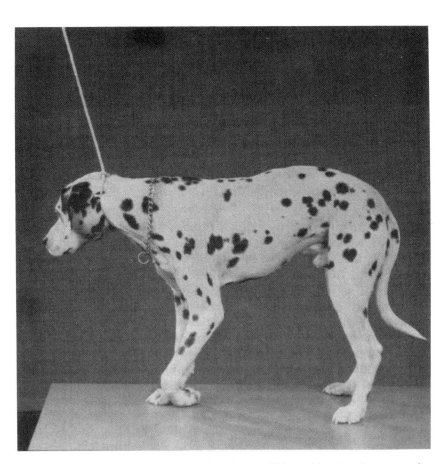

Figure 18–2. A Dalmatian with a brachial plexus injury with loss of function of suprascapular, musculocutaneous, radial, median, and ulnar nerves.

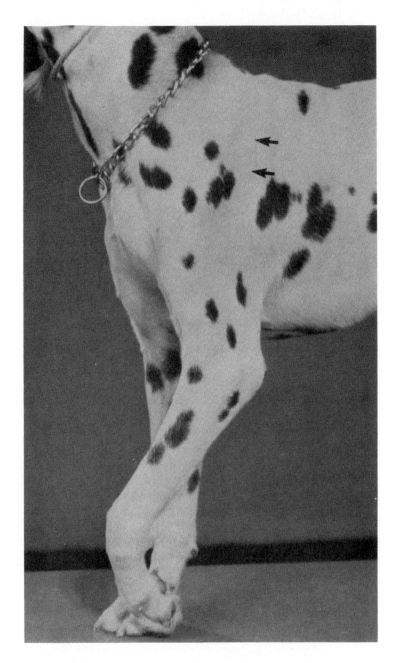

Figure 18–3. Closer view of the Dalmatian with a brachial plexus injury. Note the supraspinatus and infraspinatus muscle atrophy (arrows), along with the atrophy of the rest of the limb muscles.

is easily performed and can be useful to determine nerve integrity 72 hours after the injury.[19] If the nerve roots of C6 to T1 are torn from the spinal cord, Horner's syndrome of the eye on the same side as the injury is generally seen. The presence of Horner's syndrome indicates that the injury involves nerve roots instead of the plexus.

Each animal must be evaluated individually with serial neurologic and EMG examinations to determine the prognosis, but it is often grave in nerve root injuries as they are torn from the spinal cord (Fig. 18–4). Physical therapy as discussed previously is important, especially when multiple joints and muscles are affected.

Suprascapular nerve injury

Incidence: Frequent

The suprascapular nerve is susceptible to injury as it crosses the cranial portion of the distal scapula. Little gait deficit is seen, but the animal is presented with a cosmetic defect of atrophy of the supraspinatus and infraspinatus muscles. Coonhounds and other hunting dogs may injure this nerve by hitting the shoulder against trees.

The suprascapular nerve may be stimulated electrically at the point of the shoulder, and recordings may be taken from the supraspinatus and infraspinatus muscles to determine whether the nerve is intact. If the nerve is not intact, exploratory surgery and nerve repair may be a successful mode of therapy. Dogs function quite well with the deficit and often no therapy is needed.

Infraspinatus muscle contracture

Incidence: Occasional

An adult dog may be presented with a progressive paddling gait on one thoracic limb.[3] In some cases the thoracic limbs may be affected bilaterally. There is often a history of a painful lameness following a period of vigorous activity, which improved, and then the progressive gait abnormality

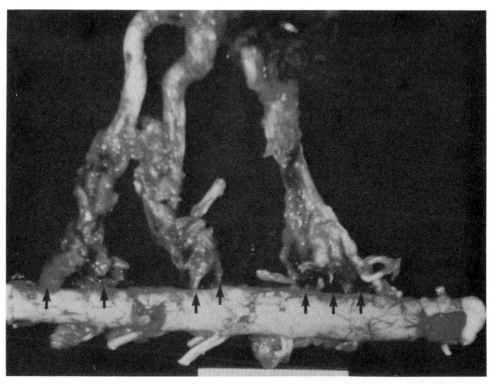

Figure 18–4. Nerve roots torn from the spinal cord in an animal with avulsion of the brachial plexus. (Courtesy of Dr. Damon Averill, Dept. of Neuropathology, Children's Hospital, Boston, Massachusetts.)

followed. Atrophy and fibrosis of the supraspinatus and infraspinatus muscles are apparent. The elbow is held adducted and the antebrachium is rotated outwardly. Tenotomy or myotenectomy may improve the range of motion of the scapulohumeral joint and improve the signs.[3] The muscle changes are permanent.

Radial nerve injury

Incidence: Frequent

Radial nerve injury alone may occur with fractures of the first rib or the humerus. With the distal radial nerve injuries, the animal may bear weight on the limb because of the ability to extend and fix the elbow, but stands knuckled over at the carpus because of the inability to actively extend the carpus or digits (see Table 18–1).

The radial nerve may be stimulated electrically on the lateral aspect of the humerus, and recordings taken from extensor muscles to determine whether the nerve is intact. The nerve should be explored and repaired surgically if there is evidence that it is severed.

Median and ulnar nerve injury

Incidence: Occasional

Fractures of the bones of the distal humerus or proximal radius and ulna, or direct blows to the nerves may damage the median and ulnar nerves. Overextension and sinking of the carpus is caused by the loss of tone in the opposing flexor muscles (see Table 18–1).

The ulnar nerve is easily stimulated at the medial aspect of the elbow and carpus, and recordings are taken from flexor muscles to determine whether the nerve is intact. If the site of injury can be determined, a severed nerve may be surgically explored and repaired.

Sciatic nerve injury

Incidence: Frequent

Sciatic nerve injury is commonly associated with fractures of the ilium or proximal femur.[8,12,23] The nerve is commonly traumatized by retraction during hip and proximal femur surgery and by improper intramuscular injections into the semimembranosus and semitendinosus muscles.[10] The signs of sciatic nerve deficit are described in Table 18–2. The sciatic nerve may be electrically stimulated at the lateral proximal femur and at the stifle, and recordings taken from the various extensor and flexor muscles to determine nerve integrity. If the nerve is severed and the site of injury is known, surgical exploration and repair may be indicated. Proximal sciatic nerve injuries in larger dogs have a poor prognosis if the nerve is severed, because of the distance the nerve must regenerate for reinnervation of distal musculature.

Semitendinosus muscle contracture

Incidence: Occasional

A nonpainful lameness of the pelvic limb may occur in dogs and cats from contracture of the semitendinosus muscle.[14,15] The exact cause is unknown, but trauma is suspected. External rotation of the hock and internal rotation of the stifle are observed as the limb is carried forward. Treatment with tenotomy and myotenectomy may temporarily improve the lameness, but fibrosis and lameness returns in 3 to 8 months.[15]

Peroneal or fibular nerve injury

Incidence: Occasional

The peroneal nerve is vulnerable to pressure, blows, or fractures affecting the lateral stifle, producing a loss of flexion of the hock and extension of the digits (see

Table 18–2). The animal stands knuckled over onto the digits (Fig. 18–5). The peroneal nerve may be electrically stimulated on the lateral aspect of the stifle and recordings taken.from the cranial tibial muscles to determine nerve integrity. The nerve may be surgically explored and repaired if necessary.

Tibial nerve injury

Incidence: Occasional

The tibial nerve may occasionally be injured along with fractures of the tibial bone or hock, producing a loss of hock extension and digit flexion (see Table 18–2).

The tibial nerve may be electrically stimulated at the hock and recordings taken from the flexor muscles of the digits or stimulated at the medial stifle and recordings taken from the gastrocnemius muscle to determine whether the nerve is intact. If the site of injury is known and the nerve is severed, exploratory surgery and repair are indicated.

Femoral nerve injury

Incidence: Rare

Femoral nerve injuries alone are relatively rare, but occasionally may be seen with trauma to the medial thigh. The nerve may be electrically stimulated with a needle placed in the medial aspect of the proximal femur and recordings taken from the quadriceps to determine whether the nerve is intact. Surgical exploration and repair may be indicated.

Quadriceps muscle contracture

Incidence: Occasional

Injury to the quadriceps muscle may produce fibrosis and contracture and the affected pelvic limb may be fixed in extension at the stifle joint. Attempts to increase mobility with surgical excision have been unsatisfactory.[2]

Lumbosacral plexus injury

Incidence: Rare

Lumbosacral plexus or nerve root injuries are much less common than brachial plexus injuries, but do occur occsionally, associated with severe proximal pelvic limb trauma. Combined femoral and sciatic nerve deficits of the pelvic limb are seen (see Table 18–2). The neurologic and EMG examinations can be used to outline the nerves affected and to determine the severity of involvement for the formulation of an accurate prognosis.

Vascular disorders

Infarcts

Incidence: Occasional

Fibrocartilaginous infarction of the spinal cord is discussed in Chapters 16 and 17. Fibrocartilaginous infarct occurring unilaterally in the low lumbar region of the spinal cord occasionally produces paralysis of one pelvic limb. Often, some weakness is apparent in the other pelvic limb also, but this may recede rapidly in a small unilateral infarct and leave a deficit caused by gray matter damage of nerve cell bodies of femoral and/or sciatic nerves. Each animal must be evaluated individually by serial neurologic and EMG examinations to determine an accurate prognosis. Many of these animals recover or compensate enough to be functional, and the diagnosis is only suspected and not confirmed. Infarction of blood vessels of peripheral nerves occurs rarely, secondary to trauma or aberrant heartworm migration.

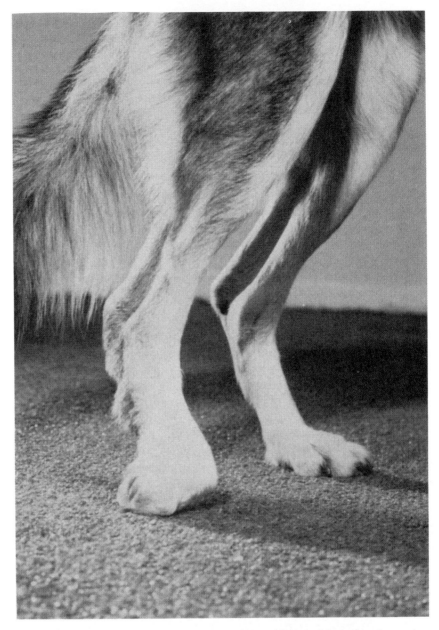

Figure 18–5. A dog with peroneal nerve injury and loss of flexion of the hock and extension of the digits.

Neoplasia

Primary peripheral nerve

Incidence: Occasional

Primary neoplasia of peripheral nerves in dogs and cats is produced from Schwann cells and supporting structures.[4,16] Schwann cells produce neurinomas, also called schwannomas or neurolemmomas. Neurofibromas and neurofibrosarcomas form from connective tissue around the nerve bundles and occur as single tumors, involving only one nerve, or as multiple tumors, involving several nerves, a plexus, or multiple nerve roots. The primary peripheral nerve tumors are slow-growing. Most commonly, adult dogs are affected. The initial presenting complaint is lameness of a limb. The brachial plexus or C6 to T2 nerve roots are common sites for neoplasia to occur, and often the animal will begin limping on one thoracic limb.[7] As the tumor enlarges over the next several months, paresis of the limb develops and atrophy of affected muscles becomes apparent. Pain is often associated with the limb movement. Ultimately, the limb may be paralyzed with decreased or no sensation below the tumor site, but extreme pain at the tumor site. Sometimes a palpable enlargement along the nerve or plexus may be found in the later stages of tumor development.

The diagnosis is suspected from the gradual progression of paresis, atrophy, and pain. If thoracic limb involvement is the primary sign, plain cervical vertebral radiographs and a myelogram should be performed to rule out a lateral herniated intervertebral disc (Chap. 17). Nerve root tumors within the spinal canal are usually seen on a cervical myelogram. Surgical exploration and removal of the tumor is the mode of therapy. The portion of the nerve containing tumor must be removed and the ends anastomosed. In the case of a brachial plexus tumor, the limb may have to be amputated because the tumor is so large that too much nervous tissue must be removed and anastomosis is impossible. The prognosis for brachial plexus neurofibromas and neurofibrosarcomas is poor. The tumors usually occur in multiples and grow along nerve roots into the spinal canal, and ultimately produce hemiplegia or quadriplegia (Fig. 18–6).

Neurofibromas and neurofibrosarcomas may affect any peripheral nerve or nerve roots and therefore can produce signs of cranial nerve deficits (Chap. 11), quadriparesis, quadriplegia, or ataxia of all four limbs (Chap. 16) or paraparesis and paraplegia (Chap. 17).

Metastatic peripheral nerve

Incidence: Occasional

Lymphosarcoma is the most common metastatic neoplasia of nerve roots. It is most

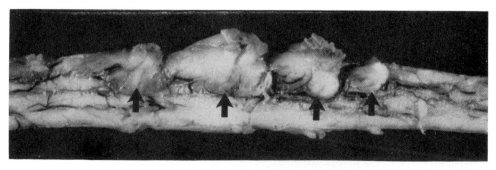

Figure 18–6. Neurofibrosarcoma of C6 to T1 nerve roots (arrows).

frequent in cats, but does occur in dogs as well.[17] Paresis of the limb and muscle atrophy occur more rapidly than with neurinomas, neurofibromas, and neurofibrosarcomas, and severe neurologic deficit may be seen within a few weeks after the onset of signs. The prognosis is poor because the nerve roots are diffusely infiltrated with abnormal lymphocytes, and surgical removal is impossible.

Other tumors of bone and muscle may not directly invade, but may entrap peripheral nerves and produce deficit in a limb. Prognosis varies with the type of tumor and the ability to remove or treat it and relieve the pressure on the nerve.

References

1. Baily, C.S.: Patterns of cutaneous anesthesia associated with brachial plexus avulsions in the dog. J. Am. Vet. Med. Assoc., *185*:889, 1984.
2. Bardet, J.F., Hohn, R. B.: Quadriceps contracture in dogs. J. Am. Vet. Med. Assoc., *183*:160, 1983.
3. Bennett, B.A.: Contracture of the infraspinatus muscle in dogs: A review of 12 cases. J. Am. Anim. Hosp. Assoc., *22*:481, 1986.
4. Braund, K.G.: Neoplasia of the nervous system. Compendium on Continuing Education, *6*:717, 1984.
5. Braund, K.G.: Clinical syndromes in veterinary neurology. Baltimore, Williams & Wilkens, 1986.
6. Braund, K.G.: Diseases of the peripheral nerves, cranial nerves and muscle. *In* Veterinary Neurology. Edited by J.E. Oliver, B.F. Hoerlein, and I.G. Mayhew. Philadelphia, W.B. Saunders, 1987.
7. Carmichael, S. and Griffith, I.R.: Brachial plexus tumors in 7 dogs. Vet. Rec., *108*:437, 1981.
8. Chambers, J.N. and Hardie, E.M.: Localization and management of sciatic nerve injury due to ischial or acetabular fracture. J. Am. Anim. Hosp. Assoc., *22*:539, 1986.
9. deLahunta, A.: Veterinary Neuroanatomy and Clinical Neurology. Philadelphia, W.B. Saunders, 1983.
10. Fanton, J.W., et al.: Sciatic nerve injury as a complication of intramedullary pin fixation of femoral fractures. J. Am. Anim. Hosp. Assoc., *19*:687, 1983.
11. Gibson, K.L. and Daniloff, J.K.: Peripheral nerve repair. Compendium on Continuing Education, *11*:938, 1989.
12. Gilmore, D.R.: Sciatic nerve injury in twenty nine dogs. J. Am. Anim. Hosp. Assoc., *20*:403, 1984.
13. Griffiths, I.R. and Duncan, I.D.: The use of electromyography and nerve conduction studies in evaluation of lower motor neuron disease and injury. J. Small Anim. Pract., *19*:328, 1978.
14. Lewis, D.D.: Fibrotic myopathy of the semitendinosis muscle in a cat. J. Am. Vet. Med. Assoc., *193*:240, 1988.
15. Moore, R.W., et al.: Fibrotic myopathy of the semitendinosus muscle in four dogs. Vet. Surg., *4*:169, 1981.
16. Patnaik, A.K., et al.: Canine malignant melanotic schwannomas: A light and electron microscopic study of two cases. Vet. Rec., *21*:483, 1984.
17. Presthus, J. and Teige, J.: Peripheral neuropathy associated with lymphosarcoma in a dog. J. Small Anim. Pract., *27*:463, 1986.
18. Raffe, M.R.: Peripheral nerve injuries in the dog (Parts I and II). Compendium on Continuing Education, *1*:269, 1979.
19. Steinberg, H.S.: The use of electrodiagnostic techniques in evaluating traumatic brachial plexus root injuries. J. Am. Anim. Hosp. Assoc., *15*:621, 1979.
20. Steinberg, H.S.: Brachial plexus injuries and dysfunction. Common Neurologic Problems. Vet. Clin. North Am., *18*:565, 1988.
21. Swaim, S.F.: Peripheral nerve surgery. *In* Veterinary Neurology. Edited by J.E. Oliver, B.F. Hoerlein, and I.G. Mayhew. Philadelphia, W.B. Saunders, 1987.
22. Van Nes, J.J.: Evaluation of traumatic forelimb paralysis of dogs. Res. Vet. Sci., *40*:144, 1986.
23. Walker, T.L.: Ischiatic nerve entrapment. J. Am. Vet. Med. Assoc., *178*:1284, 1981.
24. Wheeler, S.J., et al.: The diagnosis of brachial plexus disorders in dogs: A review of twenty two cases. J. Small Anim. Pract., *27*:147, 1986.

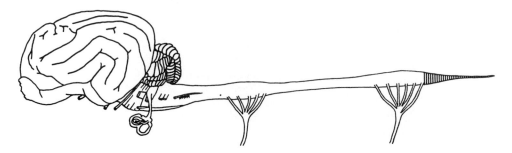

Figure 19–1. Location of lesions producing bladder distention, dilated anus, and atonic tail include the sacral and caudal spinal cord segments, nerve roots (cauda equina), and peripheral nerves (vertical lines).

Location of the lesion (Figure 19–1): *Sacral and caudal spinal cord segments and nerve roots (cauda equina) and peripheral nerves*

Mechanisms of disease and differential diagnosis

Congenital and familial disorders

Sacrocaudal agenesis and other caudal vertebral and
  spinal cord malformations

Infections and other inflammations

Bite wound abscesses
Miscellaneous nerve root infections
Vertebral infections—discospondylitis

Trauma

Lumbosacral fracture/luxation
Sacrocaudal fracture/luxation

Degeneration

Lumbosacral malarticulation and malformation

Neoplasia

Meningioma
Neurinoma
Neurofibroma
Neurofibrosarcoma
Lymphosarcoma
Vertebral neoplasia

Chapter 19

Bladder distention, dilated anus, and atonic tail

The caudal tip of the spinal cord is located at the junction of the L6–7 vertebrae in the dog and is called the conus medullaris (Fig. 19–2). The L7–Cd5 nerve roots continue in the vertebral canal, forming the cauda equina before exiting after the vertebra of the same number (Fig. 19–2).

Lesions of the sacral and caudal spinal cord segments and nerve roots often produce urinary incontinence with a flaccid, distended bladder, fecal incontinence with a dilated anus, and a paralyzed atonic tail unassociated with pelvic limb paralysis (Fig. 19–1).

The S1 to S3 spinal cord segments and nerve roots contribute to the pelvic nerve, which transmits sensory information from and parasympathetic motor innervation to the detrusor muscle, the smooth muscle of the bladder wall. The pelvic nerve also transmits sensory information from and parasympathetic motor innervation to the smooth muscle of the descending colon and rectum.

The S1 to S3 spinal cord segments and nerve roots also contribute to the pudendal nerve, which transmits sensory information from the external urethral sphincter, the anal sphincter, and the perineal region. The pudendal nerve also provides motor innervation to the external urethral sphincter (periurethral striated muscle)

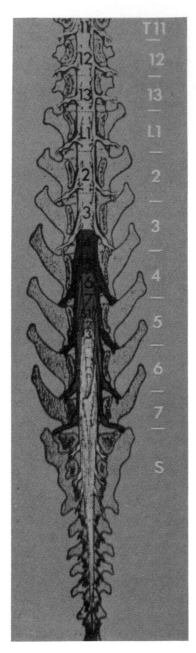

Figure 19–2. Relationship of vertebrae to spinal cord segments and nerve roots in the dog. Sacral segments are located within vertebra L5, caudal segments are located within vertebra L6, but the nerve roots continue within the canal as the cauda equina and exit after the vertebra of the same number. (After Miller, 1964.)

and the striated muscle of the anal sphincter.

Reflex contraction of the bladder is produced in a series of events involving the pelvic and pudendal nerves and S1 to S3 spinal cord segments.[10,12] When the bladder distends, afferent (sensory) nerve endings in the bladder wall and urethral sphincter are stimulated and impulses are transmitted in the pelvic and pudendal nerves to the gray matter of S1 to S3. The detrusor nuclei in the intermediolateral gray column are stimulated, efferent parasympathetic impulses are transmitted in the pelvic nerve, and the detrusor muscle contracts. Simultaneously, the pudendal nuclei in the ventral horn gray matter are inhibited, the external urethral sphincter relaxes, and urine is expelled from the bladder.

Reflex defecation involves similar pathways. Distention stimulates afferents from the rectum and the anal sphincter, which ascend to the S1 and S3 spinal cord gray matter through the pelvic and pudendal nerves, respectively. The pelvic nerves stimulate contraction of the smooth muscle of the descending colon and rectum, the pudendal nerve is inhibited, producing relaxation of the anal sphincter, and feces are expelled.

With lesions involving S1 to S3 spinal cord segments or nerve roots and pudendal or pelvic nerves, no reflex urination or defecation can occur and the sphincters are dilated. The bladder is easy to express manually. The anal sphincter is dilated, and as feces are moved along by intrinsic muscle contractions of the smooth muscle of the colon wall, the feces will drop out of the rectum. The intrinsic ability of smooth muscle to contract, even when denervated, results in some autonomous urination and defecation. The autonomous activity is not efficient, and urine usually has to be manually emptied from the bladder and occasionally feces must be removed from the rectum.

With lesions above S1 to S3 spinal cord segments, reflex urination and defecation can occur. Lower motor neuron sympathetic innervation of the bladder originates in the intermediolateral gray matter from L2 to L5, exits the spinal cord at L1 to L2 in lumbar splanchnic nerves, synapses in the caudal mesenteric ganglion, and travels to the bladder through the hypogastric nerves.[10] The sympathetic innervation to the bladder increases the threshold of the local reflex contraction and allows the detrusor muscle to stretch and increase the bladder volume before muscle contraction occurs. The hypogastric nerve also supplies sympathetic innervation to the smooth muscle of the proximal urethra and produces urethral dilatation.

In acute lesions above the S1 to S3 spinal cord segments, particularly at the T13 to L1 region, the bladder may fill and be unable to reflexly empty for 1 to 7 days. Often the bladder cannot be manually expressed because of severe spasticity in the urethra and sphincters. Attempts at manual expression may injure the muscle wall or rupture the bladder. The animal must be aseptically catheterized 3 times daily to empty urine from the bladder. Administration of diazepam (Valium) 2 to 5 mg every 8 hours orally to a 5 to 15-kg dog may produce enough muscle relaxation so manual expression may be possible. Bladder expression should be attempted 30 to 45 minutes after administration of the diazepam.

Some authors have suggested phenoxybenzamine (Dibenzyline), an alpha-blocking agent, to reduce urethral spasms.[9,12] In this author's experience, phenoxybenzamine may have grave hypotensive effects in a paraplegic dog and is not used. A urinalysis should be obtained every 3 days to monitor for cystitis. If cystitis occurs, a culture and sensitivity test should be performed and the appropriate antibotic administered. The anal sphincter may also be spastic and manual emptying of feces may be necessary. After approximately 1 week, the urethral and anal sphincters relax, and reflex urination and defecation occur. Without sympathetic inhibition of the bladder wall, reflex contraction is hyperactive and the bladder empties when filled with small amounts of urine. Whenever abdominal pressure is applied, small spurts of urine are discharged from the urethra. Reflex defecation occurs also. There is no voluntary control over urination and defecation, and the animal urinates and defecates anywhere. Residual urine may be left in the bladder, as reflex emptying may not be complete, and urinary tract infections may occur.

Urinary and fecal incontinence is a loss of voluntary control of urination and defecation, which is a complex process involving the integration of many neural responses, from the sacral spinal cord segments to the cerebral cortex. Detailed descriptions of the specific nuclei and pathways involved in the total micturition response are found elsewhere, but a summary is given here.[9,10,12] As the bladder distends with urine, sensory impulses travel up the pelvic nerves to the sacral spinal cord segments. From the sacral spinal cord, sensory impulses travel through the spinal cord and brain stem to the reticular formation of the pons, where a detrusor center is located. Some impulses also continue through the thalamus and internal capsule to the somatosensory cortex, where the feeling of the distended bladder and the need to urinate are consciously perceived. If urination is inappropriate at the time, impulses from the frontal lobe cerebral cortex descend and inhibit the detrusor center in the pons. Other impulses from the frontal lobe descend to the sacral spinal cord segments and stimulate the pudendal nuclei and nerves, which produce contraction and tightening of the external urethral sphincter. By these pathways and interactions, urination is inhibited at appropriate times, learned during housebreaking.

When the animal is taken outside, where urination is acceptable, cortical inhibition on the pontine reticular formation detrusor center is released, as is the voluntary contraction of the external urethral sphincter. Now impulses traveling up the pelvic nerves to the sacral spinal cord segments, and up the spinal cord and brain stem, effectively stimulate the detrusor center, which, influenced by the cerebellum, sends descending impulses down the brain stem and spinal cord to coordinate and modulate the local detrusor reflex at S1 to S3. Normal micturition and complete bladder emptying can then occur. Defecation has a similar pathway. Urinary and fecal incontinence may be produced by lesions anywhere along the peripheral and central nervous system pathways. Table 19–1 summarizes changes in the micturition response associated with lesions at various sites.

Only lesions of S1 to S3 that produce urinary and fecal incontinence associated with a flaccid, distended bladder and dilated anus are discussed in this chapter.

Caudal spinal cord segments, nerve roots, and nerves supply sensory and lower motor neuron (LMN) innervation to the tail. The tail may be paralyzed by upper motor neuron (UMN) or LMN lesions. A reflex tail wag is often seen in UMN lesions above the lumbosacral plexus. The tail wag reflex may become exaggerated in chronic UMN lesions because of axonal sprouting (Chap. 1). When the flexor reflex is initiated, the tail may wag excessively during and following flexion of the limb. A reflex tail wag must be differentiated from a voluntary tail wag, as the latter indicates that the spinal cord is intact. A voluntary tail wag is usually elicited by talking to the dog in a pleasant tone or offering the dog treats. The reflex tail wag may be present even if the spinal cord is severed, so long

as the lesion is above the lumbosacral plexus.

With LMN lesions of the tail, the tail is paralyzed, limp, or atonic and no reflex tail wag is seen. Lesions that produce an atonic tail are described in this chapter.

Pelvic parasympathetic nerves are also primarily involved in the vasomotor changes of penile erectile tissue. Lesions of S1 to S3 spinal cord segments or nerve roots may produce difficulty in achieving an erection or penile paralysis in male dogs.

In localizing lesions of vertebrae producing a flaccid bladder, dilated anus, and atonic tail with or without paresis or paralysis of the pelvic limbs in the dog, the relationship of spinal cord segments and nerve roots to vertebrae must be considered (Fig. 19–2). Lesions of L5 to L7 vertebrae produce flaccid paresis or paralysis of the pelvic limbs with an areflexic bladder and anus and an atonic tail. Sacral vertebral lesions affect only sacral and caudal nerve roots, and the pelvic limbs are often normal. Caudal vertebral lesions may produce only an atonic tail, with normal urination and defecation.

Patient evaluation

Signalment and history

A kitten or puppy, particularly of the tailless breeds, with bladder distention, dilated anus, and atonic tail may have a malformation of the caudal spinal cord.

A history of a cat fight with wounds around the tail-head are suggestive of ascending bacterial neuritis of sacral and caudal nerves.

Lumbosacral and sacrocaudal fractures and luxations should be considered in animals with an acute onset of a flaccid bladder, anus, and tail.

A slow, progressive onset of bladder distention, dilated anus, and atonic tail as-

Table 19–1
Location of lesions and alterations of the micturition response

Lesion site	Alteration of response
Cerebral cortex and pathways rostral to the pons	No voluntary control over micturition; loss of house-training or inability to house-train
Pons	Loss of micturition; animal must be catheterized
Cerebellum	Frequent voiding of small amounts of urine
Spinal cord above S1	Initial loss of micturition response and spasticity of sphincters (especially thoracolumbar spinal cord lesions); 1 to 7 days later, local reflex bladder contraction occurs
Spinal cord S1 to S3	Loss of bladder contraction with a large, distended bladder and dilated sphincters; no reflex bladder contraction

sociated with pain may be produced by discospondylitis, lumbosacral malarticulation, and malformation, or nerve root or vertebral neoplasia.

Physical and neurologic examinations

The perineal region and tail may be soiled with feces because of fecal incontinence. Urinary incontinence may result in urine irritation of the abdominal skin and dermatitis.

Touching the perineal region generally produces contraction of the anal sphincter, called the perineal or anal reflex. When the bulb of the penis or the vulva is pinched, the anal sphincter also contracts. This is called the bulbourethral reflex. These reflexes are mediated primarily through the pudendal nerve and spinal cord segments S1 to S2. Sensation to pin-pricking or pinching in the perineal region is decreased in the S1 to S3 skin dermatomes.

A large, flaccid, distended bladder, associated with LMN sacral lesions, is easily expressed and no spurts of urine are seen. Chronic, severe distention may result in

damage to the smooth muscle of the bladder wall, which further hinders normal micturition. A small, contracted bladder that spurts out urine when palpated is more characteristic of an UMN lesion or one above the S1 to S3 segments.

The tail may have a loss of natural curl in those breeds of dogs with a curled tail. There is little or no voluntary or reflex tail movement, and the tail hangs limp. Superficial sensation from the skin of the tail is depressed or absent. Deep pain sensation from the caudal vertebrae may also be depressed or absent. The caudal muscles may atrophy.

Ancillary diagnostic investigation

Urinalysis, blood urea nitrogen (BUN), and serum creatinine should be evaluated to detect cystitis and nephritis. Chronic cystitis may damage the muscle wall and contribute to permanent micturition problems.

Needle EMG of the anal sphincter and caudal muscles shows positive waves and fibrillation potentials 5 to 7 days after an insult to the sacral and caudal nerve roots, providing further evidence that LMN dis-

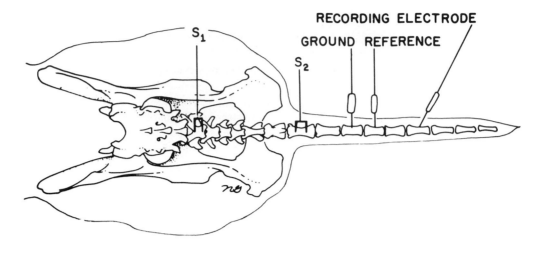

TAIL CONDUCTION VELOCITY

Figure 19-3. Tail motor nerve conduction velocity. (S1) first stimulation site; (S2) second stimulation site. An evoked response is detected by the recording electrode. The time or latency of S1 to the recording electrode is subtracted from the latency of S2 to the recording electrode. The difference in latencies is divided into the distance between S1 and S2 to give a conduction velocity expressed in meters per second (Chap. 5).

ease is present at that site. If any motor unit action potentials are seen, some integrity of the nerves is preserved (Chap. 5).

A stimulating electrode may be placed in the epidural space of the lumbosacral junction. A recording electrode can be placed in the anal sphincter or caudal muscles. Recording an evoked response in the anal sphincter or caudal muscles indicates that the pudendal and caudal nerves, respectively, are intact.

A tail nerve conduction velocity test may be performed by stimulating caudal nerves at two sites on the tail and recording an evoked response in the caudal muscles (Fig. 19–3).

A cystometrogram (CMG) is the graphic recording of intravesical pressure changes during filling and contraction of the urinary bladder. A catheter placed in the bladder is connected to a pump, a pressure transducer, and a strip-chart recorder. The animal is sedated with 2.2 mg/kg of xylazine intramuscularly or subcutaneously, and air is pumped into the bladder. A detailed description of CMG waveforms is found elsewhere.[11] The CMG provides a means of measuring bladder volume, bladder elasticity, threshold volume and pressure, the presence of a micturition reflex, and maximal contraction pressure.

An anal sphincter EMG may be recorded along with the CMG, as the anal sphincter and external urethral sphincter are both innervated by the pudendal nerve.

Pelvic nerve integrity may be evaluated by inserting a catheter containing stimulating electrodes into the bladder and placing a recording electrode in the anal sphincter. Stimulation of the bladder produces an evoked response in the anal sphincter. The pelvic nerves, sacral segments, and pudendal nerves must be intact to obtain this response.

Agenesis, discospondylitis, osteomyelitis, fractures, malformation and malarticulation, and neoplasia of sacral and caudal vertebrae may be seen on plain radiographs. Contrast radiography performed by injecting media into the epidural space or into vertebral bodies to study venous sinus arrangements gives limited success in outlining compression and tumors in this region.

Exploratory laminectomy with biopsy or removal of masses may be necessary for the diagnosis and therapy of neoplasia of nerve roots.

A summary of the approach to the evaluation of an animal with bladder distention, dilated anus, and atonic tail is outlined in Table 19–2.

Congenital and familial disorders

Sacrocaudal agenesis

Incidence: Frequent in Manx cats, occasional in others

Congenital defects of the caudal vertebral column and spinal cord produce fecal incontenence and a dilated anus, urinary incontinence associated with an areflexic bladder, and sometimes, weakness of the pelvic limbs.

Signalment and history. Manx and other tailless cats, and Old English Sheepdogs, Bulldogs, Boston terriers, and other tailless or short-tailed dogs are often affected with an agenesis of the sacrocaudal vertebrae and spinal cord.[2,8] The neurologic deficit is present from birth, but is often first noted at weaning.

Physical and neurologic examinations. Soiling and irritation of the perineal and abdominal skin are commonly found on physical examination. Spina bifida of L7 to S1 vertebrae might be palpated. A firm, cord-like mass may be palpated extending from the spinal column to the skin. In rare instances, a cleft in the skin and subcutaneous tissues may expose the caudal spinal cord segments and nerve roots.

A large, distended, easily expressed bladder is palpated in the abdomen. Feces may be retained in the rectum, and the sphincter is dilated and atonic. Stimulation of perineal, penile, and vulvar regions produces no reflex contraction in the anal sphincter, nor a behavioral response to the pain. The penis is usually paralyzed in males. Some locomotor and sensory disturbances of the pelvic limbs also may be present. Affected animals may walk with excessive flexion of the hips and hocks. Bilateral simultaneous flexion and extension of the limbs when walking produce a hopping gait, similar to that described in Weimaraner dogs with spinal dysraphia (Chap. 17). Conscious proprioception and superficial sensation on the caudal aspect of the pelvic limbs are often diminished.

In some cases, complete paralysis of the pelvic limbs with loss of pelvic limb spinal reflexes occurs.

Ancillary diagnostic investigations. Most affected animals have cystitis, apparent from the urinalysis.

Spina bifida, malformation, and complete agenesis of caudal and/or sacral vertebrae are seen on vertebral plain radiographs (Fig. 19–4); although radiographs may also be normal. An enlarged subarachnoid mass, a meningocele, or meningomyelocele may be demonstrated using myelography.

Electrical stimulation of sacral nerve roots or bladder with no response in the anal sphincter suggests a grave prognosis. Agenesis and total lack of development of sacral nerves are common.

Therapy and prognosis. With no nerve formation for innervation of the anus and bladder, no therapy can be provided and the prognosis is grave for ever gaining any bowel or bladder function. Animals may be kept alive by manually

Table 19–2
Diagnostic approach for the evaluation of animals with bladder distention, dilated anus, and atonic tail

Primary complaint: Bladder distention, dilated anus, and atonic tail

↓

Data base:

Signalment and history
Physical examination
Neurologic examination
Initial clinicopathologic tests (urinalysis, BUN, creatinine)

↓

Electrodiagnostic testing:

Needle EMG
Stimulation of cauda equina
Tail nerve conduction velocity
Stimulation of bladder wall

↓

Cystometrogram

↓

Lumbosacral or sacrocaudal radiography

↓

Exploratory laminectomy

---

emptying the bladder, controlling cystitis, and keeping the rectum and surrounding skin clean, but they rarely make acceptable pets.

Pathology. Affected animals may or may not have vertebral changes associated with the underlying spinal cord changes, but spina bifida, vertebral malformations, and agenesis of the sacrum and caudal vertebrae are most common.

The spinal cord may end in a conical-shaped mass with no obvious cauda equina (see Fig. 19–5). Sacral spinal cord segments may not be identifiable or may be threadlike. Meningocele, meningomyelocele, hydromyelia, syringomyelia, and spinal dysraphia are the changes seen in the lumbosacral and caudal spinal cord segments.

Infections and other inflammations

Bite-wound abscesses

Incidence: Occasional

Bite wounds around the tail-head can lead to abscesses and ascending bacterial neuritis and meningomyelitis of the caudal spinal cord (Fig. 19–6A,B). Less commonly, infections following tail docking can also lead to an ascending cauda equina infection.

Signalment and history. Tom cats that are allowed to roam and fight are occasionally presented for depression, anorexia, flaccid tail, anus, and areflexic bladder. Affected animals may also have pelvic limb paresis or paralysis.

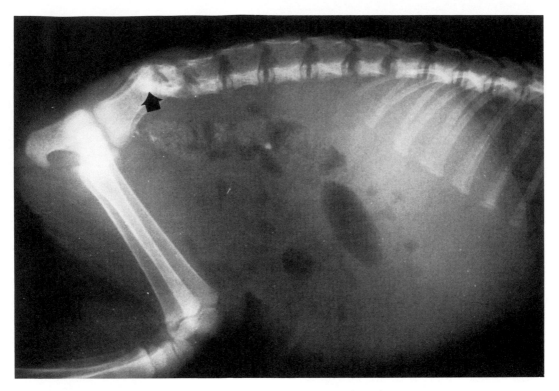

Figure 19–4. Lateral radiograph of a Manx kitten with sacrocaudal agenesis (arrow).

Physical and neurologic examinations. The body temperature is often elevated. Bite wounds and abscesses around the tail and tail-head are commonly found.

The degree of neurologic deficit varies with the severity of the nerve root involvement, but the tail is usually paralyzed and limp and has no superficial sensation. Deep sensation from the tail may also be absent in severe lesions. The anal sphincter is dilated and no perineal reflex or sensory response can be obtained. The bladder is distended and easily expressed manually. Pelvic limb paresis or paralysis with depressed or absent gastrocnemius, cranial tibial, and flexor reflexes may also be present if lumbar nerve roots are affected.

Ancillary diagnostic investigations. Neutrophilic leukocytosis is often present on the CBC. Lumbar cerebrospinal fluid analysis may show increased protein content and many neutrophils.

Radiography of the caudal and sacral vertebrae may show evidence of osteomyelitis, but is often normal. The diagnosis is suspected from the presence of bite wounds, fever, and the neurologic deficit associated with a sacrocaudal lesion.

Therapy and prognosis. Superficial skin abscesses are opened, drained, and treated with topical antibiotics. Trimethoprim sulfadiazine (Tribrissen) 15 mg/kg every 12 hours and cephradine (Velosef) 20 mg/kg every 8 hours are given orally for 3 to 4 weeks. If osteomyelitis is evident on radiographs, the antibiotic combination is continued for 6 to 8 weeks. If the animal has no obvious osteomyelitis and is diagnosed early, the neurologic deficit may im-

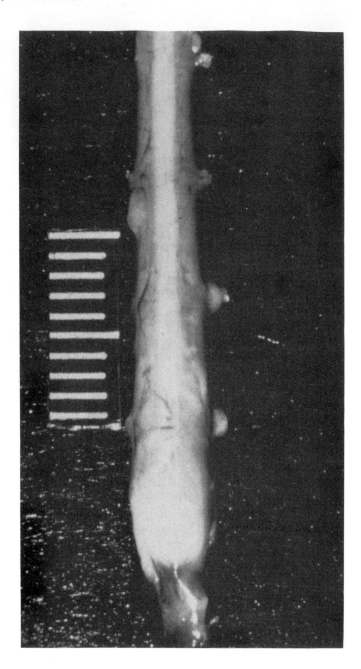

Figure 19–5. The caudal spinal cord of a Manx kitten with no sacrocaudal nerve formation and a flaccid bladder and anus. (Courtesy of Dr. Damon Averill, Dept. of Neuropathology, Children's Hospital, Boston, Mass.)

prove rapidly with antibiotic therapy. The antibiotic therapy should be continued for at least 3 weeks. In severe infections, a generalized bacterial meningomyelitis ascending to involve thoracolumbar spinal cord segments may occur, and damage to nerve roots and the spinal cord may be severe.

Pathology. Focal cellulitis around bite wounds occurs and a fistula may extend down between vertebrae, carrying infec-

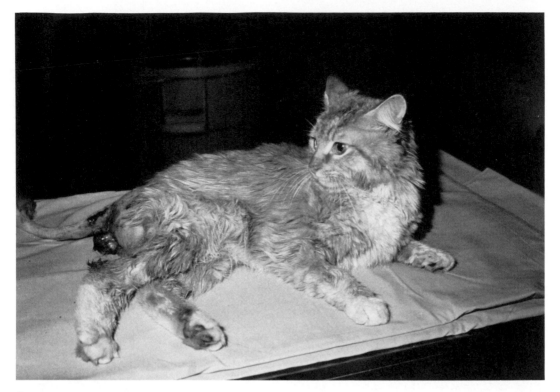

A

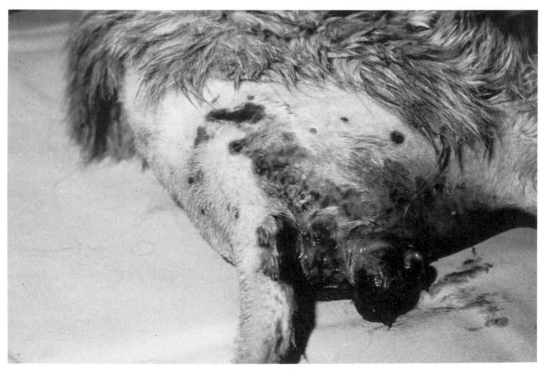

B

Figure 19–6. *(A)* Cat with bite wounds and ascending bacterial neuritis producing bladder distention, dilated anus, atonic tail, and pelvic limb paresis. *(B)* Closer view of bite wounds around the tail-head and anus.

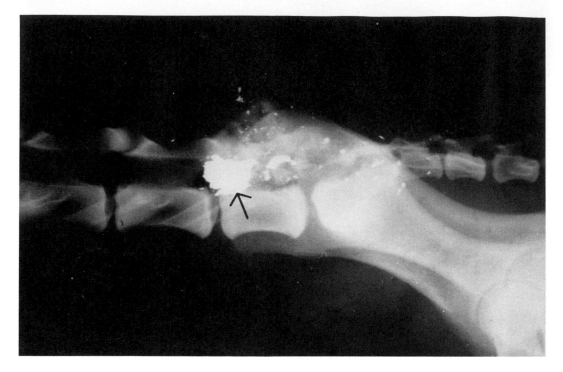

A

Figure 19–7. *(A)* A lateral radiograph of a dog with a gunshot wound. Metal appears to be in the vertebral canal at L6–7 (arrow). *(B)* A ventrodorsal radiograph confirmed the metal is located in the vertebral canal (arrow).

tion into the region of the nerve roots. Hemorrhage and purulent exudate may be found around the nerve roots and spinal cord.

Miscellaneous infections and inflammations

Incidence: Rare

Viral, protozoal, and fungal infections of the sacral and caudal spinal cord segments and nerve roots are rare. Viral myelitis most commonly affects white matter, and although sacral and caudal spinal cord segments may be involved, the gray matter is usually spared and so are the tail and anal and bladder reflexes. Granulomatous meningoencephalitis (Reticulosis) rarely

occurs in the caudal spinal cord. Spinal cord and CNS infections and inflammations in general are discussed in Chapters 7 and 16.

Vertebral infections

Incidence: Occasional

Discospondylitis, an inflammation of the intervertebral disc and adjoining vertebral bodies, may occur at the lumbosacral junction and produce inflammation and compression of sacral and caudal nerve roots.[5,13] Pain and pelvic limb weakness usually accompany bowel, bladder, and tail dysfunction. Discospondylitis is discussed in Chapters 16 and 17.

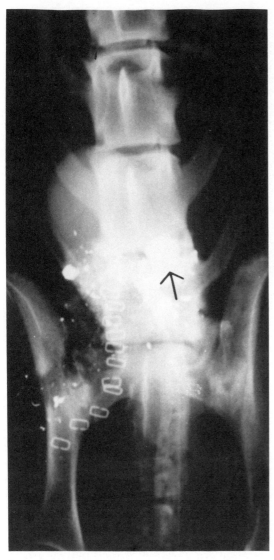

B

Trauma

Lumbosacral and sacrocaudal fracture, subluxation, and luxation

Incidence: Frequent

Lumbosacral fractures, subluxations, or luxations are common causes of distended bladder, dilated anus, and atonic tail.[1,3,7] Often the L7 nerve root is also affected, and some weakness of pelvic limb muscles in the sciatic nerve distribution occurs.

In cats especially, sacrocaudal fractures, subluxations, or luxations are commonly associated with getting their tails caught by something, which produces excess tension and separation of the sacrocaudal vertebrae. Sacral nerve roots are stretched or torn. If lumbar nerve roots are also stretched, pelvic limb paresis or

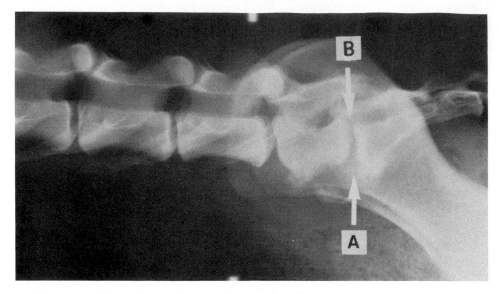

Figure 19–8. Lumbosacral malarticulation and malformation. Note ventral spondylosis (A). L7 to S1 subluxation and sacral stenosis are seen (B).

paralysis occurs, but this is less common than in lumbosacral injuries.

Peripheral nerve injury, degeneration, and regeneration are described in Chapter 18.

Critical serial evaluation of voluntary tail movement, superficial and deep sensation from the tail, perineal sensation, anal tone and reflex, and the presence of a micturition reflex can be useful in detecting any nerve root integrity and in differentiating neurapraxia (a transient loss of function) from neurotmesis (a severed nerve) (Chap. 18).

Plain radiographs of the lumbosacral or sacrocaudal vertebrae often show the site of injury, but information collected from the neurologic examination should be used to evaluate the severity of the lesion. (Fig. 19–7A,B)

Electrodiagnostic testing can provide the best information to formulate an accurate prognosis and differentiate axonotmesis, neurotmesis, and neurapraxia (see Table 18–4). Stimulation of the cauda equina in the epidural space or of the bladder by electrodes on a urinary catheter and

recording any evoked muscle response in the anal sphincter indicates whether there is some integrity to the nerve. Motor nerve conduction velocity studies on the tail can further aid in formulating an accurate prognosis for caudal nerves. The use of EMG in peripheral nerve injury is described further in Chapter 18. Surgical repair of vertebral fractures and luxations is well described elsewhere.[14]

If some integrity to the nerves is found, other ruptured axons regenerate at an average rate of 1 inch per month or 1 mm per day, and reinnervation of the muscles may be possible. It may take 2 to 4 months for improvement to be seen.

Degeneration

Lumbosacral malarticulation and malformation

Incidence: Occasional

Subluxation, stenosis, Type II IV disc protrusion, and spondylosis deformans of the

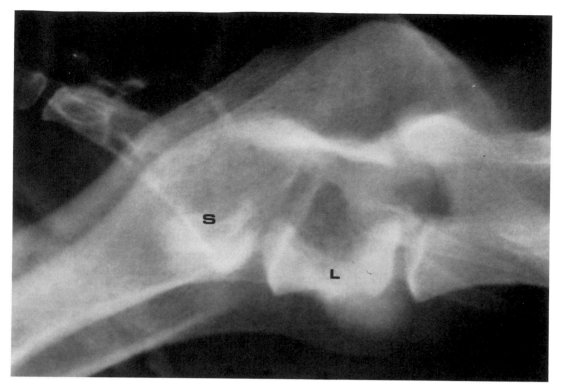

Figure 19–9. A lateral radiograph of a dog with a vertebral neoplasm involving L7 (L) and the sacrum (S).

lumbosacral vertebrae can lead to compression of the lumbosacral nerve roots.[4,6]

Signalment and history. German Shepherds and other large breeds of dogs, usually over 5 years of age but occasionally younger, may be presented for lumbosacral pain, paresis, or proprioceptive deficit in the pelvic limbs and urinary incontinence associated with a decreased micturition reflex. Fecal incontinence and tail paralysis are also complaints in some animals. Many dogs are presented at the painful stage when nerve roots are irritated, especially the L7 nerve root, and not severely compressed.

Physical and neurologic examinations. Manipulation of the tail-head or pressure on the dorsal spinous process of

L7 to S1 vertebra most commonly elicits a painful response.

Increased sensitivity in the L7 dermatome is seen when the L7 nerve is irritated. Conscious proprioceptive deficits and mild weakness in muscles of the sciatic distribution also may be seen.

A large, atonic, easily expressed bladder is commonly found on abdominal palpation. Anal tone and reflex may be depressed. Tail paresis and paralysis also may be seen.

Ancillary diagnostic investigations. Needle EMG studies are useful to confirm nerve root entrapment (Chap. 5). Positive waves and fibrillation potentials are found in the external anal sphincter and tail musculature.

Ventral spondylosis deformans of L7 to S1 vertebrae is commonly seen on plain

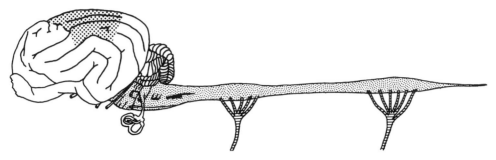

Figure 20–1. Location of lesions that might produce self-mutilation are peripheral sensory nerves (horizontal lines), sensory pathways of the spinal cord, brain stem (dense dots) and thalamus, and the somatosensory cerebral cortex (large dots).

Location of the lesion (Figure 20–1): *peripheral sensory nerves, sensory pathways through the spinal cord, brain stem, and thalamus, and the somatosensory cerebral cortex*

Mechanisms of disease and differential diagnosis

Congenital and familial disorders
Congenital sensory neuropathies

Infections
Canine distemper virus (Chaps. 7 and 16)
Herpesvirus (Aujeszky's disease or pseudorabies)

Trauma
Peripheral nerve injury (Chap. 18)
Spinal cord injury (Chap. 17)

Neoplasia
Peripheral nerve neoplasia (Chap. 18)

Idiopathic
Feline hyperesthesia syndrome
Canine hyperesthesia syndrome
Tail chasing
Chin rubbing

Chapter 20

Self-mutilation

Self-mutilation can be caused by a neurologic abnormality in the peripheral sensory nerves, sensory spinal cord, and brain stem pathways, thalamus, or somatosensory cortex of the cerebrum (Fig. 20–1).

Self-mutilation syndromes can be some of the most terrifying disorders for pet owners to endure, and the most challenging and frustrating for veterinarians to diagnose and treat.

Specific disorders known to produce self-mutilation are discussed here, but for many of the self-mutilating syndromes, the underlying cause is unknown.[6]

Patient evaluation

Signalment and history

A thorough analysis of the history of an animal with a self-mutilation syndrome is of the utmost importance, because ancillary diagnostic investigations may contribute little to the diagnosis.

Young animals that are mutilating their paws, penis, or tail may have a congenital sensory neuropathy, an infection with distemper virus, or an idiopathic syndrome. Most dogs with distemper virus infections have other signs to indicate a multifocal neurologic problem.

With an injury to a nerve, self-mutilation may be seen in certain stages of regeneration (Chap. 18).

In some animals with spinal cord injury from intervertebral disc herniation or an external source of trauma, self-mutilation is occasionally associated with paralysis of the pelvic limbs (Fig. 20–2)(Chap. 17).

Sometimes animals with progressive pelvic limb paresis or flaccid bladder, anus, and tail associated with neoplasia of the cauda equina mutilate the tail, paws, or penis (Chap. 19).

In animals presented with hysteria associated with pelvic limb and tail pain, tail chasing and mutilation, chin rubbing, and skin twitching, a thorough description of the event and frequency must be obtained to attempt to differentiate a psychomotor or sensory seizure (Chap. 8) from a disease process of the sensory spinal cord pathways or peripheral nerves.

Physical and neurologic examinations

Self-inflicted bite wounds, skin lacerations, hair loss, and dermatitis may be associated with self-mutilation. Dermatitis is often secondary to the constant chewing, licking, and rubbing. In extreme cases, an animal may actually devour its toes, paws, tail, or penis, severely hemorrhage, and become a terrifying and grotesque sight for the owner to witness.

Flaccid paresis or paralysis of a limb or limbs, with loss of spinal reflexes and muscle atrophy, along with the mutilation, indicates that the lesion is most likely in the peripheral nerve, nerve roots, or spinal cord segments to that region. Mutilation is probably associated with itching, tingling, or burning in the dermatomal regions supplied by the sensory portions of the peripheral nerves.

Spastic paralysis of the pelvic limbs with self-mutilation may be caused by disease in the sensory spinal cord pathways.

Idiopathic mutilation syndromes un-associated with any motor or other sensory deficit are difficult to localize. Episodic abnormal sensations might be caused by discharges in the somatosensory area of the parietal lobe of the cerebral cortex (see Table 8–1). Continual abnormal sensations may be associated with peripheral nerve disease affecting only the sensory portion. Sensory peripheral neuropathies in humans are associated with severe burning, itching, tingling, and aching sensations, and can lead to almost psychopathic behavior because of the intenseness of the stimulation and the lack of relief gained by scratching. Other disorders, such as habitual tail chasing and licking an area of the paw, may have no neurologic basis and may be caused by psychologic disturbances.

Ancillary diagnostic investigations

Initial cliniopathologic tests may be normal. If sensory neuritis is believed to be present, metabolic and endocrine functions should be evaluated with the appropriate serologic tests. An EEG is obtained on animals in which the behavior is episodic and a seizure disorder is suspected, or in animals thought to have viral encephalomyelitis.

If other neurologic deficits are present, such as spastic or flaccid paraplegia or monoplegia, or a flaccid tail, anus, and bladder, these problems are approached as described in Chapters 17, 18, and 19, respectively. Needle EMG may be performed, but will be normal if the motor portion of the peripheral nerves is normal. Sensory motor nerve conduction (Fig. 20–3) is the best way to effectively diagnose a sensory peripheral neuropathy. A decrease in conduction velocity or an absence of a sensory evoked response is seen in sensory nerve disease, but may be normal in sensory receptor disease. Radiography of the tail or site of self-mutilation may show vertebral or other bony abnormalities that might be contributing to the problem.

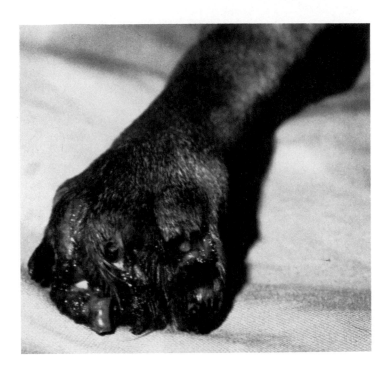

Figure 20–2. A 3-year-old paraplegic Dachshund with no deep pain in the pelvic limbs mutilated the digits on one paw.

If a sensory neuropathy is suspected, fascicular biopsy of a sensory nerve may be helpful in confirming the diagnosis.

Often no definitive location of the lesion or underlying cause can be found for the idiopathic syndromes, and trials of various therapy regimens are instituted to try to control the signs.

The diagnostic approach for the evaluation of an animal with self-mutilation syndrome is summarized in Table 20–1.

Congenital and familial disorders

Sensory neuropathies

Incidence: Rare

Congenital sensory neuropathies with self-mutilation are described in English Pointers and German Shorthair Pointers.[3–5] At 3 months of age, affected puppies begin to mutilate the digits and paws. Although the gait and spinal reflexes are normal,

there is a loss of pain sensation in the paws. The needle EMG studies are normal. Affected dogs do not recover. An autosomal recessive mode of inheritance is thought to exist.

A possible congenital sensory neuropathy has been described in Dachshunds.[7,8] Affected dogs show ataxia, conscious proprioceptive deficits, depressed patellar reflexes, incontinence, self-mutilation, and reduced sensation all over the body. Sensory nerve conduction may be absent. An autosomal recessive inheritance is believed to be the cause.

Infections

Canine distemper virus

Incidence: Occasional

Although infections of the nervous system with canine distemper virus are common, self-mutilation as a sign of disease only occurs occasionally. There may be paresis or

SUPERFICIAL RADIAL NERVE
(lateral aspect)

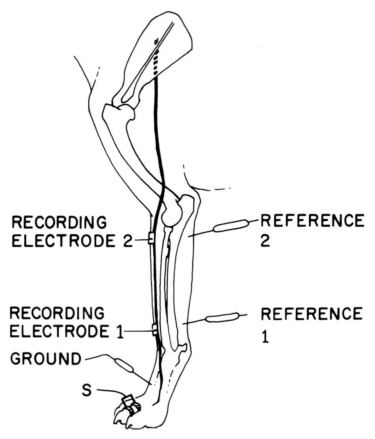

RECORDING ELECTRODE 2

RECORDING ELECTRODE 1

GROUND

S

REFERENCE 2

REFERENCE 1

Figure 20–3. Sensory nerve conduction velocity of the superficial radial nerve. (S) site of stimulation of sensory nerves of the toes. An action potential may be recorded from the nerve at recording electrode 1 and 2. The sensory nerve conduction velocity (SNCV) can be calculated in two ways:

$$SNCV = \frac{\text{Distance from S to recording electrode 1 (or 2)}}{\text{Time from S to recording electrode 1 (or 2)}} = \frac{\text{meters}}{\text{second}}$$

$$SNCV = \frac{\text{Distance between recording electrode 1 and 2}}{\text{Latency 1 - Latency 2}} = \frac{\text{meters}}{\text{second}}$$

Latency 1 is the time from S to recording electrode 1. Latency 2 is the time from S to recording electrode 2. (From Chrisman, C.L.: Electromyography in Animals. *In* Pathophysiology in Small Animal Surgery. Edited by M.J. Bojrab. Philadelphia, Lea & Febiger, 1981.)

paralysis of the limbs. The limbs and tail are the common sites of mutilation. The location of the lesion in the peripheral or central sensory pathways is unknown. The prognosis is grave, as the mutilation is often uncontrollable. Distemper virus infections are discussed in Chapters 7 and 16.

Herpesvirus (Aujeszky's disease or pseudorabies)

Incidence: *Rare*

Herpesvirus may produce an infection in dogs and cats that ascends the peripheral nerves to the spinal cord and brain stem

Table 20–1
The diagnostic approach for evaluation of an animal with self-mutilation syndrome

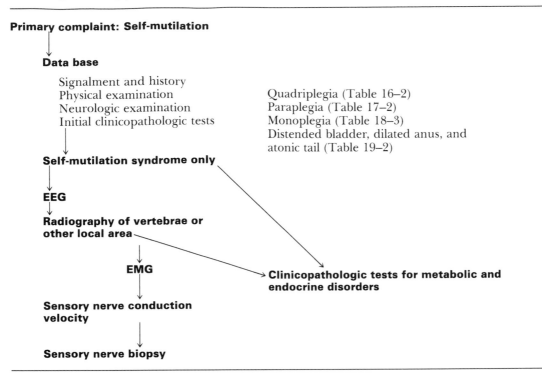

and produces cranial nerve signs, paralysis, and death in 24 to 48 hours.[9,11,13] Initially in the course of the disease, intense pruritus and mutilation of the face, swallowing deficits, and bulbar paralysis are seen, so the disorder has been referred to as "mad itch" or pseudorabies. There may be a history of cattle or pigs in the environment being affected. Pigs can act as carriers. The mode of transmission is most likely consumption of virus-contaminated tissues. Congestion and edema of dorsal root ganglia of spinal and cranial nerves are found on necropsy. Lesions are also scattered through the brain stem, cerebellum, and spinal cord, and are most severe in neurons receiving afferent fibers from affected ganglia. Intranuclear eosinophilic inclusions may be found in neurons and glial cells.

Cases of Aujeszky's disease have been reported that were not characterized by intense pruritus, but rather by severe depression, fever, and cranial nerve deficits such as ptosis, facial paralysis, depressed swallowing reflex, excessive salivation, and respiratory distress.[9] The dogs die in 24 to 48 hours. Such animals must be examined for rabies virus. The diagnosis is made at necropsy by positive fluorescent antibody in the brain for herpesvirus.

Herpes simplex and varicella-zoster viruses are known to involve portions of the peripheral nervous system and sensory ganglia in humans and produce recurrent, painful rashes and/or neuralgia. Studies in mice and rabbits indicate the virus can travel up peripheral nerves, reside in ganglion cells, and reactivate after axonal injury. Herpes zoster infections may produce pain and paresthesia for up to 3 weeks prior to vesicular eruptions on the skin. The role of other herpesvirus infections and peripheral sensory neuropathies in animals needs further study.

Trauma

Peripheral nerve injury

Incidence: Common

Self-mutilation of a desensitized region may occur following a peripheral nerve injury. Many dogs and cats may begin excessively licking or chewing a paw during certain stages of nerve regeneration. The period of mutilation may vary from a few weeks to several months. The animal must be physically kept from licking or chewing the paw by means of a large bucket or Elizabethan collar during this stage. It can be a difficult phase of nerve injury to manage. Constant monitoring, protection, and sometimes tranquilization are necessary. Often the tendency to mutilate the paw eventually decreases, but it may last several months and can be very frustrating to both the owner and veterinarian. Peripheral nerve injuries are discussed further in Chapter 18.

Spinal cord trauma

Incidence: Occasional

Although spinal cord trauma is common, the tendency for paretic or paralyzed animals to mutilate parts of their body is only occasional.

Mutilation of a limb, tail, penis, or part of the body can be a severe complication, as animals can devour a portion of their body or disembowel themselves unexpectedly. Spinal cord injuries are further discussed in Chapter 17.

Neoplasia

Peripheral nerve

Incidence: Occasional

Occasionally, animals with meningiomas, neurinomas, neurofibromas, neurofibrosarcomas, and lymphosarcomas involving sensory nerves and dorsal root ganglia mutilate the portion of the body with altered innervation. Obvious signs of motor nerve involvement are usual, as is loss of dermatome sensitivity that localizes the lesion to a specific nerve or nerves. Peripheral nerve neoplasia is discussed in Chapter 18.

Idiopathic disorders

Hyperesthesia syndromes, tail chasing, chin rubbing, and other stereotypic self-mutilation syndromes

Incidence: Frequent

Several idiopathic self-mutilation syndromes are seen in veterinary practice, characterized by hyperesthesia, tail chasing, and chin rubbing, which are frustrating and terrifying to owners, who want desperately to give their animal some relief from this obsession.

Hyperesthesia syndrome in cats, especially Siamese, Burmese, Himalayans, and Abyssinians, is characterized by twitching, rippling, or rolling of the skin along the lumbar region, which may occur spontaneously or be induced when the region is lightly touched.[1,3,10,12] The signs may begin acutely and vary in severity and frequency. Mild cases may only exhibit occasional excessive skin rippling. Other cases may have continual bouts of skin rippling and muscle spasms, and show hysterical behavior manifested by uncontrolled running, jumping, and excessive vocalization. Affected animals may attack the portion of body and hysterically bite, lick, and tear the hair from the lumbar or anal regions, flank, and tail. The disorder has also been referred to as psychogenic alopecia and dermatitis (PAD) and neuro-dermatitis.

Similar syndromes occur in dogs and may be associated with rear limb and tail hyperesthesia and mutilation.

Dogs and cats may also develop a compulsive obsession with their tails, and chase the tail continually to the point of exhaustion. They may just spin in circles or may catch the tail and chew it or suck on it.

Other dogs and cats may be obsessive about rubbing their chins. This behavior can occur periodically in mild cases, or may be manifested as continual hysterical rubbing of the chin producing severe abrasions and mutilation. These syndromes are dealt with here as a group because the diagnostic and therapeutic approach is the same (see Table 20–1), even though they may appear somewhat differently and have a different underlying cause. Most commonly, no underlying cause is found, and the veterinarian is forced to aim therapy at relief of the symptoms.

Signalment and history. Any age, breed, or sex of cat or dog may acutely develop a mutilation syndrome. The episodic behavior abnormality should be described in detail and the duration and frequency of the bouts determined. Some episodic behavior disturbances may be caused by seizure activity in the parietal and temporal lobes of the cerebral cortex. The animal may be feeling burning or tingling sensations and attack that part of the body, or run hysterically around the room vocalizing excessively, trying to escape the feelings. Seizures have a tendency to be episodic and are usually not continuous nor do they occur multiple times daily.

If the episodes are multiple daily and can be stimulated by touching the body part, an abnormality in sensory pathways in the spinal cord or sensory peripheral nerves or receptors may be present.

Diabetes mellitus, hypoglycemia or hyperinsulinism, hypothyroidism, uremia, hepatic cirrhosis, alcoholism, nutritional deficiencies, paraneoplastic syndromes secondary to carcinoma, herpesvirus infections, and many toxicities associated with fish, shellfish, heavy metals, and drugs produce polyneuropathy in humans (Chap. 16). In many cases of polyneuropathy, weakness and muscle atrophy associated with motor nerve involvement are seen (Chap. 16). In some cases, however, there are no signs of motor deficits, and the primary signs are burning, tingling, itching, and pain. Self-mutilation may occur in an attempt to relieve these abnormal sensations.

Sensory neuropathies are difficult to evaluate in animals, as they cannot directly communicate the sensations they are feeling and may exhibit hysterical behavior, which is difficult to interpret. Signs associated with systemic metabolic or endocrine disorders should be discussed. The possibility of toxicities should also be ascertained.

The role of hormonal imbalances in the production of these idiopathic self-mutilation syndromes is unknown. Behavior changes, especially during estrus in cats and pseudopregnancy in dogs, are well known. Some animals with hyperesthesia syndromes do respond to hormone therapy.

The role of psychologic disturbances in the production of these idiopathic self-mutilation syndromes is unknown. Some behaviors can become habits and be reinforced by environmental factors. Some tail-chasing syndromes may be induced by family members teasing the puppy or kitten with its own tail. Such behavior quickly ceases to be cute when the animal compulsively chases its tail continually to the point of exhaustion, and is no longer an acceptable pet because of its obsession with its tail. Some behavior modification techniques have been employed to stop the obsession.

Physical and neurologic examinations. Dermatitis found on physical examination should be evaluated for primary problems leading to pruritis, such as external parasites and allergies, but dermatitis is often secondary to the mutilation.

The neurologic examination should be performed (Chap. 3) to detect any other signs of neurologic deficit unassociated with sensory systems. Superficial and deep sensation and proprioception should be carefully evaluated. Some animals may be hyperesthetic to light touch or pin-pricking; other animals may be normal at the time of evaluation. Outlining an affected dermatomal region can be helpful in localizing the involvement to certain nerve roots.

Ancillary diagnostic investigations. Radiographs of the thoracolumbar, lumbosacral, or caudal vertebrae should be evaluated to rule out any vertebral infection, degeneration, or neoplasia that may be irritating meninges and dorsal roots, producing pain in a dermatomal region.

An EEG can detect cerebral dysrhythmia that supports the possibility of a seizure disorder. If the EEG is abnormal, a CSF analysis may be indicated to further evaluate the behavior disorder (Chap. 7).

Needle EMG and motor nerve conduction velocity may be evaluated, but are usually normal. Sensory nerve conduction studies may show a decreased conduction velocity or no evoked response in sensory neuropathies affecting the limbs. In sensory nerve receptor disease, the conduction velocity may be normal.

Biopsy and histologic examination of sensory nerves in the affected area may be used to diagnose sensory neuropathies. Further sensory nerve electrodiagnostic studies and biopsy examinations should be performed on animals with hyperesthesia syndromes.

Therapy and prognosis. If the EEG is abnormal, anticonvulsant therapy such as oral phenobarbital at 1 to 2 mg/kg every 12 hours oral starting dose and increased if needed, may be tried, to control the abnormal episodic behavior (Chap. 8).

In cases in which anticonvulsants fail or a cerebral cortex disorder is not suspected, several other therapies have been used on a trial basis, singly or in combination, to control the behavior in individual animals.

Prednisone 2 mg/kg daily divided every 12 hours orally may be tried and has relieved the signs on some occasions and not on others.

Oral phenobarbital 1 to 2 mg/kg every 12 hours, diazepam (Valium) 1 to 5 mg every 8 hours, or methocarbamol (Robaxin) 20 to 40 mg/kg every 8 hours have been given for tranquilization and muscle relaxation, and have relieved the signs in some animals and not others (Chap. 6).

Diphenylhydantoin has a stabilizing effect on peripheral nerve discharges and is given in the therapy of some sensory neuropathies in humans. The appropriate dosage of diphenylhydantoin is not known in cats and even small amounts may be toxic. A dosage of 20 to 35 mg/kg every 6 to 8 hours orally of diphenylhydantoin may be tried in dogs.

Megestrol acetate (Ovaban) has been used in cats with hyperesthetic behavior, but it is not approved for use in the cat and may produce diabetes mellitus, so special permission must be obtained from the owner. Megestrol acetate at 5 mg daily for 1 week then 2.5 mg daily or every other day for 2 weeks may be tried. If signs improve, try to reduce to once or twice a week. Monitor the cat for diabetes mellitus.

Acupuncture therapy has been used to relieve the signs in a few animals. Intralesional and nonspecific intramuscular injections of cobra venom have been used to attempt to relieve the signs in severe cases. Behavior modification, decreasing environmental stress, and obedience training have been employed in the treatment of some of these disorders.

Narcotic antagonists have improved some stereotypic self-licking, self-chewing, scratching behavior, and tail chasing in dogs. Nalmefene HCl 1 to 4 mg/kg or naltrexone 1 mg/kg subcutaneously will reduce these abnormal behaviors, but no oral form is available for longterm management.[6] One 20-kg dog improved tail-chasing behavior on a combination product containing 50 mg pentazocine and 0.5 mg naloxone given orally every 12 hours.[2]

Client communication is the most important aspect of therapy, because the owner must make a commitment to go through several different therapeutic trials to find something that might control the self-mutilation. In some instances, nothing will control the behavior and the animals are euthanized.

References

1. Braund, K.G.: Clinical Syndromes in Veterinary Neurology. Baltimore, Williams & Wilkins, 1986.
2. Brown, S.A., et al.: Naloxone-responsive compulsive tail chasing in a dog. J. Am. Vet. Med. Assoc., *190*:884, 1987.
3. Chrisman, C.L.: Clinical manifestations of multifocal peripheral nerve and muscle disorders of dogs. Compendium on Continuing Education, *7*:355, 1985.
4. Cummings, J.C., et al.: Acral mutilation and nociceptive loss in English Pointer dogs. Acta Neuropathol., *53*:119, 1981.
5. Cummings, J.C., et al.: Hereditary sensory neuropathy. Am. J. Pathol., *112*:136, 1983.
6. Dodman, N.H., et al.: Use of narcotic antagonists to modify stereotypic self licking, self chewing, and scratching behavior in dogs. J. Am. Vet. Med. Assoc., *193*:815, 1988.
7. Duncan, I.D. and Griffith, I.D.: A sensory neuropathy affecting long haired dachshund dogs. Acta Neuropathol., *23*:831, 1982.
8. Duncan, I.D. and Cuddon, P.A.: Sensory neuropathy. *In* Current Veterinary Therapy X. Edited by R.W. Kirk. Philadelphia, W.B. Saunders, 1989.
9. Howard, D.R.: Pseudorabies in dogs and cats. *In* Current Veterinary Therapy IX. Edited by R.W. Kirk. Philadelphia, W.B. Saunders, 1986.
10. Muller, G.H., Kirk, R.W., and Scott, D.W.: Psychogenic dermatoses. *In* Small Animal Dermatology. Philadelphia, W.B. Saunders, 1989.
11. Shell, L.G., et al.: Pseudorabies in a dog. J. Am. Vet. Med. Assoc., *178*:1159, 1981.
12. Tuttle, J.L. and Parker, A.: Diagnosing and treating feline hyperesthesia syndrome. D.V.M. Magazine, p. 72, February 1980.
13. Whitley, R.D. and Nelson, S.L.: Pseudorabies (Aujeszky's disease) in the canine: Two atypical cases. J. Am. Anim. Hosp. Assoc., *16*:69, 1980.

Index